METHODS IN MOLECULAR BIOLOGY™

Series Editor
John M. Walker
School of Life Sciences
University of Hertfordshire
Hatfield, Hertfordshire, AL10 9AB, UK

For further volumes:
http://www.springer.com/series/7651

Kidney Development

Methods and Protocols

Edited by

Odyssé Michos

Hammer Health Sciences Center, Department of Genetics and Development, Columbia University Medical Center, New York, NY, USA

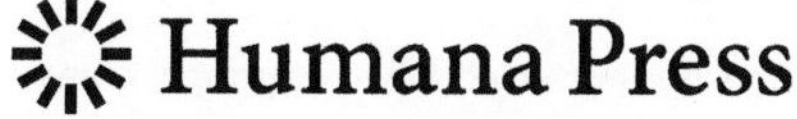

Editor
Odyssé Michos
Hammer Health Sciences Center
Department of Genetics and Development
Columbia University Medical Center
New York, NY, USA

ISSN 1064-3745 e-ISSN 1940-6029
ISBN 978-1-61779-850-4 e-ISBN 978-1-61779-851-1
DOI 10.1007/978-1-61779-851-1
Springer New York Dordrecht Heidelberg London

Library of Congress Control Number: 2012937302

© Springer Science+Business Media, LLC 2012
All rights reserved. This work may not be translated or copied in whole or in part without the written permission of the publisher (Humana Press, c/o Springer Science+Business Media, LLC, 233 Spring Street, New York, NY 10013, USA), except for brief excerpts in connection with reviews or scholarly analysis. Use in connection with any form of information storage and retrieval, electronic adaptation, computer software, or by similar or dissimilar methodology now known or hereafter developed is forbidden.
The use in this publication of trade names, trademarks, service marks, and similar terms, even if they are not identified as such, is not to be taken as an expression of opinion as to whether or not they are subject to proprietary rights.

Printed on acid-free paper

Humana Press is part of Springer Science+Business Media (www.springer.com)

Preface

Over the last decade the development of new molecular biology tools, advanced microscopy, live imaging, and systems biology approaches have revolutionized our conception of how embryonic development proceeds. One fundamental aspect of development biology is the concept of morphogenesis: understanding how a group of multipotent cells organize and differentiate into a complex organ. The mouse kidney is one of the classical model systems to study the mechanism of morphogenesis. The developing kidney has the great advantage to recapitulate many of the key process of embryonic development such as cell–cell interactions, cell movement, cell division, cell survival and death, mesenchymal to epithelial transformation, and epithelial branching morphogenesis, and also some unique features such as the formation of the glomerulus. In addition, kidney organogenesis has the great advantage to occur in ex vivo culture, which allows the study, in a dish, of many aspects of its development, particularly branching morphogenesis of the collecting duct system and nephrogenesis. Understanding the process of morphogenesis is of fundamental importance not only for studying developmental biology per se but also for regenerative medicine.

This book is divided into different chapters, written by specialists in each field, which present different approaches to tackle kidney development. The reader will be guided through the different tools that will allow her/him to study many important parts of kidney development at tissue, cellular, and molecular levels. The aim is to provide a useful and valuable bench reference for both experts and nonexpert scientists who wish to study kidney development.

Part I regroups protocols that introduce the dissection, culture, and live imaging aspects of kidney development. Part II deals on how to analyze the three-dimensional aspects of branching morphogenesis as well as nephrogenesis. Part III consists of protocols that utilize different cell types, from primary cell lines to immortalized ones, to study different aspects of cell signaling and cell migration. Parts IV and V focus on how to analyze and manipulate gene/protein expression during kidney development as well as in the adult kidney. Finally, Part VI concentrates on the adult kidney and how to assess kidney malformation and disease. It is important to note that except for Chap. 6 (zebrafish) and Chap. 11 (Xenopus), the rest of the protocols focus on mouse kidney. I believe that most protocols, especially Parts III–IV, can be adapted to other developing organs and can be very useful not only for kidney organogenesis.

In the end I would like to thank John Walker for giving me the opportunity to edit this book and all the authors for making this book a reality. It has been a great experience and I hope that this first issue of Methods in Molecular Biology focusing specifically on (kidney) organogenesis will be a success and will pave the way for future issues in this area of research. Finally, I'm grateful to Antonella Galli for her help, support, and patience.

Hinxton, UK *Odyssé Michos*

Contents

Part III Renal Primary Cell Cultures and Cell Lines

Part IV Detecting Gene/Protein Expression and Signaling

Part V Manipulating Gene Expression in Developing and Adult Kidney

Part VI Analyzing Functional Defects of the Kidney and Urinary Tract

Contributors

CHRIS ARMIT • *MRC Human Genetics Unit, Western General Hospital, Edinburgh, UK*
JAMES A. ARMITAGE • *Department of Anatomy and Developmental Biology, Monash University, Clayton, VIC, Australia*
JANE ARMSTRONG • *Hugh Robson Building, University of Edinburgh, Edinburgh, UK*
BRUCE ARONOW • *Computational Medicine Centre, Cincinnati Children's Hospital, Cincinnati, OH, USA*
RICHARD BALDOCK • *MRC Human Genetics Unit, Western General Hospital, Edinburgh, UK*
EKATERINA BATOURINA • *Department of Urology, ICRC, Columbia University, New York, NY, USA*
BRIAN BECKNELL • *Division of Nephrology and Department of Pediatrics, Ohio State University College of Medicine, Columbus, OH, USA*
JOHN F. BERTRAM • *Department of Anatomy and Developmental Biology, Monash University, Clayton, VIC, Australia*
MAXIME BOUCHARD • *Goodman Cancer Research and Department of Biochemistry, McGill University, Montreal, QC, Canada*
JANE BRENNAN • *Hugh Robson Building, University of Edinburgh, Edinburgh, UK*
ERIC W. BRUNSKILL • *Division of Developmental Biology, Children's Hospital Medical Center, Cincinnati, OH, USA*
SALLY F. BURN • *Department of Genetics and Development, Columbia University, New York, NY, USA*
KEVIN T. BUSH • *Pediatrics Department, University of California, San Diego, CA, USA*
ASHLEY R. CARPENTER • *Center for Molecular and Human Genetics, Research Institute at Nationwide Children's Hospital, Columbus, OH, USA*
CRISTINA CEBRIAN • *Department of Genetics and Development, Columbia University, New York, NY, USA*
SILVIA CEREGHINI • *INSERM U969 and CNRS-Université Pierre et Marie Curie UMR7622- Paris France*
ROBERT L. CHEVALIER • *Department of Pediatrics, University of Virginia, Charlottesville, VA, USA*
LIJUN CHI • *Program in Developmental and Stem Cell Biology, The Hospital for Sick Children, University of Toronto, Toronto, ON, Canada*
XUAN CHI • *Department of Genetics and Development, Columbia University, New York, NY, USA*
HAN SHENG CHIU • *Institute for Molecular Bioscience, The University of Queensland, Brisbane, QLD, Australia*
LUISE A. CULLEN-MCEWEN • *Department of Anatomy and Developmental Biology, Monash University, Clayton, VIC, Australia*

Duncan Davidson • *MRC Human Genetics Unit, Western General Hospital, Edinburgh, UK*
Jamie A. Davies • *Hugh Robson Building, University of Edinburgh, Edinburgh, UK*
Rebecca N. Douglas-Denton • *Department of Anatomy and Developmental Biology, Monash University, Clayton, VIC, Australia*
Iain A. Drummond • *Nephrology Division, Massachusetts General Hospital, Charlestown, MA, USA; Department of Genetics, Harvard Medical School, Boston, MA, USA*
Mark P. de Caestecker • *Division of Nephrology, Vanderbilt University Medical Center, Nashville, TN, USA*
Jesus Egido • *Renal and Vascular Research Lab, IIS-Fundacion Jimenez Diaz, Autonoma University, Madrid, Spain*
Devangini Gandhi • *Department of Urology, ICRC, Columbia University, New York, NY, USA*
Kylie M. Georgas • *Institute for Molecular Bioscience, The University of Queensland, Brisbane, QLD, Australia*
Jason P. Gleghorn • *Departments of Chemical and Biological Engineering, Princeton University, Princeton, NJ, USA*
Carmen Gomez-Guerrero • *Renal and Vascular Research Lab, IIS-Fundacion Jimenez Diaz, Autonoma University, Madrid, Spain*
David Grote • *Goodman Cancer Research Centre and Department of Biochemistry, McGill University, Montreal, QC, Canada*
Indra R. Gupta • *Department of Human Genetics and Pediatrics, Montreal Children's Hospital, McGill University, Montreal, QC, Canada*
Bernard Haggarty • *MRC Human Genetics Unit, Western General Hospital, Edinburgh, UK*
Kimmo Halt • *Department of Medical Biochemistry and Molecular Biology, Faculty of Medicine, Institute of Biomedicine, University of Oulu, Oulu, Finland*
Simon Harding • *MRC Human Genetics Unit, Western General Hospital, Edinburgh, UK*
Claire Heliot • *INSERM U969 and CNRS-Université Pierre et Marie Curie UMR7622- Paris France*
Purificacion Hernandez-Vargas • *Renal and Vascular Research Lab, IIS-Fundacion Jimenez Diaz, Autonoma University, Madrid, Spain*
Daniel A. Hirselj • *Northwest Urological Clinic, Portland, OR, USA*
Peter Hohenstein • *Institute of Genetic and Molecular Medicine, University of Edinburgh, Edinburgh, UK*
Derek Houghton • *MRC Human Genetics Unit, Western General Hospital, Edinburgh, UK*
Deborah Hyink • *Department of Medicine, Baylor College of Medicine, Houston, TX, USA*
Jessica Ineson • *Institute for Molecular Bioscience, The University of Queensland, Brisbane, QLD, Australia*
Susan E. Ingraham • *Center for Clinical and Translational Research, Research Institute at Nationwide Children's Hospital, Columbus, OH, USA; Division of Nephrology and Department of Pediatrics, Ohio State University College of Medicine, Columbus, OH, USA*

SATU KUURE • *Institute of Biotechnology, Viikki Biocenter, University of Helsinki, Helsinki, Finland*

MELISSA H. LITTLE • *Institute for Molecular Bioscience, The University of Queensland, Brisbane, QLD, Australia*

SUE LLOYD-MACGILP • *Hugh Robson Building, University of Edinburgh, Edinburgh, UK*

OSCAR LOPEZ-FRANCO • *Renal and Vascular Research Lab, IIS-Fundacion Jimenez Diaz, Autonoma University, Madrid, Spain*

JAVIER LOPEZ-RIOS • *Developmental Genetics, Department of Biomedicine, University of Basel, Basel, Switzerland*

MICHAEL LUSIS • *Institute for Molecular Bioscience, The University of Queensland, Brisbane, QLD, Australia*

BEÑAT MALLAVIA • *Renal and Vascular Research Lab, IIS-Fundacion Jimenez Diaz, Autonoma University, Madrid, Spain*

SRIRAM MANIVANNAN • *Departments of Chemical and Biological Engineering, Princeton University, Princeton, NJ, USA*

MICHAEL MARCOTTE • *Goodman Cancer Research Centre and Department of Biochemistry, McGill University, Montreal, QC, Canada*

KIRK M. MCHUGH • *Center for Molecular and Human Genetics, Research Institute at Nationwide Children's Hospital, Columbus, OH, USA*

CATHY L. MENDELSOHN • *Department of Urology, Columbia University, ICRC, New York, NY, USA*

ODYSSÉ MICHOS • *Hammer Health Sciences Center, Department of Genetics and Development, Columbia University Medical Center, New York, NY, USA*

ANDREI MOLOTKOV • *Department of Urology, ICRC, Columbia University, New York, NY, USA*

INGA J. MURAWSKI • *Department of Human Genetics, Montreal Children's Hospital, McGill University, Montreal, QC, Canada*

CELESTE M. NELSON • *Departments of Chemical and Biological Engineering, Princeton University, Princeton, NJ, USA; Department of Molecular Biology, Princeton University, Princeton, NJ, USA*

SANJAY K. NIGAM • *Pediatrics Department, University of California, San Diego, CA, USA*

JENS R. NYENGAARD • *Department of clinical medicine, Electrom Microscopy Laboratory, Aarhus university, Aarhus C, Denmark*

GUADALUPE ORTIZ-MUÑOZ • *Renal and Vascular Research Lab, IIS-Fundacion Jimenez Diaz. Autonoma University, Madrid, Spain*

LEIF OXBURGH • *Maine Medical Center Research Institute, Scarborough, ME, USA*

XINJUN PIU • *MRC Human Genetics Unit, Western General Hospital, Edinburgh, UK*

S. STEVEN POTTER • *Division of Developmental Biology, Children's Hospital Medical Center, Cincinnati, OH, USA*

PAUL N. RICCIO • *Department of Genetics and Development, Columbia University, New York, NY, USA*

DANIEL ROMAKER • *Department of Cell Biology, Lerner Research Institute/ Cleveland Clinic, Cleveland, OH, USA*

YOGMATEE ROOCHUN • *MRC Human Genetics Unit, Western General Hospital, Edinburgh, UK*

NORMAN ROSENBLUM • *Program in Developmental and Stem Cell Biology, Division of Nephrology and Department of Paediatrics, The Hospital for Sick Children, University of Toronto, Toronto, ON, Canada; Department of Laboratory Medicine and Pathobiology, University of Toronto, Toronto, ON, Canada; Department of Physiology, University of Toronto, Toronto, ON, Canada*
BREE A. RUMBALLE • *Institute for Molecular Bioscience, The University of Queensland, Brisbane, QLD, Australia*
KIERAN M. SHORT • *Department of Biochemistry and Molecular Biology, Monash University, Clayton, VIC, Australia*
SUNDER SIMS-LUCAS • *Children's Hospital of Pittsburgh, Rangos Research Institute, Pittsburgh, PA, USA*
IAN M. SMYTH • *Department of Biochemistry and Molecular Biology, Monash University, Clayton, VIC, Australia; Department of Anatomy and Developmental Biology, Monash University, Clayton, VIC, Australia*
GUANPING TAI • *Hugh Robson Building, University of Edinburgh, Edinburgh, UK*
BARBARA A. THORNHILL • *Department of Pediatrics, University of Virginia, Charlottesville, VA, USA*
SHIFAAN THOWFEEQU • *Department of Genetics and Development, Columbia University, New York, NY, USA*
ALDA TUFRO • *Department of Pediatrics and Nephrology, Yale University School of Medicine, New Haven, CT, USA*
MATHIEU UNBEKANDT • *Hugh Robson Building, University of Edinburgh, Edinburgh, UK*
SEPPO VAINIO • *Department of Medical Biochemistry and Molecular Biology, Institute of Biomedicine, Faculty of Medicine, University of Oulu, Oulu, Finland*
ALEKSANDR VASILYEV • *Nephrology Division and Department of Pathology, Charlestown , MA, USA*
CHRISTINE L. WATT • *Department of Human Genetics, Montreal Children's Hospital, McGill University, Montreal, QC, Canada*
OLIVER WESSELY • *Department of Cell Biology, Lerner Research Institute/ Cleveland Clinic, Cleveland, OH, USA*
BO ZHANG • *Department of Cell Biology, Lerner Research Institute/Cleveland Clinic, Cleveland, OH, USA; LSUHSC, Department of Cell Biology & Anatomy, New Orleans, USA*
XING ZHANG • *Pediatrics Department, University of California, San Diego, CA, USA*

Part I

Organ Culture, Tissue Manipulation, and Live Imaging

Chapter 1

Dissecting and Culturing and Imaging the Mouse Urogenital System

Paul N. Riccio and Odyssé Michos

Abstract

Current knowledge of the morphological and molecular events driving branching morphogenesis of the ureteric bud (UB) during development of the metanephric kidney has been greatly facilitated by the ability to explant this organ to culture. The UB can be further isolated from the mesenchyme and grown within a three-dimensional, collagen-based matrix when supplemented with the appropriate growth factors. The protocol presented here outlines the dissection and culture techniques necessary to dissect and culture the whole kidney and the isolated UB.

Key words: Kidney, Ureteric bud, Branching morphogenesis, Organ culture, Growth factor

1. Introduction

Epithelial–mesenchymal interactions occur during multiple steps in the development of the metanephric kidney. Instructive cues from the mesenchyme both positively regulate (e.g., GDNF) and limit (e.g., BMP4) the potential of cells in the Wolffian duct to rearrange and evaginate into the surrounding mesenchyme, ensuring that the initial ureteric bud (UB) appears at the appropriate level along the rostrocaudal axis (1). Once the primary UB has been established, mesenchymal cues are again required to sustain reiterative branching of this epithelium. This period of reiterative branching can be studied in vitro by explanting the intact metanephric kidney to culture (2). Strikingly, branching of the UB is, to some extent, intrinsic to this epithelium as the UB can be isolated from the mesenchyme and cultured independently. This protocol outlines the dissection techniques required to isolate the metanephric kidney and further isolate the UB (iUB) from the mesenchyme.

Odyssé Michos (ed.), *Kidney Development: Methods and Protocols*, Methods in Molecular Biology, vol. 886, DOI 10.1007/978-1-61779-851-1_1, © Springer Science+Business Media, LLC 2012

The intact metanephric kidney grows remarkably well at an air–medium interface, sustaining branching morphogenesis of the epithelium and differentiation of the mesenchyme into nephrons. The three-dimensional morphology of the kidney is obviously not recapitulated in this type of organ culture, and the explant assumes a flattened "pancake" shape; however, one can nonetheless use this technique to monitor the types of branching events that occur, the kinetics of branching, as well as introduce pharmacological manipulations that would not be possible in vivo. For example, the Mek inhibitor PD98059 disrupts branching, but not elongation of the epithelium (2, 3). Moreover, the development of Hoxb7-EGFP and Hoxb7-myristoylated/Venus reporter transgenes has greatly facilitated the ability to visualize and analyze the UB epithelium specifically (4, 5).

The earliest attempts to culture the iUB established branching could occur independently of cell contact with the mesenchyme. In one study, rat iUBs grew best when suspended within a type I collagen matrix, rather than sitting atop the collagen (6). Conditioned medium from cell lines derived from mesenchymal tumors proved to be mitogenic; however, it was difficult to identify which of the many factors present in such medium were responsible for the instructive signaling. A combination of conditioned medium from an immortalized metanephric mesenchyme cell line (BSN-CM) and the growth factors EGF, HGF, IGF, FGF2, and GDNF, was found to sustain branching of the iUB suspended within a collagen/Matrigel matrix (7).

The protocol outlined here, however, avoids the significant effort of collecting conditioned medium, as well as the expensive battery of recombinant proteins needed. Rosselot and Spraggon et al. reported that standard D-MEM/F12 medium supplemented with GDNF and retinoic acid (RA) was sufficient to drive branching (8). The uniform dispersal of growth factors in these iUB experiments challenges the long-standing hypothesis that gradients of mitogenic cues drive branching of the epithelium (9). While branching morphogenesis is to some extent intrinsic to the epithelium, the mesenchyme may be primarily needed to establish proper patterning. Isolated UBs recombined with lung mesenchyme, for example, assume a "lung-like" morphology, presenting a greater number of lateral branches (10).

The growth factors used in earlier iUB protocols may similarly confer specific changes in the morphology of the branching UB. Various FGF family members had unique effects on the iUB, but generally supported growth, whereas TGF-ß superfamily members generally posed an inhibitory effect (11–14). The secreted factor heregulin (HRG) has been shown to support trunk, over tip fate, in iUB experiments (15). Another notable use of the iUB protocol was the molecular dissection of downstream targets of the GDNF/Ret signaling pathway (16).

2. Materials

2.1. Isolating the Metanephric Kidney

1. Mouse embryos (E11.5 for iUB culture).
2. Surgical scissors.
3. Curved serrated forceps.
4. 2 pairs of fine watchmaker's forceps.
5. Dissection medium for organ culture: D-PBS (with Ca^{2+}, Mg^{2+}) or CO_2 independent medium.
6. 35-mm, 60-mm, 100-mm Petri dishes.
7. Stereomicroscope.

2.2. Culturing the Intact Metanephric Kidney

1. Sterile six multiwell culture plate.
2. 24-mm, 0.4 μM pore polyester membrane Transwell® filters (Corning Inc).
3. Kidney culture medium: D-MEM/F12, 10% fetal bovine serum (FBS), 1% penicillin/streptomycin, 1% L-glutamine.
4. Capillary transfer pipette such as the Wiretrol® II (Drummond).
5. Incubator set to 37°C, 5% CO_2.

2.3. Isolating and Culturing the Ureteric Bud

1. Isolated E11.5 metanephroi.
2. Capillary transfer pipette such as the Wiretrol® II (Drummond).
3. Sterile 24-multiwell culture plate.
4. Digestion medium: D-MEM/F12, 10% fetal bovine serum, 1% L-glutamine, 2 mg/mL collagenase.
5. Postdigestion medium: D-MEM/F12, 10% fetal bovine serum, 1% L-glutamine, 25 μ/mL DNase I.
6. Growth factor supplemented kidney culture medium: D-MEM/F12, 10% fetal bovine serum, 1% penicillin/streptomycin, 1% L-glutamine, 200 nM trans retinoic acid (Sigma), 200 nM cis retinoic acid (Biomol), 100 ng/mL recombinant rat GDNF (R&D).
7. Matrigel basement membrane matrix (BD Biosciences). Thaw on ice, make aliquot, and store at –20°C. Do not refreeze an aliquot after thawing. In general, we make 250 μL or 500 μL aliquots (good for 1 or 2 well in a 24-multiwell plate).
8. Incubator set to 37°C, 5% CO_2.

3. Methods

3.1. Isolating the Metanephric Kidney

1. Sacrifice the pregnant female humanely in accordance with your institutionally approved protocol and place her backside down on an absorbent bench pad. Spray the abdominal area with 70% ethanol to minimize contamination with hair in the subsequent dissection steps.
2. Make a small incision in the skin along the midline of the abdominal area. To fully separate the skin, tear from this incision by pulling towards the head and tail ends of the mouse. The peritoneum should still be intact at this point and can be cut with the forceps and surgical scissors to expose the abdominal cavity.
3. Pushing the intestines to the side, locate the uterus and pinch one of the uterine horns at the anterior end with the forceps. With the scissors, cut this anterior end free and snip along the mesometrium, leaving the horn connected at the cervical end. Pull the horn slightly taut and expose the decidua by "unzipping" the uterine wall on the side opposite the connective membrane. Decidua can then be easily pinched out of the uterus and transferred to a dish of D-PBS.
4. Tear open the extraembryonic tissues and clear them away from the embryo by pinching at the umbilicus.
5. Under the dissection microscope, lay the embryo on the side (Fig. 1a). The proper positioning of the next cut is important: several somites anterior to the hind limbs pinch the embryo

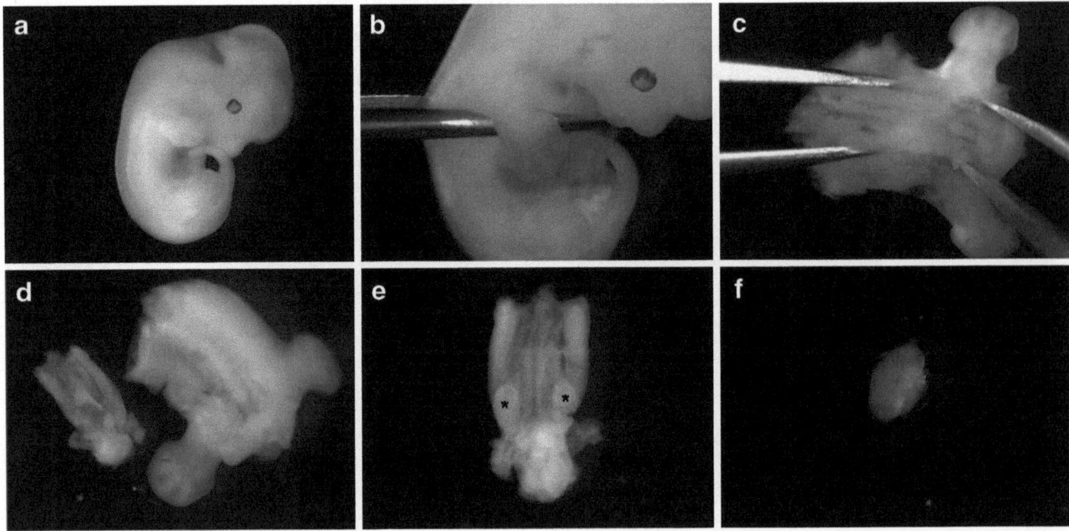

Fig. 1. Dissection step illustrating the isolation of an E12.5 metanephric kidney (*Asterisk* in (**e**): metanephric kidney).

with one pair of forceps and cleanly tear in half with the other (Fig. 1b). The anterior piece can be discarded or saved for isolation of the anterior viscera.

6. Flip the posterior piece dorsal side down. The metanephric kidneys are roughly located between the hind limb buds in a 40–60 somites embryo (E11.0-E12.5), so take care not to pierce that area.
   (a) Cut the tail and save it for genotyping if necessary.
   (b) Splay open the body wall and pin down the embryo with forceps in one hand.
   (c) Remove the gut, exposing the intermediate mesoderm (urogenital ridge).
   (d) With the other forceps, remove the urogenital ridge from the abdominal area by pulling from the rostral end down to the genital tubercle (Fig. 1c, d). The kidneys are located on the dorsal side of the urogenital ridge (Fig. 1e) and can be further dissected with tungsten needles (Fig. 1f).

3.2. Culturing the Intact Metanephric Kidney

1. Pipette 1.5 mL of kidney culture medium to the well of the 12-multiwell culture plate and insert the Transwell filter.
2. Using the capillary transfer pipette, place the isolated kidney atop of the filter. Remove any excess liquid from the top of the filter (see Note 1).
3. Replace the lid of the culture dish and incubate the isolated kidneys at 37°C, 5% CO_2. The culture can be removed periodically and photographed with a microscope outfitted with a digital camera (Fig. 2) (see Note 2).
4. For long incubations that last several days, replace the kidney culture medium every 48 h (see Note 3).

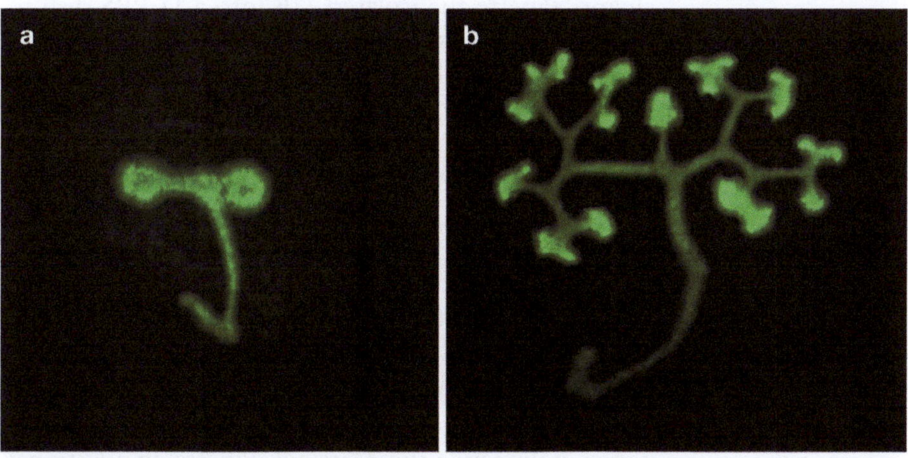

Fig. 2. Organ culture. (**a**) E11.5 HoxB7-mVenus kidney. (**b**) E11.5 HoxB7-mVenus kidney after 48 h in culture. The HoxB7 promoter drives expression of the mVenus in the UB epithelium (5).

3.3. Isolating and Culturing the Ureteric Bud

The UB can be isolated from the mesenchyme by a combination of enzymatic and mechanical dissection techniques.

1. Pipette the metanephroi (Fig. 1f) into a 35-mm dish containing 1 mL of digestion medium (collagenase solution) and incubate for 15 min at 37°C (see Note 4).
2. During the incubation period you can prepare the growth factor supplemented Matrigel solution and cast it in the well of a 24-multiwell culture plate.
   (a) Thaw the Matrigel on ice.
   (b) Prepare the growth factor supplemented kidney culture medium: add GDNF and the retinoic acid isomers to the kidney culture medium (see Note 5).
   (c) Prepare the 1:2 solution of Matrigel to medium.
   Dilute the ice-cold Matrigel with the growth factor supplemented kidney culture medium. Pipette 0.5 mL of this diluted Matrigel solution to each well of the 24-multiwell culture plate to be used.
   (d) Place the multiwell culture plate in the 37°C incubator to polymerize the Matrigel. After 30 min, the Matrigel will be sufficiently polymerized to hold a small tissue sample without it sinking (see Note 6).
3. Following the incubation in collagenase, transfer the metanephroi to a 35-mm dish containing 1 mL of postdigestion medium (DNase I solution) to halt the enzymatic digestion. The DNase I is used to keep the tissue from becoming too sticky due to the lysis of the outermost mesenchymal cells.
4. Using the tungsten needles pierce the mesenchyme close to a tip of the UB. Under optimal digestion conditions, the UB should be easily liberated through a hole torn in the mesenchyme. Pipette the isolated UB into a D-PBS dish to remove any residual mesenchyme (Fig. 3a). Identification of the T-shaped UB within the digested mesenchyme can be facilitated by adjusting the transmitted light source on the dissecting microscope to a high contrast setting.
5. Transfer the iUBs to the precast Matrigel-based medium. Position the iUB in the center of the Matrigel by gently manipulating with the tungsten needles or forceps. Ideally, the iUB should be suspended in the center of the matrix. Do not position it such that it floats to the top, or sinks to the bottom of the well.
6. Once satisfactorily positioned, incubate the iUBs in the Matrigel solution for an additional 30 min at 37°C to completely polymerize the Matrigel. Pipette an additional 0.5 mL of iUB culture medium atop the hardened Matrigel.

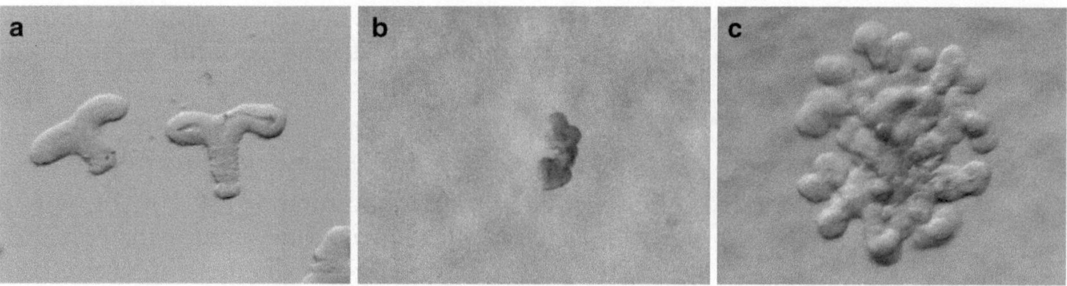

Fig. 3. In vitro culture of iUB in Matrigel. (**a**) E11.5 isolated ureteric bud (iUB) after separation with metanephric mesenchyme. (**b**) E11.5 iUB in Matrigel at 0 h of culture. (**c**) iUB after 4 days of culture in Matrigel.

7. Incubate the iUBs at 37°C, 5% CO_2 for the duration of the culture. Growth of the iUBs can be documented with a stereomicroscope outfitted with a digital camera (Fig. 3b, c) (see Note 7).

4. Notes

1. Ensuring that excess medium is pipetted off of the top of the filter is crucial to achieving organ growth in culture. Kidney rudiments that are submerged under a drop of medium, despite being adhered to the filter, will not branch well.
2. The organ explant will take approximately 1 h to fully adhere to the membrane. It will also gradually flatten during the first few hours of culture, which may require shifting the plane of focus in automated time-lapse imaging.
3. An E12.5 kidney explant can grow for up to 7 days in culture, provided the medium is changed at least every 48 h. Metanephric kidneys from older embryos (greater than E13.5) will not fare as well as the thickness of the tissue prevents proper nutrient and gas exchange for the innermost cells.
4. The actual length of the digestion period depends on the amount of mesenchyme left intact after the dissection. An appropriate collagenase digestion period should be determined empirically to avoid disrupting the epithelium as well as the mesenchyme.
5. As the final concentration of retinoic acid in the growth medium is significantly lower than stock concentrations, a serial dilution must be performed.
   (a) Prepare the kidney culture medium: D-MEM/F12 solution containing the 10% FBS, 1× L-glutamine, 1% penicillin/streptomycin.

(b) First dilution (intermediate concentration): add 10 μL of each 10 mM retinoic acid isomer to 10 mL of kidney culture medium.

(c) Working dilution (final concentration): pipette 100 μL of the first dilution to 5 mL of kidney culture medium.

(d) Add GDNF to final concentration of 100 ng/mL in growth factor supplemented kidney culture medium.

The recombinant GDNF is the most expensive component, thus rather than adding 500 ng of protein to all 5 mL, use only as much as necessary: approximately 750 μL per well.

6. Partially polymerized Matrigel is ideal for properly situating the iUB. The tissue can be moved in the matrix with forceps, and any tears created in the matrix will heal during subsequent incubation. Once fully polymerized, however, it becomes very difficult to move the iUB.

7. The extent of branching achieved will depend on many factors, but, generally, "T-shaped" UBs—from roughly 48 somite embryos—branch better than earlier rudiments that have only achieved the ampulla stage. To make meaningful comparisons of different UBs, it is necessary to carefully document the state of the tissue at the beginning of the culture.

References

1. Michos O (2009) Kidney development: from ureteric bud formation to branching morphogenesis. Curr Opin Genet Dev 19(5):484–490
2. Watanabe T, Costantini F (2004) Real-time analysis of ureteric bud branching morphogenesis in vitro. Dev Biol 271:98–108
3. Fisher CE, Michael L, Barnett MW, Davies JA (2001) Erk MAP kinase regulates branching morphogenesis in the developing mouse kidney. Development 128(21):4329–4338
4. Srinivas S, Goldberg MR, Watanabe T et al (1999) Expression of green fluorescent protein in the ureteric bud of transgenic mice: a new tool for the analysis of ureteric bud morphogenesis. Dev Genet 24:241–251
5. Chi X, Hadjantonakis AK, Wu Z, Hyink D, Costantini F (2009) A transgenic mouse that reveals cell shape and arrangement during ureteric bud branching. Genesis 47(2):61–66
6. Perantoni AO, Williams CL, Lewellyn AL (1991) Growth and branching morphogenesis of rat collecting duct anlagen in the absence of metanephrogenic mesenchyme. Differentiation 48:107–113
7. Qiao J, Dakurai H, Nigam SK (1999) Branching morphogenesis independent of mesenchymal-epithelial contact in the developing kidney. Proc Natl Acad Sci USA 96:7330–7335
8. Rosselot C, Spraggon L, Chia I et al (2010) Non-cell-autonomous retinoid signaling is crucial for renal development. Development 137:282–292
9. Sariola H, Saarma M (2003) Novel functions and signaling pathways for GDNF. J Cell Sci 116:3855–3862
10. Lin Y, Zhang S, Rehn M et al (2001) Induced repatterning of type XVIII collagen expression in ureter bud from kidney to lung type: association with sonic hedgehog and ectopic surfactant protein C. Development 128:1573–1585
11. Qiao J, Bush KT, Steer D et al (2001) Multiple fibroblast growth factors support growth of the ureteric bud but have different effects on branching morphogenesis. Mech Dev 109:123–135
12. Bush KT, Sakurai H, Steer DL et al (2004) TGF-beta superfamily members modulate growth, branching, shaping, and patterning of the ureteric bud. Dev Biol 266:285–295

13. Michos O, Gonçalves A, Lopez-Rios J et al (2007) Reduction of BMP4 activity by gremlin 1 enables ureteric bud outgrowth and GDNF/WNT11 feedback signalling during kidney branching morphogenesis. Development 134(13):2397–2405
14. Michos O, Cebrian C, Hyink D et al (2010) Kidney development in the absence of Gdnf and Spry1 requires Fgf10. PLoS Genet 6(1):e1000809
15. Sakurai H, Bush KT, Nigam SK (2005) Heregulin induces glial cell line-derived neurotrophic growth factor-independent, non-branching growth and differentiation of ureteric bud epithelia. J Biol Chem 280:42181–42187
16. Lu BC, Cebrian C, Chi X et al (2009) Etv4 and Etv5 are required downstream of GDNF and Ret for kidney branching morphogenesis. Nat Genet 41:1295–1302

Chapter 2

In Vitro Culture of Embryonic Kidney Rudiments and Isolated Ureteric Buds

Xing Zhang, Kevin T. Bush, and Sanjay K. Nigam

Abstract

In vitro culture of embryonic kidney rudiments has been utilized to study a variety of cellular processes and developmental mechanisms. Here, we describe two-dimensional (2D) culture of embryonic kidney rudiments on Transwell filters and three-dimensional (3D) cultures in collagen gels in detail, and 3D culture of isolated ureteric bud (UB) in Matrigel with BSN-conditioned media.

Key words: Microdissection, Embryonic kidney rudiments, Ureteric bud, Three-Dimensional culture

1. Introduction

The development of the metanephric kidney begins with the reciprocal inductive interactions between the ureteric bud (UB) and the metanephric mesenchyme (MM). The UB invades the surrounding MM where it undergoes branching morphogenesis giving rise to the tree-like kidney collecting system. In a reciprocal fashion, the UB signals the MM to condense near the newly formed UB tips, undergo the process of mesenchymal-to-epithelial transition (MET) followed by a series of morphological stages to form the nephrons (1). Many genes (2, 3) and molecules, including growth factors, extracellular matrix proteins, integrins, etc., have been reported to regulate these two distinct processes (4–7). A variety of such cellular processes and developmental mechanisms are capable of being studied during organogenesis. Therefore, in vitro cultures of whole embryonic kidney rudiments or progenitor tissues isolated from the embryonic kidney, including the isolated MM and UBs, have been utilized to study these mechanisms (8–12).

Odyssé Michos (ed.), *Kidney Development: Methods and Protocols*, Methods in Molecular Biology, vol. 886,
DOI 10.1007/978-1-61779-851-1_2, © Springer Science+Business Media, LLC 2012

A number of in vitro three-dimensional (3D) culture systems have been devised to obtain greater spatial growth of isolated embryonic kidneys and UBs (13–16). In this protocol, two-dimensional (2D) culture of embryonic kidney rudiments on Transwell filters and three-dimensional (3D) cultures in extracellular matrix gels are described in detail. The difference between 2D and 3D cultures are compared.

2. Materials

2.1. Reagents

1. Phosphate-Buffered Saline (PBS) without calcium or magnesium.
2. Phosphate-Buffered Saline (PBS) with calcium or magnesium.
3. 70% Ethanol.
4. Liebovitz's L-15 medium with L-glutamine.
5. Trypsin (0.1% solution in L-15 medium): dissolve powdered Trypsin (porcine pancreas; Sigma) in L-15 medium to a concentration of 1 mg/mL.
6. DNase I.
7. DMEM–F12 (50:50) mixture growth medium with L-glutamine and 15 mM HEPES.
8. 10× Dulbecco's modified Eagle's medium (DMEM).
9. Fetal Bovine Serum (FBS).
10. Type I collagen (BD Biosciences).
11. Type IV collagen (BD Biosciences).
12. Growth factor-reduced Matrigel (BD Biosciences).
13. Antibiotic-antimycotic solution.
14. Growth factors: Rat recombinant glial cell line-derived neurotrophic factor (rrGDNF) (R&D Systems); Fibroblast growth factors (FGF)—recombinant human FGF1 (Calbiochem).

2.2. Equipment

1. Stereozoom dissecting microscope.
2. Fiber-optic external light source (eliminates a potential source of heat during dissections).
3. Blunt operating scissors.
4. Potts-Smith forceps with teeth either straight or curved.
5. Dumont #55 forceps.
6. Minutien pins held in pinholder.
7. 100 × 15 mm Petri dishes.
8. Tissue culture dishes (60 × 15 mm; 35 × 10 mm).

9. Corning Transwell permeable supports 0.4 μM pore size for 12- or 24-multiwell plate.
10. Tissue culture plates: 12- or 24-multiwell plate.
11. Insert pin held in pinholder with the final ½ in. of the pin bent at ~45° angle.
12. Drummond Wiretrol I calibrated micropipettes, 50 μL and 100 μL.
13. 500 mL filter system.
14. Amicon Ultra-15 centrifugal tubes.
15. Allegra™ 25R Centrifuge.

3. Methods

3.1. Isolation of Embryonic Kidneys from Time-Pregnant Mice/Rats

1. The uterine horns from the pregnant rodents (mice—gestational day 10.5–11, or rats—gestational day 12.5–13; day 0 of gestation coincides with appearance of the vaginal plug) are dissected free from surrounding tissues and transferred to a separate 10-cm Petri dish filled with L-15 medium kept on ice.
2. The embryos are isolated and transferred to a new 10-cm Petri dish with L-15 medium kept on ice.
3. The paired embryonic urinary tracts [i.e., mesonephros, Wolffian ducts, kidneys, ureters, and urogenital sinus (under the cloacal ridge)]—which lie against the back body wall arranged in an anterior to posterior fashion running parallel to the dorsal aorta—are dissected free from surrounding tissues and the entire structure is transferred to a separate 60-mm tissue culture dish containing L-15 medium.
4. The kidneys will lie at the posterior end of the isolated urinary tract, just under the bifurcating dorsal aorta. Remove and isolate the kidneys by dissecting away the surrounding tissue. If the whole embryonic kidney is to be cultured, it should be comprised of just the ureteric bud and its surrounding metanephric mesenchyme. Transfer kidneys with a micropipette to a 35-mm tissue culture dish containing DMEM/F12 medium.

3.2. Preparation of Extracellular Matrix Gel

1. Type I collagen gel is prepared such that the final solution consists of 80% sterile type I collagen solution, 10% 10× DMEM, and 10% sterile 1 M Hepes solution. Adjust pH to 7.4 with 1 M NaOH solution and keep the solution on ice to prevent gelation before use for tissue culture (see Note 4).
2. Type IV collagen gel is prepared by mixing 75% type IV collagen, 10% 10× DMEM, 10% 1 M Hepes, 5% 20× $NaHCO_3$. Adjust pH to 7.4 with 1 M NaOH solution and keep the solution on ice to prevent gelation before use for tissue culture (see Note 4).

3. Growth factor-reduced Matrigel is obtained from BD Biosciences. A 50% Matrigel solution is prepared by diluting the original Matrigel 1:1 with 1× DMEM/F12 medium (see Note 5).

3.3. Culture of Embryonic Kidney Rudiment

1. Under the dissection microscope carefully clean away any tissues surrounding the embryonic kidney. The embryonic kidney to be cultured should be comprised of just the ureteric bud and its surrounding metanephric mesenchyme.
2. Prepare Transwell tissue culture inserts for the whole embryonic kidneys and transfer one to two whole embryonic kidneys directly onto the filter (2D culture) (see Note 2). Remove excess liquid from top of each filter and position the kidneys on the filters (see Note 3).
3. For 3D culture, pipette 600 μL type I or IV collagen solution into a 12-multiwell Transwell filter (see Note 8). Using a 50-μL Wiretrol micropipette, transfer one to two embryonic kidneys directly into the collagen gels. Using an insert pin with the angled tip position and suspend each kidney within the collagen gel; this must be done until the collagen matrix solidifies, as the kidneys will sink to the bottom of the insert (see Notes 6 and 7).
4. In the biological safety cabinet, transfer the Transwell tissue culture inserts from either the 2D or 3D culture system containing the whole embryonic kidneys cultures into the individual wells of a separate tissue culture plate containing DMEM/F12 supplemented with 10% FBS, 1× antibiotic-antimycotic solution [12-multiwell (600 μL) or 24-multiwell plate (400 μL)].
5. Culture for 7–14 days (without media changes) at 37°C with ~95% humidity. Examine and photograph the growth of the whole embryonic kidneys (Figs. 1 and 2).

3.4. Culture of Isolated UB

1. Pipette 2,000 μL of 0.1% trypsin/L-15 solution, as well as 10 μL of DNase I in a 35-mm tissue culture dish, and mix well (see Note 1).
2. Using the 50 μL Wiretrol micropipette, transfer the whole embryonic kidneys to the trypsin/DNase I solution. Place the lid on the tissue culture dish and incubate the kidneys in the trypsin/DNase I solution for 20 min at 37°C.
3. Stop the enzymatic activity by adding 200 μL of FBS to the trypsin/DNase I solution and swirl to mix (see Note 1). Remove the kidneys to a separate 35-mm tissue culture dish containing 2 mL of L-15 supplemented with 10% FBS and 10 μL of DNase I.
4. Under the dissection microscope, gently grasp the trypsinized kidney with the Dumont #55 forceps and, using the minutien

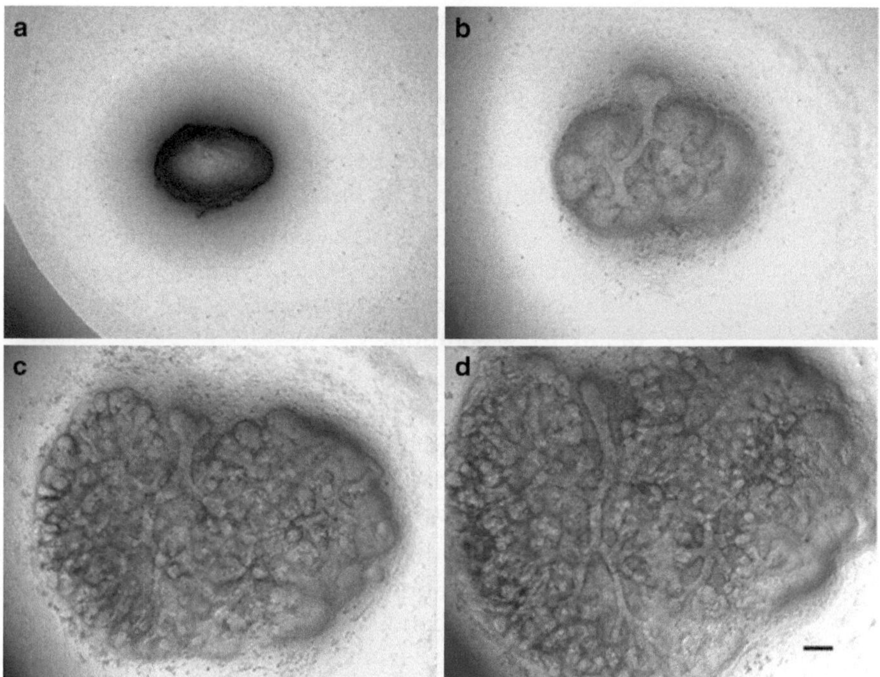

Fig. 1. Two-Dimensional (2D) in vitro rat embryonic kidney rudiments (E13) cultured on Transwell filters for different times: (**a**) control at day 0, (**b**) 2 days, (**c**) 5 days, (**d**) 7 days. All samples were cultured with DMEM/F12 medium supplemented with 10% FBS and 1× Antibiotic-antimycotic solution. Scale bar = 200 μm.

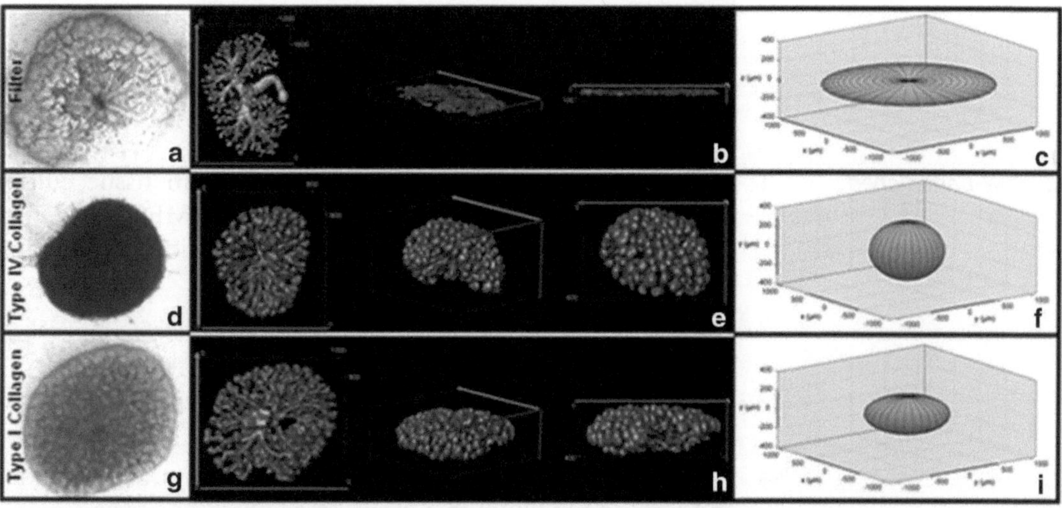

Fig. 2. 3D projection of the branching ureteric bud of E12 HoxB7-GFP mouse kidneys cultured for 7 days. Kidneys in the traditional filter culture grew flat (2D) and along the filter (**a–c**), while kidneys cultured in type IV collagen (**d–f**) or type I collagen (**g–i**) grew much thicker and in a more 3D manner (units, μm). A part of this figure is from ref. 15.

pins, carefully tease the metanephric mesenchyme away from the ureteric bud.

5. In a biological safety cabinet, prepare the 50% Matrigel solution as described above (see Note 5). Place Transwell into a separate tissue culture dish. For these studies, a 24-well tissue culture dish is typically used.
6. Pipette ~80 μL of 50% Matrigel solution directly into a Transwell filter. Using a 50-μL Wiretrol micropipette, transfer 1–2 clean iUBs with a minimum of L-15 medium directly into the Matrigel solution.
7. Under the dissection microscope, use the insert pin with the angled tip to position and suspend each iUB within the Matrigel; this must be done until the Matrigel gels, as the buds tend to sink to the bottom of the insert (see Note 6). Repeat these steps for each iUB to be cultured in 3D extracellular matrix gels.
8. Prepare the growth medium as described below. Pipette 400 μL of this BSN-conditioned medium (see Subheading 3.5 for preparation of BSN-conditioned medium) (see Note 9) into the wells of a separate 24-multiwell tissue culture plate and add 125 ng/ml each of GDNF and FGF1. The BSN conditioned media should also be supplemented with 10% FCS and 1× antibiotic/antimycotic. Transfer the Transwell tissue culture inserts into the prepared wells. Make sure that there are no air bubbles beneath the filter.
9. Place the entire setup into a CO_2 incubator and culture for 7–10 days (without medium changes) at 37°C with ~95% humidity.
10. Examine and photograph the growth and branching of the iUBs using an inverted microscope equipped with phase-contrast (Fig. 3).

3.5. BSN-Conditioned Medium

1. Culture BSN cells to confluence in 100-mm tissue culture dishes (at least 20) containing 10 mL of DMEM/F12 with 10% FBS and 1× antibiotic-antimycotic solution at 37°C in a 5% CO_2 incubator.
2. Remove the growth medium, wash the monolayers at least 3× with PBS and aspirate PBS.
3. Pipette 10 mL of serum-free DMEM/F12 to the culture dishes and maintain the culture at 37°C in a 5% CO_2 incubator.
4. Collect the serum-free medium after 2–3 days of incubation and pool the medium in a clean, sterile flask or bottle.
5. Apply the ~200 mL of BSN-conditioned medium to a 0.22-μm membrane filter to remove cellular debris and further concentrate the medium 30-fold with a Centricon (Millipore) filter with an 8-kDa nominal molecular mass cutoff.

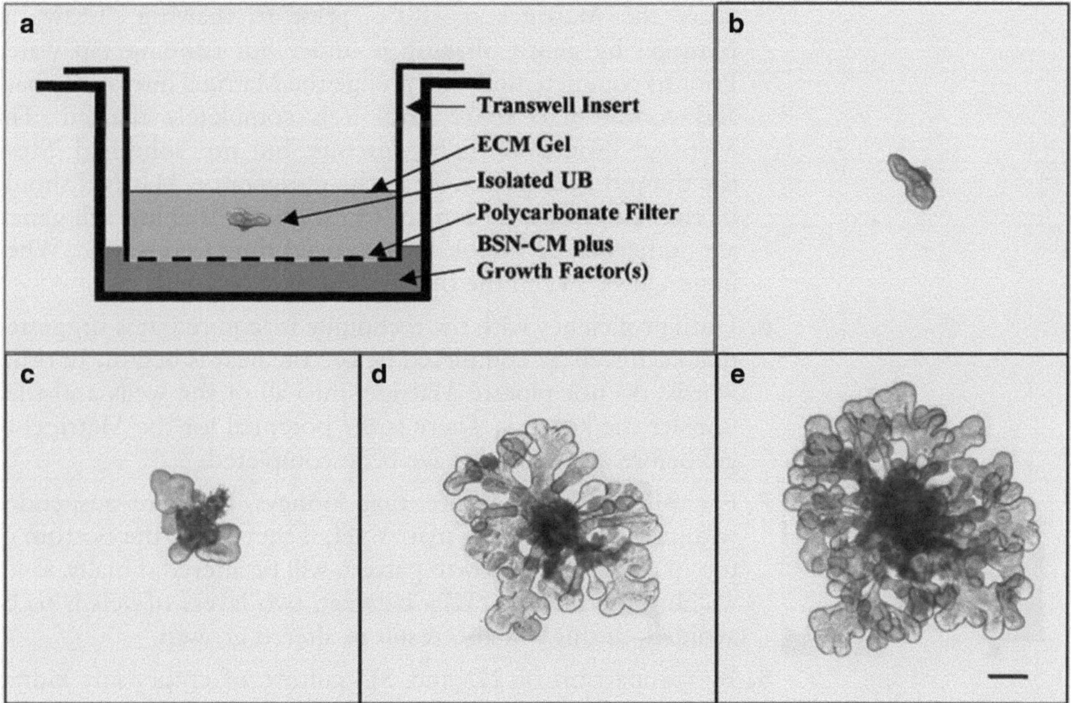

Fig. 3. Schematic drawing of in vitro culture of iUB in Matrigel (**a**), and phase contrast images of iUB culture for different time: (**b**) control at day 0, (**c**) 2 days, (**d**) 5 days, (**e**) 7 days. Isolated UB samples were cultured with BSN-conditioned medium supplemented with 10% FBS and 1× Antibiotic-antimycotic solution, and 125 ng/mL FGF1 and 125 ng/mL GDNF. Scale bar = 200 μm. A part of this figure is from Ref. 14.

4. Notes

1. Do not forget to add the FBS or DNase I solution during separation of UB and MM. Without these supplements added to the L-15 medium, the kidneys will become extremely sticky and will adhere to each other as well as the bottom of the tissue culture dish.
2. After placing the kidneys/UBs on the Transwell filters, the inserts must remain moist throughout the remaining steps of the protocol; otherwise, the applied organs/tissues may dry to the filter during the following transfer and positioning steps.
3. The tissues/organs are cultured on the top of the filter at the air–media interface. If excess media/moisture accumulates on the filter, it should be removed. The growth of the tissue/organs is adversely affected if they are completely covered by liquid.
4. For preparation of type I or IV collagen solutions, keep all reagents on ice during the process. First, mix all other reagents, and then add type I or IV collagen to the above mixture. Gently pipette to obtain a homogeneous solution (avoid bubbles).

5. Store the Matrigel at −80°C prior to thawing. Thaw the Matrigel by gently shaking it under hot running tap water. Prior to complete thawing, plunge the Matrigel into an ice-bath and continue to shake until it is completely thawed. The Matrigel should be highly viscous, but not solidified. Store the thawed Matrigel on ice in the refrigerator. Matrigel should be thawed at least 24 h prior to use, as the shaking will generate numerous air bubbles which need time to dissipate. When in use, always keep the thawed Matrigel on ice.
6. Until proficiency with the technique is acquired, it is suggested that each well be completed before the next is begun. In other words, do not pipette Matrigel into all of the wells and then transfer the kidneys. There is the potential for the Matrigel to gel before all the wells have been completed.
7. For 3D cultures, ensure that kidneys/UBs are suspended within the extracellular matrix gel; if they are at the bottom or top of the gel, the growth pattern will be altered. Finally, sandwiching the kidneys/UBs between two layers of gels is to be avoided, as this will also result in altered growth.
8. By comparison of 2D and 3D culture of embryonic kidney rudiments (Fig. 2), we found that type IV collagen supports the deepest tissue growth and the largest kidney volume, followed by type I collagen culture and the filter culture system. Furthermore, only kidneys in type IV collagen exhibited a 3D umbrella-like branching pattern characteristic as in vivo kidney development.
9. If BSN-conditioned media is unavailable growth and branching of the isolated UB can be achieved by supplementation of DMEM/F12 with purified growth factors. For example, pleiotrophin (17) or heregulin (18) can be added to the media along with GDNF and FGF1.

Acknowledgment

This work was supported by National Institute of Diabetes and Digestive and Kidney Diseases grants (to S.K.N). The care and use of animals described in this investigation conform to the procedures of the laboratory's Animal Protocol approved by the Animal Subjects Program and the IACUC of the University of California, San Diego. We thank Eran Rosines for creating the 3D projection of the branching ureteric buds (Fig. 2) from 2-photon images.

References

1. Shah MM, Sampogna RV, Sakurai H, Bush KT, Nigam SK (2004) Branching morphogenesis and kidney disease. Development 131: 1449–1462
2. Dressler GR (1995) The genetic control of renal development. Curr Opin Nephrol Hypertens 4:253–257
3. Sampogna RV, Nigam SK (2004) Implications of gene networks for understanding resilience and vulnerability in the kidney branching program. Physiology 19:339–347
4. Pohl M, Stuart RO, Sakurai H, Nigam SK (2000) Branching morphogenesis during kidney development. Annu Rev Physiol 62:595–620
5. Costantini F, Kopan R (2010) Patterning a complex organ: branching morphogenesis and nephron segmentation in kidney development. Dev Cell 18:698–712
6. Lelongt B, Ronco P (2003) Role of extracellular matrix in kidney development and repair. Pediatr Nephrol 18:731–742
7. Lechner MS, Dressler GR (1997) The molecular basis of embryonic kidney development. Mech Dev 62:105–120
8. Bard JB, Ross AS (1991) LIF, the ES-cell inhibition factor, reversibly blocks nephrogenesis in cultured mouse kidney rudiments. Development 113:193–198
9. Davies J (1994) Control of calbindin-D28K expression in developing mouse kidney. Dev Dyn 199:45–51
10. Michos O, Gonçalves A, Lopez-Rios J et al (2007) Reduction of BMP4 activity by gremlin 1 enables ureteric bud outgrowth and GDNF/WNT11 feedback signalling during kidney branching morphogenesis. Development 134: 2397–2405
11. Thesleff I, Ekblom P (1984) Role of transferrin in branching morphogenesis, growth and differentiation of the embryonic kidney. J Embryol Exp Morphol 82:147–161
12. Sebinger DD, Unbekandt M, Ganeva VV et al (2010) A novel, low-volume method for organ culture of embryonic kidneys that allows development of cortico-medullary anatomical organization. PLoS One 5:e10550
13. Steer DL, Bush KT, Meyer TN, Schwesinger C, Nigam SK (2002) A strategy for in vitro propagation of rat nephrons. Kidney Int 62:1958–1965
14. Qiao J, Sakurai H, Nigam SK (1999) Branching morphogenesis independent of mesenchymal-epithelial contact in the developing kidney. Proc Natl Acad Sci USA 96:7330–7335
15. Rosines E, Schmidt HJ, Nigam SK (2007) The effect of hyaluronic acid size and concentration on branching morphogenesis and tubule differentiation in developing kidney culture systems: potential applications to engineering of renal tissues. Biomaterials 28:4806–4817
16. Rosines E, Johkura K, Zhang X et al (2010) Constructing kidney-like tissues from cells based on programs for organ development: toward a method of in vitro tissue engineering of the kidney. Tissue Eng Part A 16:2441–2455
17. Sakurai H, Bush KT, Nigam SK (2001) Identification of pleiotrophin as a mesenchymal factor involved in ureteric bud branching morphogeneisis. Development 128:3283–3293
18. Sakurai H, Bush KT, Nigam SK (2005) Heregulin induces glial cell line-derived neurotrophic growth factor-independent, non-branching growth and differentiation of ureteric bud epithelia. J Biol Chem 280:42181–42187

Chapter 3

In Vitro Induction of Nephrogenesis in Mouse Metanephric Mesenchyme with Lithium Introduction and Ureteric Bud Recombination

Kimmo Halt and Seppo Vainio

Abstract

The organ culture setup of embryonic kidney has served as a model of nephrogenesis for several decades. In vitro culture of the mouse metanephric mesenchyme enables easy manipulation and analysis of the tissue and provides information of cellular interactions, morphogenesis, cell differentiation, and molecular biology of the developmental process. The advantages of the tissue culture method include enhanced representativeness of situation in living organism compared to cell culture assays and less demanding and time-consuming possibilities to experimental work compared with in vivo research.

Key words: Kidney development, Nephrogenesis, Organ culture, Metanephros, Metanephric mesenchyme, Ureteric bud, Induction

1. Introduction

The permanent kidney of amniotes originates from the intermediate mesoderm giving rise to the ureteric bud (UB) and the metanephric mesenchyme (MM) (1, 2). Together, these two components make up the metanephros that undergoes development into a mature kidney through iterative steps (1, 2). Reciprocal interactions between the UB and MM cause successive dichotomous branching of the UB while the MM is induced to condensate and epithelialize adjacent to the tips of the UB (1, 2). Epithelialized vesicles undergo morphogenesis into mature nephrons forming a connection with the UB-derived collecting duct system in distal end and basement membrane delineated filtration unit with the glomerular epithelium in proximal head (1, 2). At the molecular

Odyssé Michos (ed.), *Kidney Development: Methods and Protocols*, Methods in Molecular Biology, vol. 886,
DOI 10.1007/978-1-61779-851-1_3, © Springer Science+Business Media, LLC 2012

level, activation of Wnt pathway has been demonstrated both sufficient and required for nephrogenic induction. Namely, *Wnt9b* (3) expressed in the UB tip acts upstream of *Wnt4*, which plays an essential role in the epithelization of a presumptive nephron (4, 5). The organ culture assay of the MM has been used for decades to uncover the cellular and molecular interplay associated to nephrogenesis. Grobstein (1955) was the first to introduce a method to induce nephrogenesis in mammalian MM using embryonic spinal cord as a nephrogenic inductor (6). Since then, the organ culture setup has been used and modified while the basic principle has remained the same, including microsurgical dissection of metanephros, subsequent removal of the UB, and finally induction of nephrogenesis in MM. Induction of nephrogenesis in plain MM can be achieved with various means. Lithium, a chemical Wnt pathway activator (7), was found to induce presumptive nephron condensation recapitulating the early steps of traditional embryonic spinal cord induction (8). However, the lithium induction assay does not seem to promote further epithelization of nephrons (8), which restricts the analysis to very early events of nephrogenesis. To support further differentiation of the MM, the natural inducer, UB, can be recombined with MM (9, 10). Recombination assay enables separate manipulation of the MM and UB and resembles more the anatomy of the living organism. The subcultured tissue can be subject to analysis by, for example, (immuno)-histology, protein or mRNA measurements, and time-lapse follow-up. In this chapter, we describe the methods to induce nephrogenesis in MM with lithium and recombination of the natural inducer, the UB, with MM.

2. Materials

2.1. Pancreatin–Trypsin Solution

1. Dissolve 0.25 g of pancreatin from porcine pancreas (Sigma) and 0.17 g NaCl into 20 mL of sterile water and keep 3–4 h in magnetic stirring at room temperature.
2. Leave solution at 4°C overnight.
3. Centrifuge at 2,700 × *g* for 10 min and aliquot the supernatant for storing at −20°C.
4. Dissolve 0.45 g of trypsin from porcine pancreas (Sigma) in 2 mL of pancreatin solution (see above) and 18 mL Tyrode's solution on ice.
5. Make sure that the pH value is 7.2–7.8.
6. Put the solution in 0.5-mL aliquots and store at −20°C.

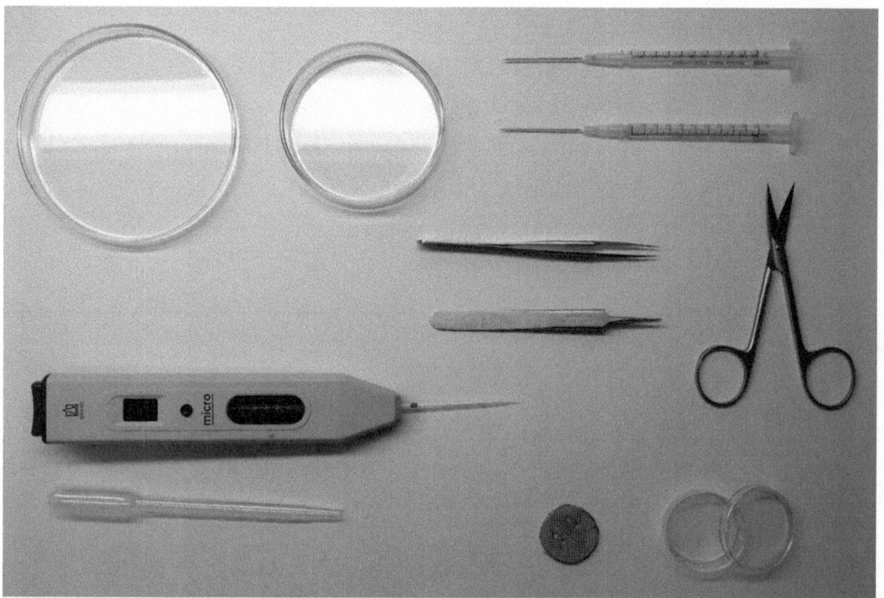

Fig. 1. Overview of the instruments. Petri dishes, hypodermic needles attached to syringes, Dumont #5 fine tip forceps, 11-cm surgical scissors, micropipette controller with stretched glass capillary, cut Pasteur pipette, metal grid, and a 35-mm tissue culture plate.

2.2. Preparation and Dissection of Embryos

See Fig. 1.

1. Dumont #5 forceps, fine tip.
2. Surgical scissors, 10–12 cm.
3. Plastic Pasteur pipettes.
4. 20-gauge hypodermic needles.
5. 1-mL syringes.
6. Zoom stereomicroscope with transmitted light.
7. Dulbecco's Phosphate-Buffered Saline (PBS): 0.901 mM $CaCl_2$, 0.493 mM $MgCl_2 \cdot 6\ H_2O$, 2.67 mM KCl, 1.47 mM KH_2PO_4, 137.93 mM NaCl, 8.06 mM $Na_2HPO_4 \cdot 7\ H_2O$.
8. 6- and 10-cm glass petri dishes.
9. Micropipettes.
10. Pancreatin–trypsin solution (see Subheading 2.1).
11. Growth media: Dulbecco's modified Eagle's medium (DMEM) with GlutaMAX-I and 1,000 mg/mL glucose (Gibco), 10% FBS, 100 μ/mL penicillin, 0.1 mg/mL streptomycin.

2.3. Organ Culture

See Fig. 1.

1. Incubator.
2. 35-mm plastic tissue culture dishes.
3. 30-mm metal grid.

4. Micropipettes.
5. Micropipette controller (Brand).
6. Growth medium.
7. Polycarbonate filters with 0.1–1.0 μm pore size (Whatman).
8. 5 M lithium chloride.
9. 100-μL glass capillaries.

3. Methods

All procedures can be performed in room temperature unless otherwise stated. See Note 1 for the amount of the embryonic material and see Note 2 for the timescale of the procedure.

3.1. Dissection of the Embryonic Tissues

1. Obtain mouse embryos 11.5 days post coitum, when the ureteric bud has invaded into the metanephric mesenchyme (see Note 3).
2. After removal of the uterus, cut it open in Dulbecco's PBS using scissors and forceps.
3. Transfer the embryos on a clean 10-cm glass petri filled half full with Dulbecco's PBS using plastic Pasteur pipette (Fig. 2a). To avoid any damage to embryos, cut the Pasteur pipette tip wide enough to permit the suction of the embryo (Fig. 1).
4. Cut the embryonic membranes open under a stereomicroscope using needles attached to syringes (Fig. 1) and expose the embryo (Fig. 2b). For technical tips for the cutting, see Note 4.

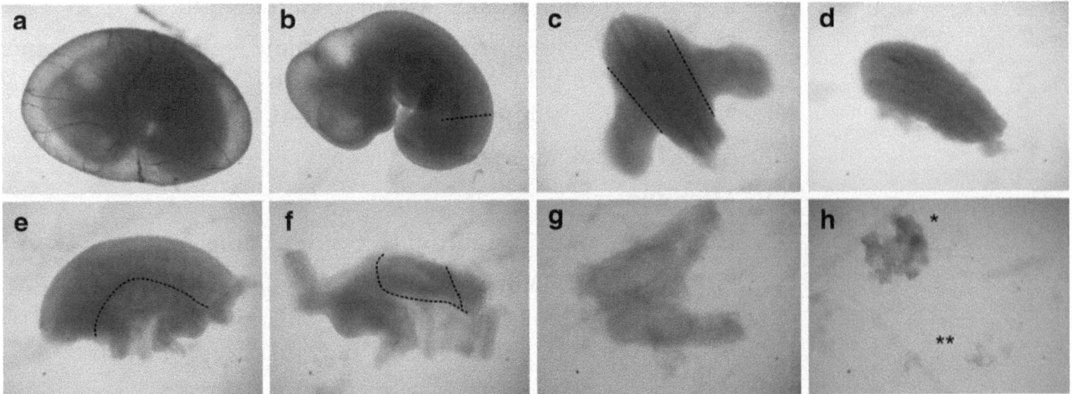

Fig. 2. Sequential presentation of the dissection procedure. (**a**) Embryo detached from the uterus. (**b**) Exposed embryo. (**c**) Caudal part of the embryo containing hind limbs, *dorsal view*. (**d**) Hind limbs removed. (**e**) Lateral view of caudal part of the embryo, hind limbs removed. (**f**) Spinal cord and somites removed, *lateral view* showing metanephros as a more translucent area in the middle of the dorsal part. (**g**) Remaining tissue removed around metanephroi, dorsal view. (**h**) The MM (*) and UBs (**) separated.

5. Cut the embryo half cranial to the hind limbs and shorten the tail (Fig. 2b, c).
6. Put the caudal part of the embryo ventrally towards the bottom of the dish and remove the hind limbs medially (Fig. 2c, d).
7. Place the remaining part of the caudal embryo on its side and cut the dorsal part off just ventral to the spinal cord (Fig. 2e, f).
8. Remove any remaining tissue around the exposed metanephroi (Fig. 2f, g).
9. Collect the metanephroi with micropipette into 50 μL of Dulbecco's PBS and place them into a 35-mm plastic dish. Hold the dish in tipped position to keep the metanephroi on one side of the dish.
10. Put growth medium into a 5-cm glass petri dish to cover the bottom of the dish completely.
11. Melt the pancreatin–trypsin solution and immediately apply 0.5 mL of it onto the metanephroi in plastic dish (see Note 5).
12. Keep the metanephroi in pancreatin–trypsin for 30–40 s and transfer them into growth medium (see Note 6).
13. Remove any remaining Wolffian duct and by scratching the mesenchyme gently with one needle expose the ureteric bud and pull it out while holding the tissue in place with the other needle (Fig. 2h, see Notes 7 and 8).
14. Collect the ureteric buds and metanephric mesenchymes in separate dishes containing Dulbecco's PBS.

3.2. Induction of Nephrogenesis in MM with Lithium in Organ Culture Setup

1. Prepare growth medium with 15 mM lithium chloride by diluting 3 μL 5 M lithium chloride in 1 mL of growth medium (see Note 9).
2. Dip the metal grid in growth media and place it into tissue culture dish (Fig. 3).
3. Put growth medium containing lithium under the metal grid to fill the space underneath it completely (Fig. 3).
4. Wash for a few seconds the polycarbonate filter in 70% ethanol, Dulbecco's PBS, and growth medium and put it onto metal grid.
5. Transfer the MMs onto plate with 10-μL micropipette. Usually, a volume of 3 μL is sufficient (see Note 9).
6. Put the plate with lid into incubator and culture up to 48 h at 37°C in humidified air supplemented with 5% CO_2 (Fig. 4a, b, see Note 10).

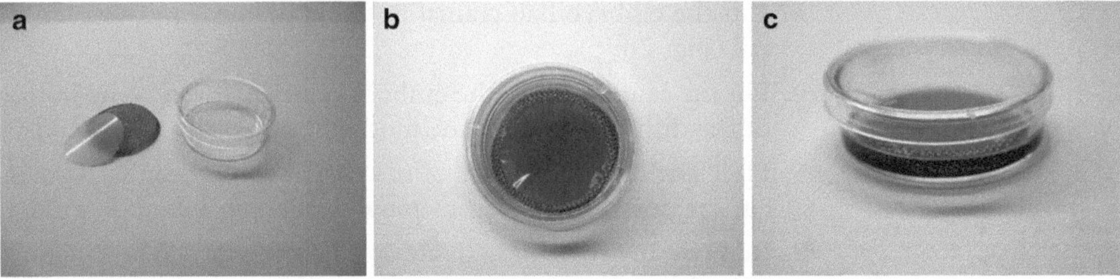

Fig. 3. Preparation of the tissue culture plate. (**a**) A polycarbonate filter, metal grid, and a 35-mm tissue culture plate. (**b**) Top and (**c**) side views of ready organ culture plates, where tissues can be inserted on the filter.

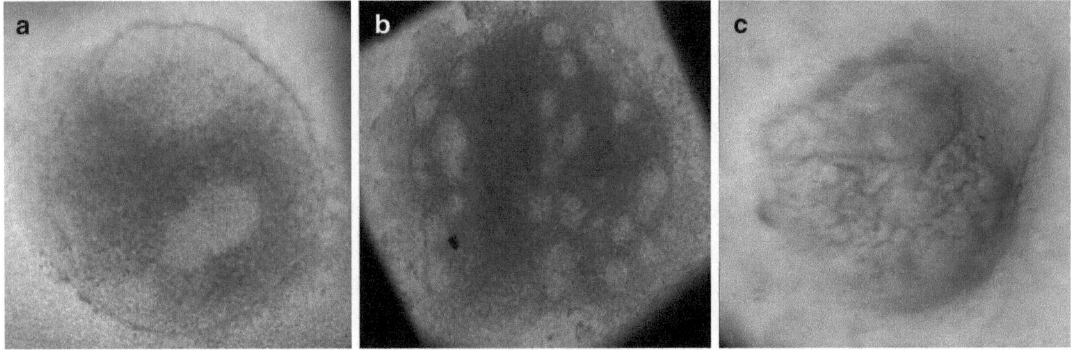

Fig. 4. Isolated MM in culture induced by lithium. (**a**) Typical appearance of 24-h lithium-induced MM. Note the appearance of the translucent areas in the light microscope. (**b**) After 48 h of culturing, translucent areas have specified into smaller spots representing the pre-epithelialized nephron vesicles. (**c**) UB recombined with MM and cultured for 5 days. Note the extensive branching of the UB and MM and precise border of the tissue.

3.3. Induction with the UB

1. Prepare 2 mL growth medium with 15 mM lithium chloride by diluting 6 μL 5 M lithium chloride in it.
2. Transfer the UBs into prepared solution in a 35-mm tissue culture plate and place it into incubator for 30 min.
3. Prepare tissue culture plate with metal grid, polycarbonate filter, and MMs as described above.
4. Stretch a glass capillary into thin tube with flame and attach it into micropipette controller (Fig. 1).
5. Transfer the lithium-incubated UBs next to the MMs using the stretched glass capillary and micropipette controller. Then, poke the UBs under or otherwise in contact with the MM using hypodermic needle.
6. Put the tissues into incubator at 37°C with normal air supplemented with 5% CO_2. The tissue can be cultured at least for 7 days. During the first couple of days, branching of the UB and condensation of MM should be visible in light microscope (Fig. 4c, see Note 9).
7. Change the medium every 2 days (see Note 10).

4. Notes

1. Depending on your experiment, you need various amount of tissue. Usually, one CD-1 female carries 10–15 embryos. This varies between different strains.
2. Dissection of the embryos is time consuming. Reserve at least half working day for the experiment. The dissected tissues retain their competence for nephrogenesis over this time.
3. Correct timing of embryonic development is essential. Especially, too old embryos have UBs that have branched over the "T-bud" stage, making it extremely difficult to remove. We consider the next noon at the day of appearance of vaginal plug to be E0.5.
4. Cutting with hypodermic needles demands practice. A good technique is to use the cutting blades of the needles as in scissors to slash the tissue between them instead of more intuitive way to tear and pull.
5. Temperature of the enzyme solution affects the outcome. Use the enzyme solution immediately after it has melted completely. You can also try carrying out the treatment on ice.
6. The duration of the enzyme treatment is critical for the rest of the procedure. Both too short and too long exposures to enzymes make the tissue difficult to dissect further. 30 s is considered as a safe starting time. If you experience sticky and stretchy tissues, you should try shortening the treatment.
7. To make sure that the UB has been removed completely, try to remove the whole UB as one block. If the UB gets broken during removal, it is difficult to see some remaining parts of UB in MM.
8. Cutting the MM accidently into pieces does not compromise its competence for nephrogenesis. Just collect the parts of the MM when inserting it onto culture and place them close to each other. They will gain contact and develop normally.
9. Several explants can be put in one tissue culture dish. Taking advantage of the widened holes in metal grid, you can follow their development with light microscope. Usually, 1.0–1.5 mL of medium is sufficient amount for one plate.
10. Supposing that the dissection has been carried out carefully and correct tissues have been obtained, the rate of the successful induction of nephrogenesis is close to 100%. Usually, the failure of nephrogenesis is due to faulty contents of growth medium, accidental lack of the inducer (lithium), long delays (over 8 h) in tissue processing, dehydration of the explant (especially, be careful when handling plates containing tissues

onto filters exposed to room air), and too long culture time (see protocol). A good indicator for tissue viability is the sharpness of the border of the explant. A viable tissue shows a distinct border and slightly uplifted profile (Fig. 4).

References

1. Saxén L (1987) Organogenesis of the kidney. Cambridge University Press, Cambridge, UK
2. Gilbert SF (2000) Paraxial and intermediate mesoderm. In: Gilbert SF (ed) Developmental biology, 6th edn. Sinauer Associated, Inc, Sunderland, MA, p 470
3. Carroll TJ, Park JS, Hayashi S, Majumdar A, McMahon AP (2005) Wnt9b plays a central role in the regulation of mesenchymal to epithelial transitions underlying organogenesis of the mammalian urogenital system. Dev Cell 9:283–293
4. Stark K, Vainio S, Vassileva G, McMahon AP (1994) Epithelial transformation of metanephric mesenchyme in the developing kidney regulated by Wnt-4. Nature 372:679–683
5. Kispert A, Vainio S, McMahon AP (1998) Wnt-4 is a mesenchymal signal for epithelial transformation of metanephric mesenchyme in the developing kidney. Development 125:4225–4234
6. Grobstein B (1955) Inductive interaction in the development of the mouse metanephros. J Exp Zool 130:319–340
7. Hedgepeth CM, Conrad LJ, Zhang J et al (1997) Activation of Wnt signalling pathway: a molecular mechanism for lithium activation. Dev Biol 185:82–91
8. Davies JA, Garrod DR (1995) Induction of early stages of kidney tubule differentiation by lithium ions. Dev Biol 167:50–60
9. Lin Y, Liu A, Zhang S et al (2001) Induction of ureter bud branching as a response to Wnt-2b signalling during early kidney organogenesis. Dev Dyn 222:26–39
10. Lin Y, Zhang S, Tuukkanen J et al (2003) Patterning parameters associated with the branching of the ureteric bud regulated by epithelial-mesenchymal interactions. Int J Dev Biol 47:3–13

Chapter 4

Live Imaging of the Developing Mouse Mesonephros

David Grote, Michael Marcotte, and Maxime Bouchard

Abstract

Embryonic development is a highly dynamic process involving complex tissue interactions and movements. Recent progress in cell labeling, image acquisition, and image processing technologies has brought the study of embryo morphogenesis to another level. It is now possible to visualize in real time the dynamic morphogenetic changes occurring in vivo and to reconstitute and quantify them in 4D rendering. However, extended live embryo imaging remains challenging in terms of embryo survival and minimization of phototoxicity. Here, we describe a procedure to image the developing mesonephros for up to 16 h in intact mouse embryos. This method can easily be adapted to the imaging of other structures at similar developmental stages.

Key words: Live imaging, Confocal microscopy, Embryonic development, Kidney development, Embryo culture, Mouse

1. Introduction

In the past 3 decades, the characterization of developmental phenotypes has largely relied on the use of marker analysis on fixed embryos. As powerful and informative as this approach can be, it is inherently limited by the fact that the dynamic nature of embryonic development is lost in fixed tissues. In addition, fine cellular structures can also be affected during the fixation process. In recent years, major improvements in imaging, cell labeling, and computer technologies have opened the way to performing developmental studies in live embryos.

To obtain high-quality data, confocal imaging is the method of choice, as it allows optical sectioning of a sample and imaging of deep structures without physically altering the tissue. This is achieved by controlling the pinhole that transmits light emitted

Odyssé Michos (ed.), *Kidney Development: Methods and Protocols*, Methods in Molecular Biology, vol. 886, DOI 10.1007/978-1-61779-851-1_4, © Springer Science+Business Media, LLC 2012

from a given focal plane but blocks light emitted from other focal planes. Serial imaging of adjacent focal planes can be used to reconstitute the morphological changes of three-dimensional (3D) structures in time. Different types of confocal microscopes are available to image developing embryos. Scanning confocal microscopes are most common and can be used for live imaging, but their relatively low speed of image capture can be detrimental for embryo survival (phototoxicity) and fluorescence signals (photobleaching). The alternative spinning disk confocal microscopes are better adapted to live imaging due to their high rate of image acquisition (1, 2). However, spinning disk microscopes have fixed pinhole widths leading to cross talk between pinholes, lower spatial resolution, and limited objective selection (1). Newer technologies, such as swept field confocal microscopes, use innovative approaches (i.e., separated excitation and emission light paths and linear pinhole arrays) to overcome the limitation of faster confocal microscopes and are thus optimal for high-resolution live imaging.

Live imaging of embryos can be performed on several species. The two major limitations are embryo size and embryo viability under the microscope. As the embryo gets bigger, the depth covered by confocal imaging becomes limiting. The depth of clear focal planes one can reach within a tissue depends primarily on the transparency of the embryo and the working distance of the objective. In an optimized confocal system, depths of up to 200 μm can be imaged (3). This corresponds roughly to a complete embryonic day (E) 8.5 mouse embryo but becomes progressively limiting for more central structures past this stage.

Among the species commonly used as model systems, the mouse is especially relevant to human disease and offers robust genetic tools such as the Cre/lox technology, suitable for tissue-specific manipulation of gene expression. Transgenic technology also allows for the generation of mouse lines expressing fluorescent proteins in specific tissues, which is ideal for live imaging (4). However, in contrast to many other common model systems such as Xenopus or Zebrafish, mouse embryos develop in utero and are thus less amenable to high-resolution live imaging. To circumvent this problem, culture conditions used for whole embryo roller culture can be adapted for extended embryo survival under static conditions on the microscope stage. Temperature, humidity, CO_2, and O_2 levels must be tightly regulated and the embryos must be kept in rich culture media (5).

High-resolution 3D live imaging can generate a massive amount of data, which requires high computing power to perform image acquisition and processing. Among the basic image processing functions, deconvolution and 3D rendering are usually the most useful when analyzing data generated from live imaging experiments. Deconvolution improves image resolution using an algorithm to reassign out-of-focus light to the plane from which it originated (6).

3D rendering creates a three-dimensional representation of a structure from a stack of 2D images. This is usually very informative when studying developmental processes that occur in three dimensions. Other functions can be used to perform data analysis, such as cell counting or cell tracking. Several software packages are available that can be used for deconvolution, rendering, and other types of processing.

Imaging the developing kidney has been a scientific interest for some time. Excellent reports have been published on zebrafish kidney development (7) and imaging of ex vivo kidney cultures (8–10). Here, we describe a method for imaging the developing embryonic kidney (mesonephros) within the living mouse embryos at E8.75 to E9.5. This method has been developed on a spinning disk confocal microscope using a BAC transgenic line specifically expressing GFP in mesonephric tissues under the control of the *Pax2* genomic locus (11). This protocol can easily be adapted to other developing organs, culture conditions, and confocal microscopes.

2. Materials

2.1. Media

1. Fetal bovine serum.
2. ddH$_2$O.
3. 1 M Hepes, pH 7.2.
4. DMEM/F12 1:1 nutrient mix (without Hepes, without phenol red, with L-glutamine).
5. 200 mM L-Glutamine.
6. Penicillin–streptomycin (pen–strep) (penicillin 10,000 units/mL and streptomycin 10,000 μg/mL).
7. Rat serum: Rat serum can be purchased commercially; however, we recommend preparing your own rat serum as we have met with limited success using commercially available products. Rat serum should be prepared according to institutional and national animal care regulations. In our institution, rat serum is prepared as follows.
   (a) Male rats (see Note 1) are anesthetized with isoflurane in a controlled flow anesthesia chamber until unresponsive and not flinching when pinched on the foot with forceps. When unresponsive, lay the rat on its back and continue to dispense anesthesia using a nose cone.
   (b) Make an inverted V-shaped incision in the abdomen to open the abdominal cavity. Move the intestines to reveal the dorsal aorta and vena cava (see Note 2). Carefully

remove fat and connective tissue from the dorsal aorta and vena cava to create an opening over the vessels.

(c) Using a 20-mL syringe and a beveled 21-gauge needle, insert the needle bevel down into the dorsal aorta. Keep the needle in line with the aorta. Draw plunger back slowly to match the rate of blood flow (see Note 3). Each rat should yield about 15 mL of blood.

(d) Collect blood in 15-mL conical tubes and put on ice.

(e) Ensure that rat is dead by severing the heart completely.

(f) Spin tubes at 1,500 × *g* for 5 min to pellet red blood cells.

(g) Using curved forceps, pinch and squeeze fibrin clot to release serum.

(h) Spin again and remove fibrin clot.

(i) Pool serum into 50-mL conical tubes and spin again to remove any remaining red blood cells.

(j) Aliquot into 5-mL aliquots in 15-mL tubes and freeze at -80°C.

8. Dissecting medium:

   (a) Add 4 mL of heat-inactivated fetal bovine serum (30 min, 56°C) to 45 mL of DMEM/F12 in a 50-mL conical tube.

   (b) Add 500 μL of 1 M Hepes buffer, pH 7.2.

   (c) Add 500 μL of penicillin–streptomycin.

   (d) If the DMEM/F12 mix is more than 6 weeks old, add 500 μL of 200 mM L-glutamine.

   (e) Mix by inversion. Filter through a 0.2-μm filter.

9. Culture medium:

   1. Add 4.9 mL of heat-inactivated rat serum (30 min, 56°C) to 4.9 mL of DMEM/F12.
   2. Add 100 μL of 1 M Hepes, pH 7.2.
   3. Add 100 μL of penicillin–streptomycin.
   4. If DMEM/F12 is more than 6 weeks old, add 100 μL of 200 mM L-glutamine.
   5. Filter through a 0.2-μm filter.

2.2. Equipment and Materials

1. On-stage incubation chamber (e.g., Chamlide TC with TC adaptor for chambered coverglass from Live Cell Instruments) (see Note 4) (Fig. 1a).
2. Gas flow and temperature regulator for on-stage incubation chamber (e.g., CU-105 gas flow and temperature controller from Live Cell Instruments).

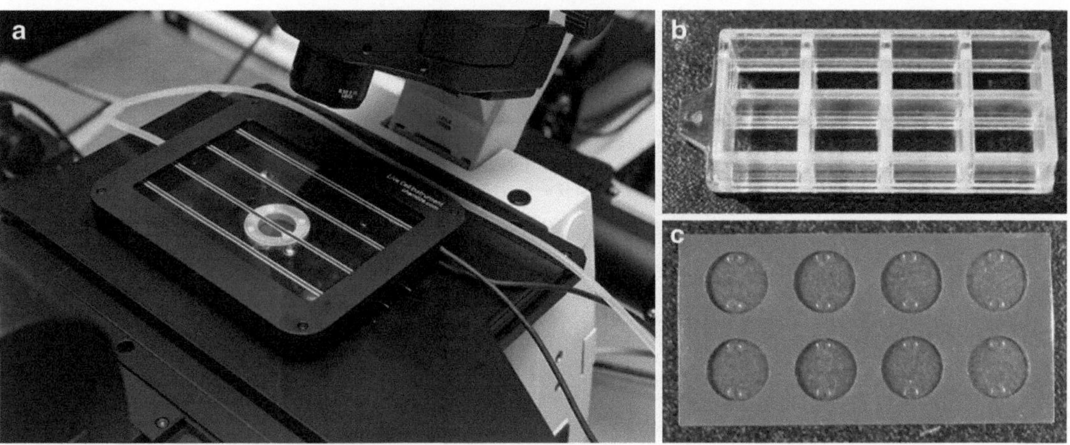

Fig. 1. Basic imaging supplies. (**a**) On-stage incubator setup. (**b**) Lab-tek II 8 well chambered coverglass. (**c**) 8-well cell perfusion gaskets.

3. 8-well-chambered cover glasses (e.g., Lab Tek II chambered coverglass system from NUNC) (Fig. 1b).
4. CoverWell perfusion chamber gaskets, eight chambers, 9 mm diameter, 1 mm deep (Invitrogen) (Fig. 1c).
5. CoverWell perfusion chamber gaskets, eight chambers, 9 mm diameter, 0.5 mm deep (Invitrogen).
6. Confocal microscope: Leica DMI 6000 B with a 20× plan-apochromat air objective (see Note 5) Quorum WaveFX Spinning Disc confocal system, Hammamatsu image EM camera (see Note 6), and 491 nm 25 mW diode Laser (see Note 7).
7. Gas mixture: 40% O_2, 5% CO_2, 55% N_2.
8. Dissecting microscope (e.g., Stemi-2000 stereo microscope from Zeiss).
9. Heating plate for dissections (e.g., Heatable universal mounting frame KH-L from PeCon).
10. Temperature regulator for heating plate for dissections (e.g., Tempcontrol 37 analog 1 channel temperature regulator from PeCon).
11. Cell culture incubator (37°C, 5% CO_2).
12. Digital Monitoring thermometer with a cable and small probe suitable to measure temperature within chambered cover glass wells.
13. Pyrex petri dish, 60 × 15 mm (see Note 8).
14. Cell culture dish, 35 × 10 mm.
15. Hair tool: To make the hair tool, sterilize a piece of hair about 4-cm long in 70% ethanol, break the end of a glass Pasteur

pipette to shorten it, and use melted paraffin to attach the hair to the end of the pipette.

16. 37°C water bath.
17. Two pairs of Dumont #5 forceps.
18. Fine iris scissors—Straight.
19. Sharp Surgical Scissors—Straight.
20. Plastic transfer pipettes.
21. Mineral oil certified for embryo culture.

3. Methods

3.1. Preparative Steps

The following steps must be performed a minimum of 4 h in advance or the night before the experiment.

1. Prepare dissecting medium and culture medium and store at 4°C if prepared the night before.
2. Turn on the microscope and calibrate the stage.
3. Fill the humidifier with ddH_2O.
4. Place the live imaging chamber on the microscope with the adaptor for chambered slides.
5. Put 500 μL of sterile distilled water in each well of an 8-well-chambered cover glass and place it in the incubation chamber on the microscope stage. This is to allow the microscope stage to equilibrate while a second chambered cover glass is being prepared for imaging.
6. Turn on the heating unit for the on-stage incubation chamber (see Notes 9 and 10), humidifier, and objective warmer (see Note 11).
7. Open the gas mixture and set the flow rate at 10 lb per square inch (psi) (see Note 12).
8. Prepare an embryo holder for each well of a second 8-well-chambered cover glass. To prepare the embryo holder:
   (a) Cut out one quarter of a cell perfusion gasket well (Fig. 2a, b). Use 0.5-mm-deep wells for E8.75–E9.0 embryos and 1-mm-deep wells for E9.0–E9.5 embryos.
   (b) Make a V-shaped cut in the plastic surface of this quarter well about 1 mm by 3 mm (Fig. 2c) (see Note 13).
   (c) Remove the strip of plastic from the gasket to expose the adhesive and place it on the bottom of the chambered cover glass.

The following preparatory steps should be performed at least 1 h in advance.

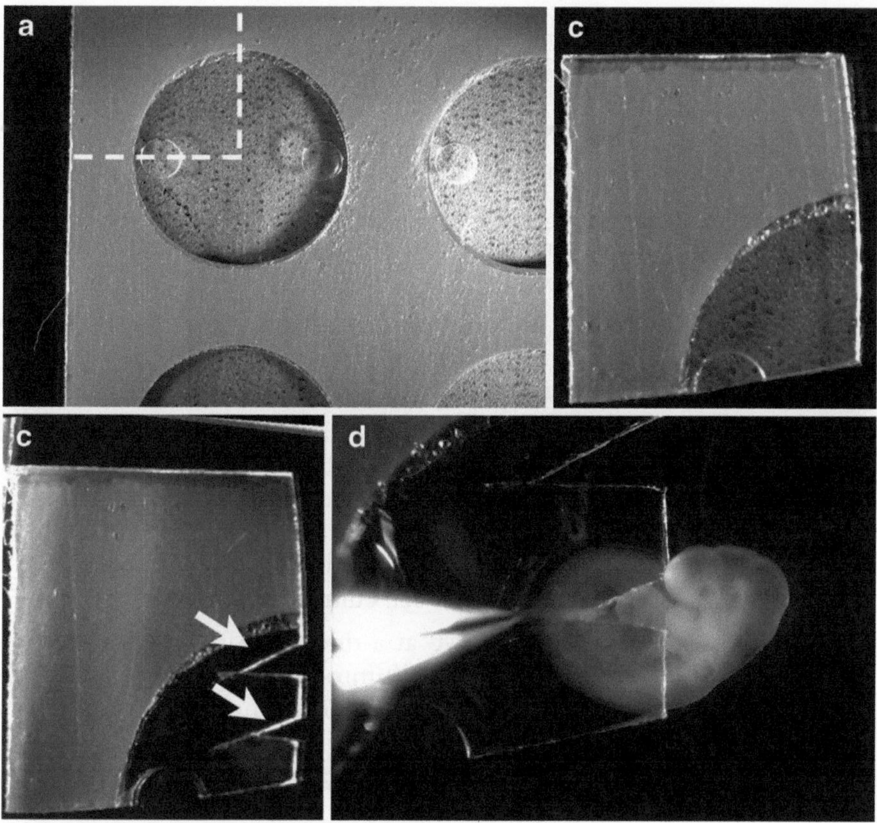

Fig. 2. Preparation of embryo holder. (**a**) Cell perfusion gaskets, cut a quarter of a well (*dashed line*) to make holder for embryo. (**b**) A quarter of one cell perfusion gasket well. (**c**) Use iris scissors to make small V-shaped cuts (*white arrows*) in the plastic surface of the cell perfusion gasket. (**d**) Place the embryo under the plastic surface of the gasket using the hair tool. Then, grasp the amniotic membrane with forceps and carefully wedge it into the V-shaped cut.

9. Check the temperature and water levels in the cell culture incubator and water bath (should be exactly 37°C).
10. Place the mineral oil in 37°C water bath to pre-warm.
11. Add 500 μL of culture media to each well of an 8-well-chambered cover glass. Place the chambered cover glass in the cell culture incubator to pre-warm.
12. Place the remaining culture media in a 35-mm cell culture dish. Place the dish in the cell culture incubator.
13. Fill a 60-mm Pyrex petri dish with dissecting media and place it on the heatable universal mounting frame. Adjust the media temperature to 37°C using the digital thermometer to monitor the temperature.
14. Place the remaining dissecting medium in the cell culture incubator to pre-warm.
15. Turn on the 491-nm laser.

3.2. Dissection

1. Set up mattings of the desired mice and check females for plugs to determine the first day of pregnancy.
2. Sacrifice the pregnant mouse by cervical dislocation at the desired embryonic stage (see Notes 14 and 15).
3. Spray the abdomen with 70% ethanol to sterilize.
4. Use surgical scissors to cut an inverted V incision in the abdomen, and move aside intestines to expose uterine horns (see Note 16).
5. Cut out the uterine horns from the mother. Place the uterine horns in pre-warmed dissecting media. From this point on, keep the embryos at 37°C.
6. Separate the embryos within the uterus under the dissecting scope. To do this, place scissors on the uterine horn between embryos, use tweezers to push uterus up between scissor blades, and cut the uterus. Place individual embryos in a 35-mm cell culture dish and add pre-warmed dissecting media. Place them in the cell culture incubator.
7. Take one embryo at a time and dissect it in pre-warmed dissecting media in a 60-mm glass-dissecting dish (see Note 17). Keep the dissecting dish on the heating plate and use the digital thermometer to monitor the temperature of the media. Maintain the temperature as close to 37°C as possible (see Note 18).
8. Carefully remove embryos from uterus. Insert fine forceps in the hole in the uterus made when embryos were separated. Insert a second set of forceps and make a small tear in the uterus (see Note 19). Continue to tear open the uterus until the placenta can be removed from the uterus easily.
9. Being careful not to damage the embryo, use fine forceps to tear open the placenta and remove the yolk sac with the embryo inside.
10. Remove the yolk sac, rinse it in PBS, and keep it for genotyping if required.
11. Open the amniotic membrane, but leave it attached to the embryo at the primitive gut.
12. Count the number of somites of the embryo to determine the exact developmental stage (for stages E8.0–E9.5).
13. Check for fluorescence, either using a fluorescent dissecting scope or the confocal microscope to be used.
14. Place the embryos that express fluorescence in culture media. If the genotype of the embryos is needed, use the pre-warmed chambered cover glass with culture media to isolate the embryos. Otherwise, pool embryos in the 35-mm cell culture dish with pre-warmed culture media. Place the embryos in the cell culture incubator.

3.3. Embryo Placement

1. Using a plastic pipette, transfer the embryo to the pre-warmed 8-well-chambered cover glass that contains 0.5 mL of culture media (see Note 20). Place the chamber on the dissecting microscope in the heating plate for dissections.
2. Use the hair tool to place the embryo under the clear plastic surface of the embryo holder next to the V-shaped cut, with the amniotic membrane facing the cut.
3. Use fine forceps to grasp the amniotic membrane and the hair tool to manipulate the embryo (see Note 21). Carefully wedge the amniotic membrane into the cut in the plastic surface of the embryo holder gasket (Fig. 2d).
4. Position each embryo as above in separate wells of the chambered cover glass.
5. Add 60 μL of mineral oil on the surface of each well.
6. Carefully mount the chambered cover glass in the on-stage incubator.

3.4. Imaging

1. Once embryos are mounted on the stage, open the image acquisition software (see Note 22).
2. In order to deconvolve the image and to be able to make a 3D reconstruction of the structure, a Z-spacing of 1:3 nyquist sampling rate (see Note 23) must be used. The Z-spacing should also extend several frames above and below the sample.
3. Set the interval between time points. The desired interval should depend on the nature of the processes being studied. The minimum interval time possible depends on the number of samples being imaged and the capacity of the system being used. We use 10–20 time points/h for mesonephros' development.
4. Locate the embryo and the structure of interest in bright field.
5. Switch to the 491-nm laser and focus on the structure of interest (see Note 24). Adjust the laser intensity, exposure time, and camera sensitivity to improve image quality (see Note 25).
6. If using an automated stage, program in the location of each embryo to be imaged.
7. Review the coordinates of each embryo and start image acquisition.
8. Once image acquisition is started, check on the experiment every 30–60 min to verify that the structure of interest remains in frame (see Notes 26 and 27) and that the embryos are surviving. To monitor survival, check for heartbeat and verify that there are no signs of necrosis. Under these conditions, embryos can survive up to 18 h.

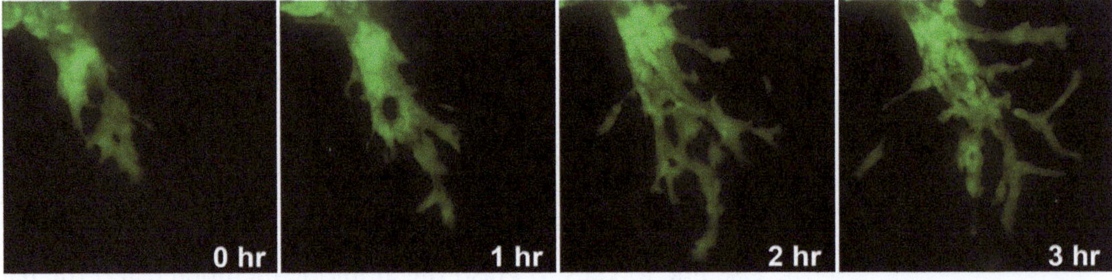

Fig. 3. Time-lapse imaging of developing pro/mesonephros. Pictures were extracted from time-lapse imaging of the growing mesonephros in E9.5 embryos. Fluorescence is obtained by GFP expression in mesonephric tissue using the Pax2BACGFP transgenic line.

9. After image acquisition is complete (see Note 28), count the somites of each embryo and compare it with the count before the experiment to assess embryo growth.

3.5. Image Processing

1. Basic image processing can be done with specialized imaging software, such as Volocity (Improvision). Delete non-informative time points, such as out-of-frame images or unhealthy embryos. If embryos moved out of frame and the position needed to be reprogrammed in, images can be spliced together. 2D movies can be generated from a depth projection of z-stacks (Fig. 3).
2. Deconvolution is done in Autoquant (MediaCybernetics) using blind iterative deconvolution (see Note 29).
3. Deconvolved data can then be rendered with Imaris (Bitplane) to produce a 3D image or movie

4. Notes

1. Retired male breeders are good for this use. Females should be avoided as their hormones can impair embryo survival.
2. The vena cava and dorsal aorta run parallel down the back of the abdominal cavity. The dorsal aorta is the pinker of the two.
3. Drawing the plunger too quickly may result in hemolysis. High levels of hemolysis strongly affect serum quality.
4. Two main types of incubation system are available: incubators that fit on the stage and those that enclose the optics system. Those that enclose the optics system provide greater environmental stability but are more expensive and take longer to equilibrate.

5. The choice of objective will affect resolution and the depth into the tissue that can be imaged. Objectives with higher numerical apertures will have better resolution but generally will have a shorter working distance and will not be able to image as deep into the tissue.
6. Many microscope systems are available. Point scanners comparable to the Zeiss LSM 710 are good when imaging multiple colors; however, they are limited in their maximum speed. Line scanning microscopes, such as the Nikon live scan swept field confocal, and spinning disk microscopes, such as the system described in Subheading 2.2, can be used for high-speed imaging. This is ideal for imaging events that occur on short timescales. It is also useful if imaging a large number of Z-stacks and a large number of embryos, as it will lower the minimum interval between time points. Two photon excitation systems and selective plane illumination systems are optimal for imaging structures deep within the embryo.
7. The frequency of the laser light being used can influence embryo viability. Higher frequency light is more phototoxic. However, infrared light may harm the sample by heating it.
8. Glass dissecting dishes are used as glass cannot be scratched and will not damage dissecting tools.
9. Ambient temperature can affect the temperature on the stage. Check room temperature before each experiment. Use the digital thermometer inserted in one of the water-filled wells of the chambered cover glass in order to check that the temperature on the stage is 37°C.
10. The temperature on the stage will likely be lower than the temperature settings on the instruments. The first time the experiment is done, the correct operating temperatures will need to be determined. Set instruments at about 38°C and allow the temperature on the stage to equilibrate. Adjust the temperature such that the system equilibrates at 37°C.
11. If using an oil immersion objective, be sure to use oil designed for use at 37°C and to pre-warm the oil.
12. Keep the flow rate to a minimum to minimize evaporation of culture medium, which will strongly impact embryo viability.
13. Depending on the stage of the embryo, the size of v-shaped cut needed in the embryo holder may vary; if possible, cut two triangles of different sizes per embryo holder.
14. Ensure that all preparations are complete before sacrificing the mother.
15. Euthanize mice in accordance with institutional and national animal care regulations. Ask to be trained to do cervical dislocation from your animal facility. Cervical dislocation is

preferred as other methods of euthanasia may affect embryo development.

16. Occasionally, female mice that have plugged will not be pregnant. If possible, one should start multiple plug checks such that a second experimental mouse will be available on the day of the experiment should the first not be pregnant. If mice regularly plug but are not pregnant, the male may be infertile or conditions in the animal facility may be stressful to the mice, preventing them from becoming pregnant.
17. It is essential to do the dissection quickly to ensure embryo viability. However, it is equally important not to damage the embryos. If unfamiliar with dissecting out embryos at this stage, it may be helpful to practice on less valuable samples.
18. Blood and placental tissue will accumulate in the dissecting media. This may make dissections difficult. Use a small dissecting dish to conserve media so that the media can be changed for clean pre-warmed dissecting media when necessary.
19. Be careful not to apply pressure on the uterus: this may cause embryos to pop out of the yolk sac, which will damage the embryo.
20. To prevent damage to the embryo, cut the tip and pre-flush pipette with medium.
21. Proper positioning of embryo is critical for obtaining good image quality. The closer the structure of interest is to the cover glass, the better the resolution will be. Additionally, proper positioning will ensure that the embryo does not become dislodged during imaging.
22. This experiment generates a large amount of data. Before starting image acquisition, verify that there is sufficient storage capacity available. This depends on the number of embryos imaged, the size of the z-stack, the resolution of the images, and the length of the experiment. When first performing this experiment, ensure that there is ample storage capacity available on the destination drive. Upwards of 30 GB is recommended.
23. The required Nyquist sampling rate can be calculated online at http://www.svi.nl/NyquistCalculator.
24. Use autocontrast if available: this will help make the image easily visible.
25. In order to avoid harming the embryos, laser intensity and exposure time should be minimized. Using lower laser power and exposure time may decrease resolution but could be necessary to keep embryos alive. Camera sensitivity can also be adjusted to improve resolution. Binning may also be used to decrease laser intensity and exposure time but at the expense of resolution.

26. If using an automated stage to image multiple embryos, there may be stage drift if the stage is not properly calibrated. This will cause embryos to move out of frame. For this reason, the stage should be properly calibrated. If the problem occurs, the experiment can be stopped and the position of each embryo can be reprogrammed in.
27. Due to the motion of the automated stage and due to heart beating, embryos may become dislodged from the cell perfusion gasket. If this occurs, image acquisition can be stopped, the chambered cover glass removed, and the embryo repositioned.
28. Back up data as soon as possible after the experiment.
29. Try different deconvolution settings to identify what works best. Given that the distance of the embryo from the cover glass and the depth of the structure of interest within the embryo will vary for different embryos, the best settings may vary from sample to sample.

Acknowledgments

This work was supported by an operating grant from the Canadian Institutes for Health Research (CIHR; MOP-84470). M.B. holds a Canada Research Chair in Developmental Genetics of the Urogenital System.

References

1. Conchello JA, Lichtman JW (2005) Optical sectioning microscopy. Nat Methods 2:920–931
2. Wang E, Babbey CM, Dunn KW (2005) Performance comparison between the high-speed Yokogawa spinning disc confocal system and single-point scanning confocal systems. J Microsc 218:148–159
3. Megason SG, Fraser SE (2003) Digitizing life at the level of the cell: high-performance laser-scanning microscopy and image analysis for in toto imaging of development. Mech Dev 120:1407–1420
4. Nowotschin S, Eakin GS, Hadjantonakis AK (2009) Live-imaging fluorescent proteins in mouse embryos: multi-dimensional, multi-spectral perspectives. Trends Biotechnol 27:266–276
5. Martin P, Cockroft DL (2008) Culture of post-implantation mouse embryos. Methods Mol Biol 461:7–22
6. Biggs DS (2010) 3D deconvolution microscopy. Curr Protoc Cytom Chapter 12, Unit 12.19.11–12.19.20
7. Vasilyev A, Liu Y, Mudumana S et al (2009) Collective cell migration drives morphogenesis of the kidney nephron. PLoS Biol 7:e9
8. Barak H, Boyle SC (2011) Organ culture and immunostaining of mouse embryonic kidneys. Cold Spring Harb Protoc 2011, pdb prot5558
9. Costantini F, Watanabe T, Lu B, Chi X, Srinivas S (2011) Imaging kidney development. Cold Spring Harb Protoc 2011
10. Watanabe T, Costantini F (2004) Real-time analysis of ureteric bud branching morphogenesis in vitro. Dev Biol 271:98–108
11. Pfeffer PL, Payer B, Reim G, di Magliano MP, Busslinger M (2002) The activation and maintenance of Pax2 expression at the mid-hindbrain boundary is controlled by separate enhancers. Development 129:307–318

Chapter 5

Organotypic Culture of the Urogenital Tract

Ekaterina Batourina, Devangini Gandhi, Cathy L. Mendelsohn, and Andrei Molotkov

Abstract

Organotypic culture is an invaluable technique that allows researchers with the tool to analyze a tissue development in an isolated and well-defined environment. This technique also permits one to study the roles of different signaling systems/signaling molecules and to take advantage of the modern real-time imaging techniques, including confocal microscopy. With great success, our lab has used organotypic culture of the urogenital tract (UGT) to study growth and extension of the mesonephric (Wolffian) duct and its cloaca connection, ureter maturation, and bladder urothelium development (Batourina et al. Nat Genet 32:109, 2002; Batourina et al. Nat Genet 37:1082, 2005; Mendelsohn Organogenesis 5:306, 2009).

Key words: Organotypic culture, Urogenital tract, Bladder urothelium, Ureter connection, Bladder development, Urogenital development

1. Introduction

Urinary tract abnormalities comprise a complex syndrome of malformations that include some of the most common birth defects in humans (4). Despite the frequent occurrence of these abnormalities, little is known about their cause or about the events that normally control ureter maturation (5, 6). Development of the urogenital tract (UGT) begins with Wolffian ducts, which are paired epithelial tubes that form in both sexes but persist only in males, where they differentiate into the vas deferens, seminal vesicles, and epididymis. Wolffian ducts extend along the anterior–posterior embryonic axis, and at embryonic day 9 (E9) integrate into the primitive urogenital sinus–the primordium of the bladder and urethra. The ureteric bud, an epithelial outgrowth that sprouts from the base of the Wolffian ducts, forms at E10. The ureteric bud tips

Odyssé Michos (ed.), *Kidney Development: Methods and Protocols*, Methods in Molecular Biology, vol. 886, DOI 10.1007/978-1-61779-851-1_5, © Springer Science+Business Media, LLC 2012

invade the metanephric blastema on E11, where they differentiate into the renal collecting duct system; the portion of the ureteric bud that lies outside the kidney becomes the ureter–the tube that will connect the kidney with the bladder. At this stage, the upper ureter joins the kidney and the lower (distal) ureter is in an immature configuration attached to the Wolffian duct. Mature connections are established during ureter maturation, a poorly understood process in which distal ureters detach from the Wolffian ducts and migrate up to their final integration site at the base of the bladder.

Urinary bladder develops from the terminal portion of the hindgut endoderm, which begins around E10.5 when the terminal portion of the hindgut dilates to form the cloaca (7). At E11–E12, the cloaca divides into dorsal and ventral parts by the urorectal septum. The dorsal part, known as the anorectal canal, gives rise to the epithelial linings of rectum and anus, while the ventral part–urogenital sinus (UGS)—forms the urethra and bladder (7). At E12–E13, the most cranial part of UGS starts to grow and forms the urothelium of the bladder, with the surrounding mesenchyme giving rise to mesodermal components of the bladder, such as blood vessels, smooth muscle, and connective tissue. Bladder urothelium is a transitional epithelium of endodermal origin (8, 9) consisting of the three main layers–basal layer, intermediate layers, and a superficial specialized layer of the umbrella cells (10). The exact cellular mechanisms of the umbrella cells formation is a poorly understood process in which the simple epithelial lining of the UGS stratifies and forms multilayer structure of the mature bladder urothelium lining.

2. Materials

1. All-trans retinoic acid (atRA, Sigma, R-2625, 50 mg); prepare stock solution of 10 mM of atRA by dissolving 50 mg of RA (use the whole ampoule) in 1.6 mL of DMSO and adding 15 mL of 100% alcohol, store at –20°C.
2. Fibronectin (Invitrogen, 33010-018); working solution–200 μg/mL in PBS.
3. OPTI-MEM cell culture medium.
4. Sterile phosphate-buffered saline (PBS), 10× solution.
5. Matrigel: BD Matrigel Matrix (BD Biosciences).
6. Rat serum: SD MALE.
7. DMEM/F12.
8. Antibiotic: Penicillin and streptomycin.

9. Culture dishes with glass bottom (MatTeK corporation, P35G-0-20-C); the day before experiment–coat the inside glass bottom of the dishes with the fibronectin (200 μg/mL solution in PBS), keep the plate at 4°C.
10. Sterilized culture plate inserts: 0.4 μm culture membrane (Millipore, PICMORG50).
11. GDNF (R&D system).
12. HGF (R&D system).
13. FGF7 (R&D system).
14. Mineral oil (Sigma, M8410).

2.1. Medium Composition

1. E9 embryonic culture medium: OPTI-MEM with 50–75% of rat serum.
2. E12 embryonic culture medium: DMEM/F12 serum-free medium, with 5 μg/mL of insulin, 5 μg/mL of holo-transferrin, and 5 ng/mL of selenium.
3. E14 embryonic culture medium: DMEM/F12 medium containing 10% fetal calf serum, 5 μg/mL of insulin, 5 μg/mL of holo-transferrin, 5 ng/mL of selenium, and antibiotics (1/100). Immediately before use, add 100 ng/mL each of FGF7, HGF, and GDNF.

2.2. Embryo Preparation

1. Embryo collection:
   (a) Dissecting stereomicroscope.
   (b) Petri dishes (100 × 15 mm).
   (c) DMEM/F12 or OPTI-MEM kept at room temperature (RT).
2. Embryo dissection:
   (a) Dissecting stereomicroscope with fluorescent light.
   (b) Petri dishes (100 × 15 mm).
   (c) Forceps (Dumont #55).
   (d) Scissors.

2.3. Imagine Equipment

1. Dissecting stereomicroscope with fluorescent light for dissecting the embryos, and for handling, positioning, and embedding embryos or bladder tissue in agarose.
2. Inverted fluorescent microscope (Ziess Axiovert 200 M) equipped with environmental controlled chamber and motorized stage for long-term tissue culture imaging.
3. Long focus objectives 10×, 20×, and 40×.

3. Methods

3.1. Embryonic Culture of Whole Mount E9 Mouse Embryos

1. Obtain a timed pregnant female mouse (see Note 1).
2. Sacrifice animals by CO_2 asphyxiation at the embryonic development day 9 between 10 a.m. and 1 p.m. (the stage of the embryonic development is counted from the time when vaginal plug was registered, which is a E0.5 time point).
3. By standard technique, dissect embryos using fine surgical scissors and forceps and place them in DMEM/F12 medium solution kept at room temperature; if genotyping is required, collect yolk sacs for PCR analysis.
4. Under fluorescent dissecting microscope, cut embryos at the level of 10th somite and place the caudal part of the embryos sagittally on the glass plate pre-covered with fibronectin. Put the glass plate into cell culture incubator (37°C, 5% CO_2) and allow at least 30 min for the embryos to firmly attach to the plate.

   Important: Do not add medium to the glass culture plate at this time.
5. After a 30-min incubation, add matrigel to prevent liquid evaporation and drying of the embryo and enough to cover the whole embryo (about 15–30 μL) (see Note 2).

   Important: In order to prevent tissue damage, allow enough time for the matrigel to polymerize; the exact time may need to be adjusted to your conditions and often might be less than 30 min.
6. Add 1.5–2 mL of culture medium–enough to cover the embryo.
7. At this time, the embryo is ready for imaging.
8. Best results for live imaging are obtained using environmentally controlled live imaging system. It is also possible to use a non-confocal fluorescent microscope (for example, Zeiss Axiovert 200 M); however, imaging time must be reduced to as short as possible. If you are not using an environmentally controlled chamber–return the culture to the tissue incubator as soon as possible; you may also have to limit how often you take images to just one every few hours to prevent temperature and environmental stress to the embryo.
9. Images were taken every 30 min for 4–8 h using an environmentally controlled live imaging system (for example, we have used Zeiss Axiovert 200 M equipped with microscopy top stage system set at 37°C, 5% CO_2, and Hamamatsu ORKA-ER camera). Following standard microscope protocol, we were able to reliably obtain images and maintain a live culture for up to 20 h (Fig. 1).
10. See also Notes 3–6.

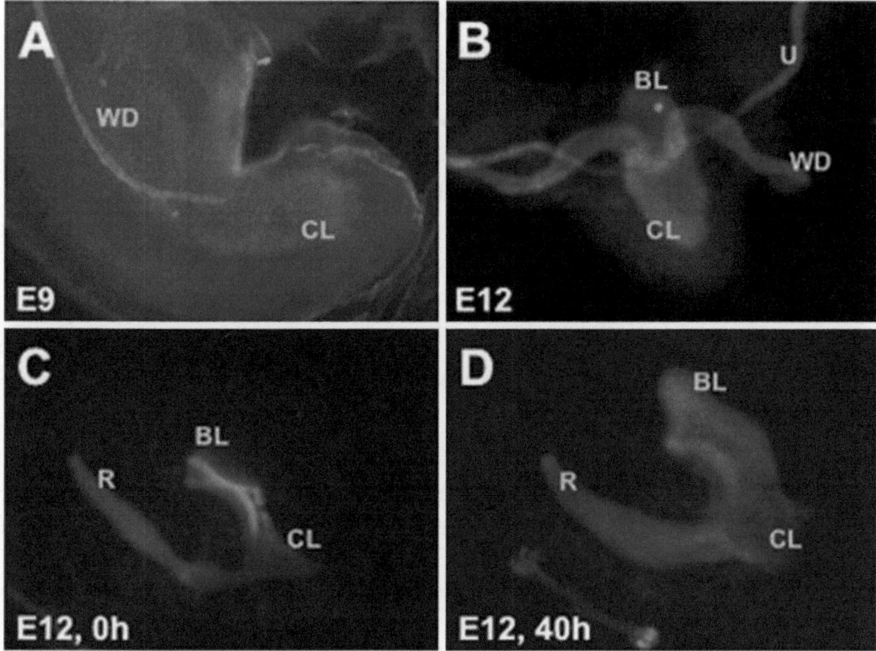

Fig. 1. Examples of the E9 and E12 embryonic cultures are shown. (**a**) E9 Hoxb7GFP/wt embryo was cultured for 24 h, fixed in PFA, and co-stained with antibodies to cadherin to study the formation of Wolffian duct–cloaca joining. Hoxb7 promoter was used to drive GFP expression in the Wolffian duct. (**b**) Example of E12 ShhCre/wt;R26 GFP/wt embryo shows whole-mount preparation of the urogenital tract (UGT) culture; picture is taken after UGT dissection; UGT is placed onto a filter ready for the culture. (**c**, **d**) Example of E12 embryonic culture of UGT; ShhCre/wt mice were crossed with the R26GFP/wt reporter mice to visualize development of the UGT. Note a growth of the urinary bladder (BL) after 40 h in culture. *WD* Wolffian duct, *CL* cloaca, *U* ureter, *BL* urinary bladder, *R* rectum.

3.2. Whole Mount E12 Embryonic Culture of UGT

1. Obtain timed E12 embryos following procedures described in Subheading 3.1.
2. *Important*: Use a medium for the E12 embryos described in Subheading 2.
3. Add 1–1.5 mL of medium to a small 3-cm Petri dish and place embryo on its back into the Petri dish; adjust the volume of the medium so that the embryo is not floating.
4. Using fine-tip forceps, carefully dissect all extra tissues around UGT such as spinal cord, limbs, intestine, etc. without damaging the UGT. Avoid removing any extra mesenchymal tissues at that time.
5. Transfer the UGT into a clean 3-cm Petri dish containing 1–1.5 mL of medium. Using dissecting needle or fine-tip forceps, carefully clean extra mesenchymal tissues around the ducts and cloaca. If you are using forceps–work with the closed tips.
6. Transfer the UGT on the filter, add about 1–1.5 mL of the medium, and place the tissue in the incubator for 2 h. After 2 h, add 30–50 μL of the mineral oil to prevent tissue from drying. At this step, tissue is ready for imaging (Fig. 1). Follow procedures and tips described in Subheading 3.1.

3.3. Whole Mount Embryonic Slice Culture of E16.5 Bladders

1. Obtain a timed pregnant female mouse.
2. Before beginning, prepare 4% agarose by dissolving 4 g of agarose in 100 mL PBS and heat it in the microwave until all the agarose dissolves while taking special care to prevent excessive evaporation of the liquid.

   Important: Cool the agarose solution by placing it into the water bath preset at 50°C for at least 30 min to prevent heat damage to the tissues.
3. Sacrifice animals by CO_2 asphyxia.
4. By conventional technique, dissect embryos and place them into ice-cold DMEM medium. If embryo genotyping is required, collect yolk sacs and store them at –20°C for PCR analysis.
5. Under dissecting microscope, carefully dissect urine bladder with the surrounding tissues and genital tubercle while taking special attention to remove skin and bones; leaving skin and bones with the sample might hamper sectioning of the tissue on a vibratome; collect the tissues into individual wells of 12-multi-well plate and keep them in ice-cold DMEM medium.
6. Pour agarose into the small plastic weigh dishes and under a dissecting microscope place bladder samples into it; position the samples to make sure that the sample is in the right plane for the future vibratome sectioning; we normally place two to three bladder samples in one dish.
7. After embedding tissues, place the dish inside of the 10-cm Petri dishes, cover it, and keep samples at 4°C until agarose is set which normally takes about 15–20 min to solidify; after agarose solidifies, pour a small amount of PBS on top of the agarose to prevent it from drying; keep the samples at 4°C at all time.
8. Take one dish and remove agarose block; under dissecting microscope using the shaving blade, cut the agarose block around the samples making sure that you have about 3–4 mm of agarose around the tissue (see Note 7). Pick one agarose block with the sample for the sectioning and return the rest of the blocks to 4°C.

   Important: To prevent tissue from drying, always keep the blocks you are not currently using covered inside Petri dishes.
9. Prepare vibratome by cleaning the chamber with alcohol; put a small drop of the tissue glue on a vibratome stage and place the agarose block on it; make sure that the block is positioned for the desired sectioning plane; after about 20 s, fill the chamber

with the ice-cold PBS; allow 5 min for the glue to set. According to manufacturer's instruction, adjust the vibratome control for a very slow forward movement and set vibration control to a maximum (see Note 8). Section the block at desired thickness (see Note 9).

10. Collect individual sections into 24-multi-well plate filled with DMEM solution; keep the 24-multi-well plate with the sections at room temperature.

    Verify sections under dissecting microscope and mark wells, which contain bladder sections. We are typically able to get one to two good sagittal bladder sections from the single E16 embryonic bladder.

11. Pick samples with the bladder tissue and place them onto a filter membrane; add about 1.2 mL of the culture medium under the filter; do not add medium on top of the filter or directly inside chamber with the samples; you should have enough medium for the filter chamber to slightly float; put the dish with the sample into tissue incubator (see Note 10).
12. *Important*: After you have all the sections you plan to put on the membrane done, cover the samples with the small volume of the mineral oil. Use 30–50 μL of the oil–just enough to form a thin oil membrane on the surface of the filter and bladder sections. Oil prevents tissues from drying and medium from evaporating which greatly improves the tissue survival and also keeps the stable medium composition.
13. Section the rest of the samples and place them onto filter membranes. Keep the culture samples inside the tissue incubator when you are not working with them.
14. Allow 2 h for the tissues to stabilize.
15. To take a live movie of the bladder culture, place the culture dishes inside the environmentally controlled microscope chamber set at 37°C, 5% CO_2 (Fig. 2).

    Important: To prevent tissue medium from evaporation and tissue from drying, insure that CO_2 is saturated with water and place inside one to two extra dishes filled with water. To prevent tissue damage when taking images, limit the exposure time to the minimal possible (see Notes 11–13).

16. If histological analysis is desired, stop bladder culture at different time points by picking the sections from the tissue membrane using fine forceps and fixing them in 4% PFA; after fixation, follow the standard protocols for tissue processing/IHC staining and analysis (Fig. 2). The sections can also be used for gene expression analysis using standard RT-PCR or real-time PCR protocols.

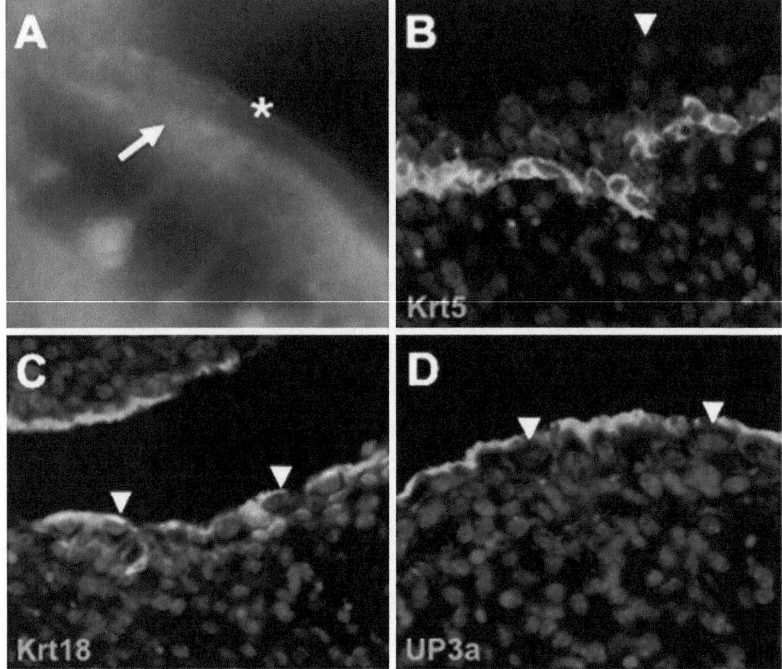

Fig. 2. Example of the whole-mount culture of urinary bladder vibratome sections. (**a**) E16 bladder of Gli1CreER/wt;R26gfp/wt embryo was sectioned on a vibratome and placed in the culture. Note that Gli1-gfp-labeled cells (*arrow*) are located immediately beneath urothelium (*asterisk*), which is well preserved and distinguishable. (**b**–**d**) Frozen sections of the cultured E16 bladder (**a**) were prepared after 72 h in culture and stained with antibodies to Krt5 (**b**), Krt18 (**c**), and UP3a (**d**). Note that the expression pattern of the urothelium cell type-specific markers was identical to found in normal embryonic urothelium at E16-E17, where Krt5 is expressed in basal cells and Krt18 and UP3a are expressed in top-layer umbrella cells (*arrow heads* on **b**–**d**).

4. Notes

1. For our studies, we routinely use reporter lines with the GFP expression targeted to the mesonephric ducts or cloaca to simplify dissection and imaging.
2. As an alternative to matrigel, we have also successfully used mineral oil to cover the embryo. If you are using Matrigel, allow 30–60 min for Matrigel to polymerize.
3. Using mineral oil to prevent culture from drying can substantially increase the time the embryo will survive in the culture.
4. If high-quality imaging is not required, good results can also be obtained by placing embryos on a filter membrane, which will ensure better penetration and exchange of the medium; use the mineral oil to cover the embryo.

5. If long-term imaging is required, insure that CO_2 is saturated with water and place few dishes containing water inside the chamber to insure that culture medium is not evaporated and tissue is not drying.
6. If IHC analysis of the cultured tissue is desired, pick the embryo from the culture dish using fine forceps or pipette with the wide tip and place it into 4% PFA; follow the standard protocol for the tissue sectioning/antibody staining.
7. We found that for the future sectioning on the vibratome the square or rectangular blocks work the best.
8. We normally set forward control at 1–2 and vibration at 8–9; you may have to adjust these controls for the best results.
9. We found that the thickness of 300 μm works best for us.
10. We normally place three to four bladder sections on a single tissue filter membrane. We have also positioned the sections in a rhombic or square pattern and labeled the position of the first section.
11. We found that due to tissue growing, the area of the interest goes out of the focus plan as fast as after 3–4 h; for a long-term imaging, it is generally a good idea to do a Z-stack. We normally limit the number of the focus planes to 20 and take them at 10 μm.
12. In our experiments, we found that the tissue fluorescence increases during the course of the culture, which may result in over-exposure; to prevent this, we adjust exposure time using the brightest focus plane and after that decrease it somewhat.
13. We are normally able to grow bladder sections in the culture for up to 72–96 h.

References

1. Batourina E, Choi C, Paragas N et al (2002) Distal ureter morphogenesis depends on epithelial cell remodeling mediated by vitamin A and Ret. Nat Genet 32:109
2. Batourina E, Tsai S, Lambert S et al (2005) Apoptosis induced by vitamin A signaling is crucial for connecting the ureters to the bladder. Nat Genet 37:1082
3. Mendelsohn C (2009) Using mouse models to understand normal and abnormal urogenital tract development. Organogenesis 5:306
4. Scott JE (1987) Fetal ureteric reflux. Br J Urol 59:291
5. Bernstein GT, Mandell J, Lebowitz RL et al (1988) Ureteropelvic junction obstruction in the neonate. J Urol 140:1216
6. Kaefer M, Tobin MS, Hendren WH et al (1997) Continent urinary diversion: the Children's Hospital experience. J Urol 157:1394
7. Staack A, Hayward SW, Baskin LS, Cunha GR (2005) Molecular, cellular and developmental biology of urothelium as a basis of bladder regeneration. Differentiation 73:121
8. Baskin LS, Hayward SW, Sutherland RA et al (1997) Cellular signaling in the bladder. Front Biosci 2:d592
9. Seifert AW, Harfe BD, Cohn MJ (2008) Cell lineage analysis demonstrates an endodermal origin of the distal urethra and perineum. Dev Biol 318:143
10. Lewis SA (2000) Everything you wanted to know about the bladder epithelium but were afraid to ask. Am J Physiol Renal Physiol 278:F867

Chapter 6

Live Imaging Kidney Development in Zebrafish

Aleksandr Vasilyev and Iain A. Drummond

Abstract

The zebrafish has emerged as a powerful model to study organ development and regeneration. It has a number of advantages over other vertebrate model systems. The embryo can be kept transparent throughout embryonic development, which allows direct visualization of the developing organs. In addition, embryos can be easily manipulated surgically, genetically, or chemically. Furthermore, because nephron shape and function are remarkably conserved among vertebrates, zebrafish findings can directly inform human studies. Here, we describe a simple procedure that can be used by laboratories to investigate the development of zebrafish kidney and other organs by time-lapse microscopy.

Key words: Zebrafish, Live cell imaging, Time lapse, Kidney, Migration

1. Introduction

Zebrafish has emerged as a powerful system to study tissue and organ development. This vertebrate model has optical properties (due to transparency and rapid external development) rivaling those of *Caenorhabditis elegans.* At the same time, zebrafish body plan and organ architecture are much closer to those of human than any invertebrate model. Hence, it can be more informative with respect to human organ development and physiology.

A number of studies have examined organ development in zebrafish by using time-lapse microscopy (1–3). Such studies significantly improve our understanding of organ development by placing the relevant cellular and molecular processes in a context of time and space, thus allowing quantitative models and predictions to be directly tested. We recently discovered that collective epithelial migration is a central process in pronephric morphogenesis and it is governed by the onset of fluid flow within the kidney (4).

Odyssé Michos (ed.), *Kidney Development: Methods and Protocols*, Methods in Molecular Biology, vol. 886, DOI 10.1007/978-1-61779-851-1_6, © Springer Science+Business Media, LLC 2012

Here, we describe a simple method of imaging kidney development in zebrafish by time-lapse microscopy, but first we briefly introduce zebrafish kidney structure and development. In the course of vertebrate evolution, three distinct kidneys of increasing complexity have been generated: the pronephros, mesonephros, and metanephros (5). Despite some differences in organ morphology between the various kidney forms, the structure of the nephron (the functional unit of the kidney) is largely preserved from pronephros to metanephros.

The nephron has two principal functions: metabolic waste removal and maintenance of water and solute balance (6). The nephron performs these functions by first filtering the blood in the glomerulus and then recovering useful ions and small molecules by epithelial transport.

In zebrafish, the larval kidney consists of two nephrons with fused glomeruli (7). Two pronephric tubules connect the glomerulus to the pronephric ducts that fuse before making an exit at the level of the cloaca (Fig. 1). During the first 48 h of development, most components of the pronephros are established, including the pronephric duct, tubule, and eventually the glomerulus (8).

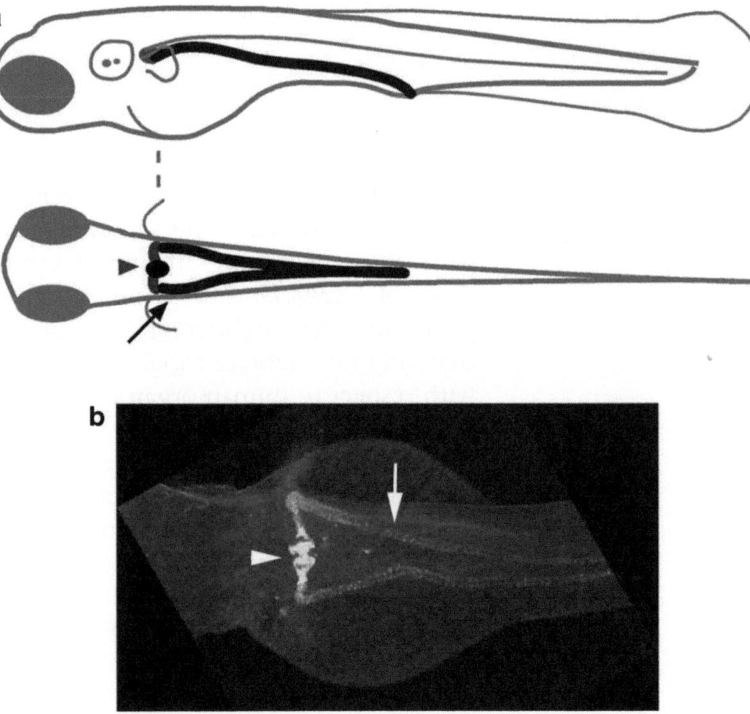

Fig. 1. The zebrafish pronephric kidney. (**a**) Cartoon of the zebrafish embryo highlighting the pronephric kidney. *Arrowhead* points to the glomerulus. *Arrow* points to the proximal tubule. (**b**) Confocal projection of a 3dpf Tg(wt1b:GFP) transgenic embryo stained against GFP (anti-GFP, *arrowhead*) and against alpha subunit of the Na/K ATPase, *arrow*.

After specification of the segmented pronephric nephron, the development of the kidney continues through complex movements, at the center of which is a collective migration of kidney epithelial cells. These epithelial movements lead to continuous morphogenesis until the final form of the larval kidney is attained at around 5 dpf. After a short period of a relative developmental quiescence, at about 2 weeks post fertilization, kidney morphogenesis continues through induction of new nephrons in a rostral-to-caudal direction. This process presumably continues throughout the life of an animal as the body mass increases (9, 10).

All the processes involved in kidney morphogenesis can be visualized in live assays through the use of fluorescent protein-expressing transgenics. A number of transgenics are now available for researchers interested in live studies of kidney development in zebrafish. They include, among others, Tg(wt1b:GFP) (11), Tg(atp1a1a.4:GFP), (12), Tg(cdh17:GFP) (9, 10), Tg(ret1:GFP) (13), Tg(enpep:GFP) (14), Tg(pod:mCherry) (10), and Tg(cd41:GFP) (4, 15) (Table 1). In addition, a number of Tol2 enhancer trap insertional transgenics have been generated to allow visualization of different segments and cell types of the kidney ET(krt8:EGFP)sqet11-9, ET(krt8:EGFP)sqet33-d10 (16, 17). Methods to generate fluorescent transgenics are outside the scope of this review; however, a few excellent texts exist on this subject for those interested (18, 19).

Here, we describe a method of imaging live zebrafish in time-lapse series. This simple method allows for 24 h of continuous observation without significant experimental artifact. Certain limitations apply to the potential applicability of this basic method.

Table 1
Kidney fluorescent zebrafish lines

Transgenic	Expression pattern	References
Tg(wt1b:GFP)	Glomerulus, PT[a]	(11)
Tg(atp1a1a.4:GFP)	Distal to glomerulus	(12)
Tg(cdh17:GFP)	Distal to glomerulus	(9, 10)
Tg(ret1:GFP)	Pronephric duct	(13)
Tg(enpep:GFP)	Distal to glomerulus	(14)
Tg(pod:mCherry)	Glomerulus	(10)
Tg(cd41:GFP)	Multiciliated cells	(15)
ET(krt8:EGFP)sqet11-9	Straight PT[a], DT[b]	(16, 17)
ET(krt8:EGFP)sqet33-d10	Convoluted PT[a]	(16, 17)

[a] *PT* proximal tubule
[b] *DT* distal tubule

It cannot be used when long periods (days) of observation are required. It also becomes less useful in observing younger embryos undergoing significant global morphogenic movements; however, shorter series (up to a few hours) are still possible in these embryos.

2. Materials

2.1. Fluorescent Transgenics

1. The Tg(atp1a1a.4:GFP) transgenic line was generated as described in ref. 12.
2. The ET(krt8:EGFP)sqet11-9 line and the ET(krt8:EGFP) sqet33-d10 line were a gift from Dr. Vladimir Korzh (16, 17).
3. The ret1:GFP line was a gift from Dr. Shannon Fisher (13).
4. cd41:GFP line was a gift from Drs. H.F. Lin and R.I. Handin (15).
5. All the fish lines were raised and maintained as described in refs. 4, 20. The embryos were obtained by in-crossing the heterozygous transgenic fish.

2.2. General Embryo Care

1. E3 medium: 5 mM NaCl, 0.17 mM KCl, 0.33 mM $CaCl_2$, 0.33 mM $MgSO_4$. Methylene blue (0.2%) can be added to the medium to limit fungal and bacterial growth. For the imaging, the embryos are moved into methylene blue-free medium, +/− PTU (below), depending on the stage of the embryo.
2. E3-PTU medium: 0.003% N-phenylthiourea (PTU—Sigma) is added to the E3 solution (no methylene blue). We normally make 10× stock of E3-PTU by overnight dissolution on a stir plate. The pH is adjusted to 7.0–7.2 by adding 7.5% $NaHCO_3$.
3. Temperature controlled incubator FTC90i (VELP Scientifica).
4. Plastic Petri dishes, 100 mm (Falcon).

2.3. Morpholino Treatment of the Embryos

1. E3 medium: 5 mM NaCl, 0.17 mM KCl, 0.33 mM $CaCl_2$, 0.33 mM $MgSO_4$, 0.2% methylene blue.
2. Morpholinos: ift88 (NM_001001725) morpholino exon1: 5′-AGCAGATGCAAAATGACTCACTGGG-3′ (Gene Tools), 0.2 mM. ATG tnnt2 (NM_152893) morpholino: 5′-CATGTTTGCTCTGATCTGACACGCA-3′ (Gene Tools), 0.125 mM.
3. Morpholinos are diluted in 100 mM KCl, 10 mM HEPES, 0.1% Phenol Red (4× stock of the injection medium is used to dilute morpholinos).
4. Nanoliter2000 microinjector (World Precision Instruments).

5. Glass capillaries for Nanoliter 2000 (World Precision Instruments).
6. Narishige PP83 pipet puller (Narishige).
7. Dissecting microscope (SMZ645, Nikon).
8. Wide microscope slide, 3×2 in. (Fisher).
9. Regular microscope slide, 3×1 in. (Fisher).
10. Plastic transfer pipette (Fisher).
11. Pulled glass probe (Fig. 4b).

2.4. Mounting Zebrafish for Live Imaging

1. E3 medium: 5 mM NaCl, 0.17 mM KCl, 0.33 mM $CaCl_2$, 0.33 mM $MgSO_4$. Methylene blue (0.2%) can be added to the medium to limit fungal and bacterial growth. For the imaging, the embryos are moved into methylene blue-free medium containing PTU (below).
2. E3-PTU medium: 0.003% N-phenylthiourea (PTU—Sigma) is added to the E3 solution (no methylene blue). We normally make 10× stock of E3-PTU by overnight dissolution on a stir plate. The pH is adjusted to 7.0–7.2 by adding 7.5% $NaHCO_3$.
3. LMP Agarose. 1–2% Low melting point agarose (Invitrogen) is prepared by heating 200–400 mg of agarose in 20 mL E3 (no methylene blue, no PTU) in a microwave. The E3 agarose gel can be reused a number of times by reheating it in a microwave.
4. 20× (4 mg/mL) stock solution of Tricaine (Tricaine methanesulfonate, Sigma), buffered to neutral pH with 7.5% $NaHCO_3$. This solution is kept at 4°C.
5. The final imaging solution is obtained by 1:20 dilution of 20× Tricaine stock in E3-PTU medium. If a chemical is tested in live assay, we use 1% DMSO in the imaging solution to improve penetration of the chemical.
6. Plastic Petri dish, 35 mm (Falcon).
7. Forceps (Dumont #5).
8. Pulled glass probe (Fig. 4b).
9. Plastic microcentrifuge tube.
10. Dissecting microscope (SMZ645, Nikon).
11. Plastic transfer pipette (Fisher).

2.5. Imaging

1. E3-PTU medium: 0.003% N-phenylthiourea (PTU—Sigma) is added to the E3 solution (no methylene blue).
2. Glass slide 3×1 in. (Fisher).
3. Plasticine modeling clay.
4. Zeiss Pascal LSM5 upright scanning confocal microscope with 40× or 60× water dipping lens.

5. Pascal image acquisition software.
6. Plastic cover with an imaging window (65 mm).
7. (Optional) Miniature Incubator for Petri Dishes (Bioscience Tools).
8. (Optional) Precision Temperature controller (Bioscience Tools).
9. (Optional) Temperature probe (Bioscience Tools).

2.6. Image Processing and Morphometry

1. ImageJ software (NIH, http://rsbweb.nih.gov/ij/).

3. Methods

3.1. General Embryo Care

1. The embryos are collected as described in ref. 20 and kept in E3 medium in 100-mm dishes at 28.5°C until used for imaging. Dead embryos should be removed and the total number of embryos per dish should be kept below 100 for the optimal rate of development.
2. At 24 hpf, the E3 medium is removed and replaced with E3-PTU medium to prevent pigmentation, which can significantly interfere with imaging fluorescent signals.

3.2. Morpholino Treatment of the Embryos

Morpholino knockdown is a powerful way to examine the role of different genes in zebrafish kidney development. Here, we illustrate the technique using cardiac troponin T (tnnt2) and intraflagellar transport protein 88 (ift88) morpholinos. tnnt2 morpholino has no direct effect on the kidney, but has profound secondary effect on kidney architecture due to altered glomerular filtration and luminal fluid flow (21). Ift88 morpholino interferes with cilia assembly and results in kidney tubule dilatation and cystic change (22).

1. To inject a one- to two-cell-stage embryos, we use the nanoinjector assembly as illustrated in Fig. 2a.
2. The embryos are positioned in a groove created by placing a 3 × 1-in. microscope slide on top of a 2 × 3-in. wide microscope slide (Fig. 2b, inset). After placing the embryos, most fluid is removed to create sufficient surface tension to hold embryos in place (Fig. 2b). About 50 embryos can be lined up this way for a round of injection.
3. A fixed volume (4.6 nL) of a morpholino-containing solution (Fig. 2a, inset) is injected into each embryo. The exact amount of the effective dose may vary slightly from morpholino to morpholino (0.5–2pmol). Morpholino efficacy can be later confirmed by RT PCR (in case of ift88) or by observing absent heart contractions (tnnt2) and kidney cyst formation (ift88).

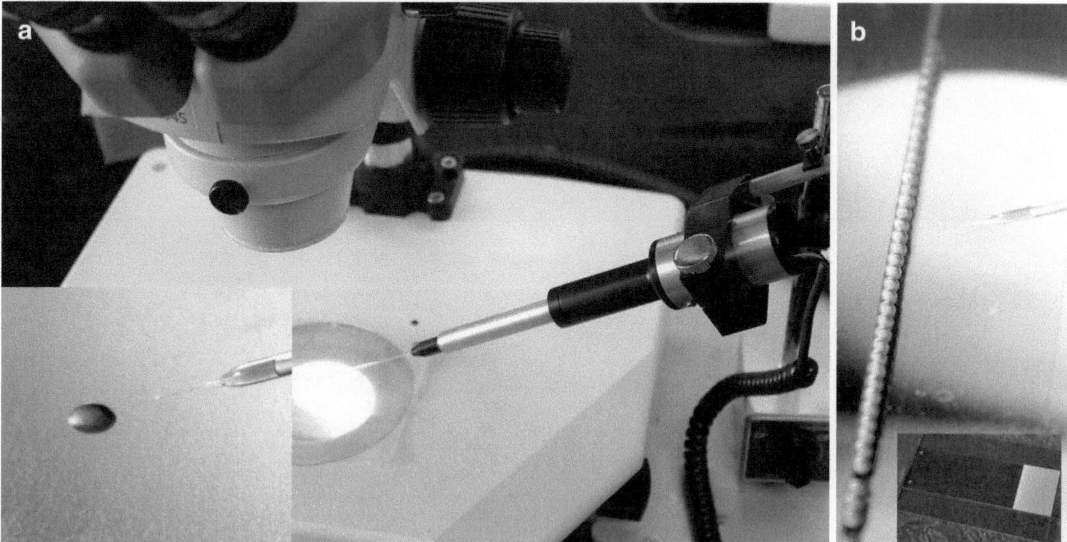

Fig. 2. Morpholino injection setup. (**a**) The injection setup consists of a dissecting microscope and Drummond nanoinjector. Injection solution is drawn into the injection pipette from a 3–4-μL drop placed on top of parafilm (**a**, inset). A 3 × 1-in. microscope slide is placed on top of a larger 3 × 2-in. slide to create a grove, where one- to two-cell-stage embryos will be positioned (**b**, inset). The embryos are placed with a plastic pipette and the excess fluid is removed. The embryos are lined up using pulled glass probe and much of the remaining fluid is drawn out by capillary force (can be done with a corner of a paper napkin) to leave just enough medium to prevent embryo dehydration. The embryos are injected with 4.6 nL of morpholino solution (**b**).

When injecting one- to two-cell-stage embryos, one should aim at the zone of cytoplasmic streaming to ensure delivery of morpholino solution from the yolk to the embryo (see Note 1). The success of injection can be monitored in a couple of hours by observing pink color change of the developing embryo (due to the presence of phenol red in injection solution).

4. The injected embryos are carefully flushed down into a 100-mm Petri dish containing fresh E3 medium and placed into a 28.5°C incubator.
5. Dead embryos should be removed after a few hours to prevent excessive bacterial and protozoal proliferation.

3.3. Mounting Zebrafish for Live Imaging

1. The embryos should be removed from chorions for optimal imaging results. Pronase treatment can be employed; however, we prefer manual dechorionation with a pair of fine forceps. Even the youngest embryos can be easily dechorionated without prior chemical treatment after a short practice.
2. The embryos are placed in a 100-mm Petri dish and covered with E3 or E3-PTU depending on the stage.
3. To dechorionate the embryo, the chorion should be grabbed with fine forceps as shown in Fig. 3a, b. The chorion can then be gently pulled apart to release the embryo (Fig. 3c, d).

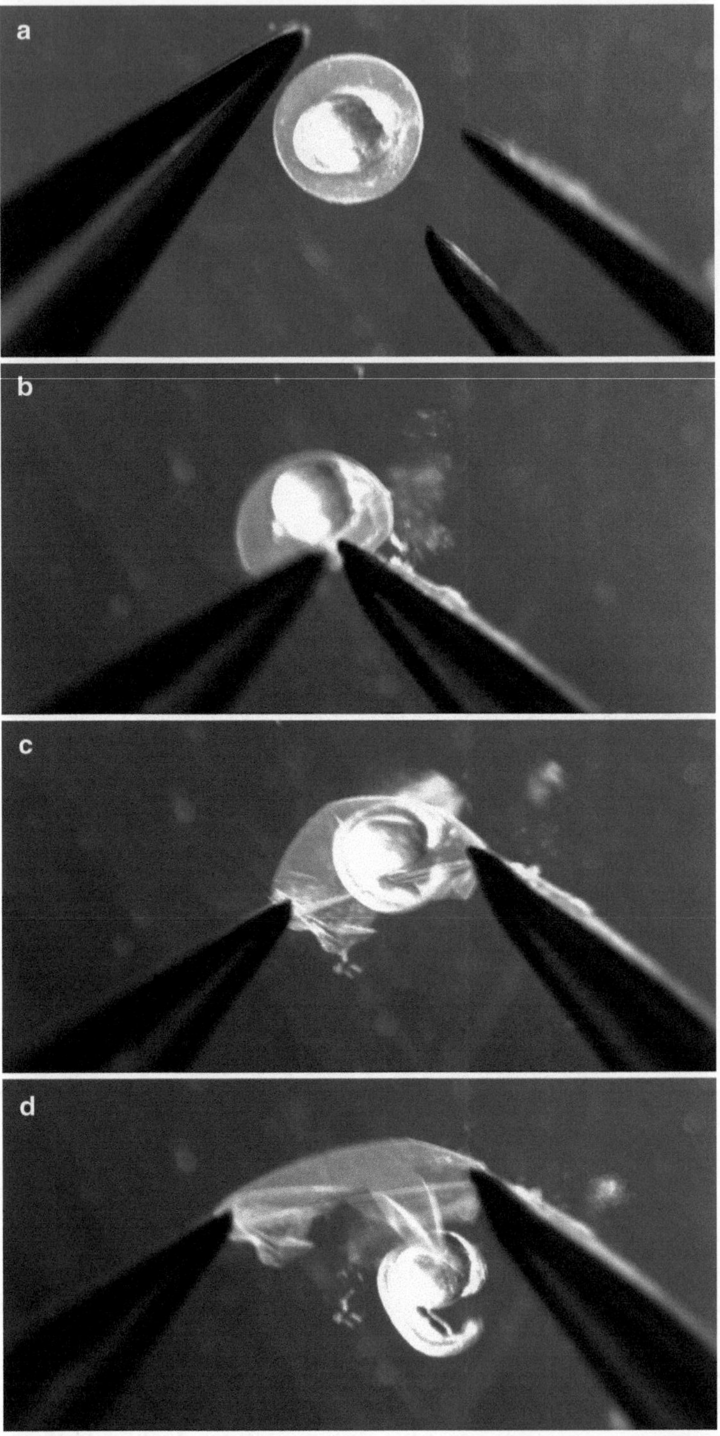

Fig. 3. Dechorionation of the embryo. (**a–c**) Successive steps in dechorionation of the embryo are shown. At the end, the chorion should be opened like a book to release the embryo. (**a**) The chorion is grabbed with the forceps while the second pair is used to support the embryo and the chorion. (**b**) The second pair is used to grab the chorion near the position of the first forceps. (**c**) The chorion is gently pulled apart to produce a tear. If needed, chorion can be re-grabbed so that the forceps are again near each other; thus, the tear is extended until the embryo freely falls out of the chorion (**d**).

4. When working with very young embryos (pre-somitogenesis), the Petri dish should be first prepared by covering the bottom with agarose (regular- or low-melting-point agarose can be used). Because embryos are fragile at these early stages, chorions should be opened carefully by re-grabbing the chorion and carefully opening it until the embryo falls out of it freely.
5. LMP agarose should be reheated to melt it. 1 mL of melted LMP agarose is placed into a microcentrifuge tube. This speeds up cooling of the agarose. To this volume, 50 μl of 20× Tricaine is added. The mixture is allowed to cool down to about the human body temperature. It is essential to properly anesthetize the embryos for the duration of the imaging. Under-anesthetized embryos will spontaneously twitch, compromising the experiment (see Note 2).
6. By this time, a 35-mm plastic Petri dish should be positioned on a dissecting microscope and a pulled glass probe placed nearby. It is important to have everything in place because one needs to be able to orient the embryo before agarose begins to solidify, which takes about 1–3 min.
7. The embryo is drawn into a plastic or glass transfer pipette with just enough solution to cover it, and transferred into cooled down melted agarose–tricaine solution. The agarose containing the embryo is then redrawn into the transfer pipette and placed in the center of the 35-mm dish (Fig. 4a). When introducing the embryo to the agarose, one needs to make sure that it is sufficiently cool (body temperature, see Note 3). Applying agarose that is too warm may result in embryo death or cardiac arrest. We find that applying 1 mL of agarose to a 35-mm dish will allow optimal spreading of the agarose to evenly fill the bottom of the dish. Covering the entire bottom of the dish improves mechanical stability of the system and prevents potential horizontal travel (see Note 4).
8. The glass probe (Fig. 4b) is used to spread the agarose to evenly cover the bottom of the dish (Fig. 4c). The embryo is then reoriented by gentle manipulation with glass probe until it is in the desired position for optimal imaging. The best position varies from application to application. In general, we like the kidney segment of interest and the skin surface to be perpendicular to the beam path. In most circumstances, this can be achieved by placing the embryo as shown in Fig. 4d. Early-stage embryos are significantly curved, but the same principle applies: the beam path should be perpendicular to the skin surface and to the long axis of the structure of interest. Having the skin surface perpendicular to the beam path allows us to minimize light scatter, thus improving image quality. Having the long axis of the structure of interest perpendicular to the beam path allows us to minimize total z-stack depth, thus

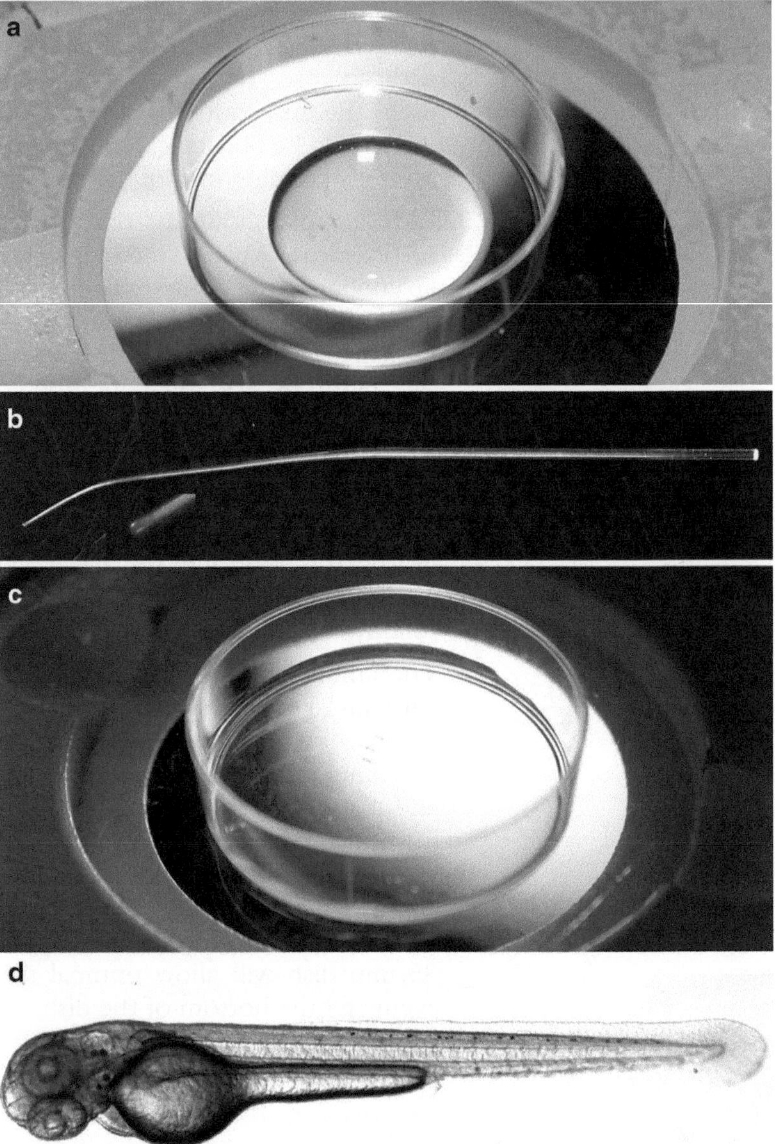

Fig. 4. Embryo immobilization for time-lapse imaging. (**a**) 1 mL of low-melting-point agarose containing anesthetized embryos is placed in the center of a 35-mm plastic dish. (**b**) Glass capillary is pulled over the flame to produce a smooth polished tip (inset) for embryo manipulation. (**c**) Glass manipulator is used to spread the agarose to evenly cover the bottom of the Petri dish. After that, embryos are oriented in the center of the dish. (**d**) 2.5 dpf zebrafish embryo immobilized in agarose for kidney imaging. Note that the trunk is slightly elevated above horizontal (evidenced by eyes not being lined up).

reducing the acquisition time and minimizing bleaching of the embryos. After applying agarose (containing the embryos) to the dish, one typically has about a minute to properly orient the embryos (see Note 5). The embryos should be continuously kept in that orientation by using pulled glass probe under the dissecting microscope until they stop moving, at which point the probe should be removed and the agarose allowed to solidify. Lower percent agarose (<1%) will require longer period of continued embryo adjustment before it stops moving due to gravity. Because it is difficult to obtain an optimal imaging orientation, we like to embed two to three embryos in a dish and then select the one with the optimal orientation.

9. The embryos should be maintained in the optimal position until they stop moving due to gravity. The agarose is still soft at this point and the surface of the agarose will remain flat after removing the glass probe.
10. The Petri dish is covered to limit the evaporation and the agarose is allowed to completely solidify (which takes about 15 min). At that point, the embryo is ready for imaging.

3.4. Imaging

1. The Petri dish containing the immobilized embryo is placed on top of a microscope slide and secured with modeling plasticine. The glass slide is positioned on the stage of a confocal microscope (Fig. 5a).
2. The imaging solution (E3-PTU with tricaine) is carefully added to cover three-fourths of the dish volume. The solution covering the agarose should only be applied after agarose is sufficiently hardened (we allow at least 15 min at room temperature), and the dish is positioned for imaging (see Note 6). Transporting the dish with solution covering the agarose may sufficiently disturb the agarose to render the imaging session unusable. Global embryo movement can also be a significant obstacle to time-lapse imaging. Agarose has a restrictive effect on embryo growth, thus generating additional, unnatural forces. This may not be an issue for short time intervals, but can compromise the interpretation of results in long (hours) recordings. By knowing the most prominent global morphogenic movements, one can partially relieve the constraints of the agarose by cutting out small "windows" to allow tissue extension. For example, agarose can be removed from around the tip of the tail to allow tail extension. However, early embryo morphogenesis consists of many global movements that may require alternative methods of imaging (23).
3. An imaging cover consisting of a Petri dish lid with the center drilled out to accommodate the microscope lens is placed on top of the Petri dish (see Note 7). The hole should be about 1 mm wider than the diameter of the objective: this virtually eliminates evaporation while allowing vertical travel of the objective with respect to the stage for z-stacked time series. The plastic cover should be flat, and freely travel on top of the dish containing embryo. This allows free lateral displacement

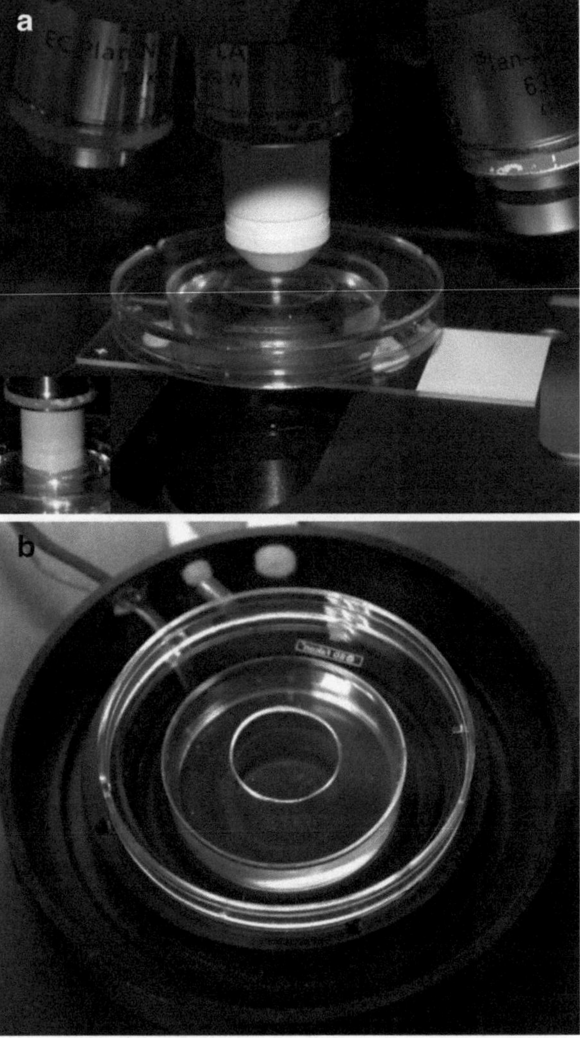

Fig. 5. Time-lapse imaging of fluorescent zebrafish. (**a**) Covered dish, mounted for imaging on a confocal microscope using 3 × 1-in. microscope slide as a support. The dish is secured on a slide using small amount of plasticine. (**a**, inset) 40× confocal objective is shown in the working position inside the cover. (**b**) Imaging dish mounted inside the heated chamber. Movie S1 Dechorionation of early embryos. The chorion is re-grabbed a few times and small successive tears are made to open the chorion and allow the embryo to fall out of the chorion by gravity. Note that no force is applied directly to the embryo. Because of that, even the earliest stage embryos can be successfully manually dechorionated. Movie S2 Circumferential epithelial migration in obstructed kidney tubules. The ET(krt8:EGFP)sqet33-d10 embryos were injected with a combination of tnnt2 and ift88 morpholino. The 3dpf embryo was then imaged in a 30-min per interval time lapse. The maximal intensity projection is generated using Zeiss Pascal software and reoriented using ImageJ. Significant tubule distension is seen here even in the absence of heart contractions. Additionally, segmental circumferential migration is seen. At the same time, local vortex currents are observed in distended lumina due to beating motile cilia. Head is to the left. Number of frames = 18.

of the cover and optimal horizontal positioning of the embryo for imaging (see Note 8). The desired water-dipping objective is lowered to visualize the region of interest (Fig. 5a, inset, also see Note 9). To prevent a bubble from forming at the water-lens interface, lower the lens into the medium slightly off vertical. If an air bubble forms, wipe the objective with lens paper and lower it again. This usually solves the problem. When a lower magnification is desired and air lenses are used in the upright configuration, a glass coverslip is needed to interface with the imaging solution.

4. To produce time-lapse images, we use an upright Zeiss LSM5 Pascal confocal microscope. In our experience, an upright configuration allows for optimal visualization of the embryo in live assays. Water-dipping lenses have a long working distance, and agarose-embedded zebrafish embryos provide clear visualization of the tissue of interest if oriented properly. Inverted systems can also be utilized, but they may present some challenges because of the short working distance of conventional oil lenses and a need to maintain the water interface of water-immersion lens for potentially long periods of time lapse. Also, using dry lenses on an inverted system introduces significant spherical aberration and point spread in the *Z* axis due to index of refraction mismatch (air:glass:water).

5. We normally use the following parameters for image acquisition (40× water-dipping objective): Virtual slice thickness of 4 μm, z-stack interval = 2 μm (Nyquist sampling), pixel dwell time = 4 μs, image dimension = 512 × 512, acquisition type = frame, averaging = 2. These parameters allow continuous 20-min interval recording with minimal photobleaching of the sample. To achieve long stability of the sample, we set the time-lapse interval (from the beginning of a given z-stack to the beginning of the next z-stack) to be at least twice the stack acquisition time. If shorter time-lapse intervals are required, pixel dwell time, frame pixel size, or the number of frames used for averaging can be reduced (see Note 10).

6. Maximum intensity projections of each stack can be generated using Pascal software. The flattened time-lapse projections or the original stacks can be further processed and analyzed using ImageJ (NIH).

7. Because zebrafish can develop normally at room temperature, a temperature-controlled stage is not required for observing most relevant developmental phenomena as long as room temperature is maintained reasonably high (we keep it at 25°C). However, the absolute rates of development may be altered in cooler conditions. If precise temperature control is critical, temperature-controlled incubator for Petri dishes can be used. We use miniature incubator for Petri dishes by Bioscience tools (Fig. 5b).

The imaging setup described here is adequate for most practical situations. Very long time-lapse imaging may require a more elaborate experimental design (24).

3.5. Image Processing and Morphometry

1. The images can be initially processed using Zeiss Pascal software, which can be used to generate flattened confocal stacks of a timed series of images (time-lapse movies) or perform simple morphometry (such as distance measurement, etc.).
2. The images can be further imported into ImageJ (NIH) for further processing and analysis. Some compilations of ImageJ, such as Fiji (http://fiji.sc/wiki/index.php/Fiji), have additional features (through plug-in libraries) that allow advanced image manipulation, such as derivation of a three-dimensional structure from image stacks.
3. Matlab (http://www.mathworks.com/products/matlab/) can also be interfaced with common imaging formats, such as LSM files, to allow almost unlimited number of ways to process and analyze the acquired data.

4. Notes

1. When injecting one- to two-cell-stage embryos, one should aim at the zone of cytoplasmic streaming.
2. Under-anesthetized embryos will spontaneously twitch, compromising the experiment.
3. When adding agarose, make sure that it is sufficiently cool (body temperature).
4. Covering the entire bottom of the imaging dish with agarose improves mechanical stability of the system and prevents potential horizontal travel.
5. After applying agarose (containing the embryos) to the dish, one typically has about a minute to properly orient the embryos. The embryos should be continuously kept in that orientation until they stop moving. Lower percent agarose (<1%) will require longer period of continued embryo adjustment before it stops moving due to gravity.
6. Allow about 15 min for agarose to solidify before adding imaging solution. Add imaging solution only after the dish is positioned on a microscope.
7. When using an upright imaging system, evaporation of the recording medium should be limited by using a flat plastic cover that has a hole drilled in it to allow access of a water-dipping lens. One easy way to make such a cover is to use a 65-mm Petri dish cover and drill a hole of a desired diameter

using drill press, drill bit (starter), and a router bit (to extend to a desired dimension). Alternatively, the hole can be cut out using a blade. Care should be taken to prevent injury.

8. The plastic cover should be flat and larger than the imaging dish to allow free lateral displacement of the cover and optimal horizontal positioning of the embryo for imaging.
9. When lowering the objective, keep it slightly off vertical to prevent air bubble formation.
10. Global embryo movement can create an obstacle to time-lapse imaging. Agarose has a restrictive effect on the embryo, thus generating unnatural forces. One can partially relieve the constraints of the agarose by cutting out small "windows" to allow for tissue extension.

Acknowledgment

The authors thank Dr. Shannon Fisher for sharing the retl/zcs:GFP transgenic, Dr. Vladimir Korzh for sharing ET(krt8:EGFP) sqet11-9 and ET(krt8:EGFP)sqet33-d10 transgenics, as well as Drs. H.F. Lin and R.I. Handin for sharing cd41:GFP transgenic. We also thank Dr. Gromoslaw Smolen and Yan Liu for the useful advice. This work was supported by National Institutes of Health Grant K08DK082782 and HSCI Pilot grant to AV and NIH DK053093, DK071041, and DK070263 grants to IAD.

References

1. Gutzman JH, Graeden EG, Lowery LA, Holley HS, Sive H (2008) Formation of the zebrafish midbrain-hindbrain boundary constriction requires laminin-dependent basal constriction. Mech Dev 125:974–983
2. Hall C, Flores MV, Crosier K, Crosier P (2009) Live cell imaging of zebrafish leukocytes. Methods Mol Biol 546:255–271
3. Aman A, Piotrowski T (2008) Wnt/beta-catenin and Fgf signaling control collective cell migration by restricting chemokine receptor expression. Dev Cell 15:749–761
4. Vasilyev A, Liu Y, Mudumana S et al (2009) Collective cell migration drives morphogenesis of the kidney nephron. PLoS Biol 7:e9
5. Saxen L, Sariola H (1987) Early organogenesis of the kidney. Pediatr Nephrol 1:385–392
6. Vize PD, Woolf AS, Bard JBL (2002) The kidney: from normal development to congenital diseases. Academic, Boston
7. Drummond IA, Majumdar A, Hentschel H et al (1998) Early development of the zebrafish pronephros and analysis of mutations affecting pronephric function. Development 125: 4655–4667
8. Kramer-Zucker AG, Wiessner S, Jensen AM, Drummond IA (2005) Organization of the pronephric filtration apparatus in zebrafish requires Nephrin, Podocin and the FERM domain protein Mosaic eyes. Dev Biol 285: 316–329
9. Diep CQ, Ma D, Deo RC et al (2011) Identification of adult nephron progenitors capable of kidney regeneration in zebrafish. Nature 470:95–100
10. Zhou W, Boucher RC, Bollig F, Englert C, Hildebrandt F (2010) Characterization of mesonephric development and regeneration using transgenic zebrafish. Am J Physiol 299: F1040–F1047

11. Bollig F, Mehringer R, Perner B et al (2006) Identification and comparative expression analysis of a second wt1 gene in zebrafish. Dev Dyn 235:554–561
12. Liu Y, Pathak N, Kramer-Zucker A, Drummond IA (2007) Notch signaling controls the differentiation of transporting epithelia and multiciliated cells in the zebrafish pronephros. Development 134:1111–1122
13. Fisher S, Grice EA, Vinton RM, Bessling SL, McCallion AS (2006) Conservation of RET regulatory function from human to zebrafish without sequence similarity. Science 312:276–279
14. Seiler C, Pack M (2011) Transgenic labeling of the zebrafish pronephric duct and tubules using a promoter from the enpep gene. Gene Expr Patterns 11:118–121
15. Lin HF, Traver D, Zhu H et al (2005) Analysis of thrombocyte development in CD41-GFP transgenic zebrafish. Blood 106:3803–3810
16. Choo BG, Kondrichin I, Parinov S et al (2006) Zebrafish transgenic Enhancer TRAP line database (ZETRAP). BMC Dev Biol 6:5
17. Parinov S, Kondrichin I, Korzh V, Emelyanov A (2004) Tol2 transposon-mediated enhancer trap to identify developmentally regulated zebrafish genes in vivo. Dev Dyn 231:449–459
18. Kwan KM, Fujimoto E, Grabher C et al (2007) The Tol2kit: a multisite gateway-based construction kit for Tol2 transposon transgenesis constructs. Dev Dyn 236: 3088–3099
19. Kikuta H, Kawakami K (2009) Transient and stable transgenesis using tol2 transposon vectors. Methods Mol Biol 546:69–84
20. Westerfield M (2000) The zebrafish book. A guide for the laboratory use of zebrafish (*Danio rerio*). University of Oregon, Eugene
21. Serluca FC, Drummond IA, Fishman MC (2002) Endothelial signaling in kidney morphogenesis: a role for hemodynamic forces. Curr Biol 12:492–497
22. Kramer-Zucker AG, Olale F, Haycraft CJ et al (2005) Cilia-driven fluid flow in the zebrafish pronephros, brain and Kupffer's vesicle is required for normal organogenesis. Development 132:1907–1921
23. Carvalho L, Heisenberg CP (2009) Imaging zebrafish embryos by two-photon excitation time-lapse microscopy. Methods Mol Biol 546:273–287
24. Kamei M, Weinstein BM (2005) Long-term time-lapse fluorescence imaging of developing zebrafish. Zebrafish 2:113–123

Part II

Analyzing Ureteric Bud Branching and Nephrogenesis

Chapter 7

Analysis of 3D Branching Pattern: Hematoxylin and Eosin Method

Sunder Sims-Lucas

Abstract

Accurate analysis of the three-dimensional (3D) architecture of developing organs is critical to understanding how developmental defects can be linked with structural abnormalities. Here, we describe a 3D reconstruction technique of the developing kidney including the outer kidney capsule, ureteric epithelium, and developing nephrons. This 3D reconstructive process involves generating serial sections of the developing kidney, followed by histological staining. Each serial image is projected on the monitor and each tissue lineage or structure is traced. The kidney tracings are aligned and a 3D image is rendered. Each reconstructed tissue/ lineage can then be subjected to quantitative analysis (e.g., surface area or volume). The reconstructed ureteric epithelium can be skeletonized to determine the branching architecture.

Key words: Kidney development, 3D reconstruction, Histology, Hematoxylin and eosin, Branching morphogenesis

1. Introduction

Development of the permanent kidney requires reciprocal interactions of the metanephric mesenchyme and the ureteric bud (1, 2). Following the initial outgrowth from the Wolffian duct, the ureteric bud undergoes a series of dichotomous branching events at the ampullary tips. At the same time, the developing nephrons are induced to condense around the tips of the ureteric epithelium and undergo a parallel series of differentiation events ultimately forming mature glomeruli. The ureteric epithelium ends as a complex 3-dimensional (3D) structure draining thousands (rodent) to millions (humans) of nephrons in each kidney through single ureters (3). Inappropriate ureteric branching can result in an under-endowment of nephrons, which predisposes the kidney to disease (4, 5). Concurrent with ureteric branching is nephron differentiation/maturation (nephrogenesis). Initially,

Odyssé Michos (ed.), *Kidney Development: Methods and Protocols*, Methods in Molecular Biology, vol. 886, DOI 10.1007/978-1-61779-851-1_7, © Springer Science+Business Media, LLC 2012

nephrogenic mesenchyme condenses around ureteric tips and converts into epithelial vesicles (the most immature "nephrons"). Vesicles differentiate into comma and then S-shaped bodies that join with the collecting ducts before maturing into functional nephrons (glomeruli and tubules) (6–9).

Characterizing ureteric branching in 3D kidneys has been challenging. It is largely undertaken in cultured kidney explants that flatten, allowing for visualization of branching by whole mount immunofluorescent staining or transgenic green fluorescent protein expression. Counting ureteric tips or branch points in whole mount specimens quantitates branching. Recently, investigators have used confocal microscopy to quantify ureteric branch lengths in cultured kidney explants (10). Despite the elegant studies, these approaches are limited in that explants are removed from their physiological environment and fail to grow in 3 dimensions. There is also significant variability due to operator skill, culture conditions (media, incubator conditions), and in precise ages of the explants.

Recent reports have focused on ureteric branching in kidneys that developed in vivo. One study estimated branch lengths and tips in fluorescently labeled serial ultra-thick murine cryosections (11). Despite the elegant study, the technique was limited by the need for special stains and potential sampling errors caused by the thick sections. Others have generated 3D images of fluorescently labeled ureteric trees using confocal microscopy without quantitating branching (11, 12). A comprehensive assessment of branching morphogenesis in kidneys was achieved using optical projection tomography (OPT) (13). Despite producing high-fidelity images of immunohistochemically stained ureteric trees, OPT is limited by the size of the kidneys and the penetration of the stain (as mentioned in the following chapter).

Quantitation of nephron formation in utero has been labor intensive and restricted to estimates. Rigorous quantitative assessment has only been achieved in vitro utilizing immunohistochemical staining in cultured kidney explants. Thus, relative distribution, 3D structure, and size of developing nephrons (vesicles through mature nephrons) have not been determined to our knowledge. Given limitations of the aforementioned techniques, we developed a 3-dimensional procedure to quantify ureteric branching morphogenesis and nephrogenesis of developing murine kidneys in vivo (14, 15).

2. Materials

2.1. Equipment

1. Standard automated histological paraffin processor.
2. Tissue cassettes.

3. Standard embedding station with hot and cold plate areas.
4. Microtome.
5. Water bath set at 45°C.
6. Shandon Paratrimmer.
7. Razor blades.
8. Micromaster microscope.
9. Metal staining racks.
10. Pyrex glass dishes with metal lids (at least 20).
11. Coverslips.

2.2. Staining Supplies of Slides

1. Solutions for dewaxing slides:
   (a) 100% Ethanol (EtOH).
   (b) Xylene.
   (c) Distilled water.
2. Hematoxylin and eosin solutions:
   (a) Hematoxylin.
   (b) Running water.
   (c) Clarifier.
   (d) Bluing reagent.
   (e) 95% EtOH.
   (f) Eosin.
   (g) 100% EtOH.
   (h) Xylene.
3. Periodic acid Schiff solutions:
   (a) 0.5% Periodic acid solution.
   (b) Schiff reagent.
   (c) Hematoxylin.
   (d) Running water.
4. Masson's trichrome staining:
   (a) Weigert's Iron hematoxylin solution (equal parts Stock solution A and B): stock solution A (1 g hematoxylin, 95% EtOH), stock solution B (4 mL 29% ferric chloride in water, 95 mL distilled water, 1 mL concentrated hydrochloric acid).
   (b) Biebrich scarlet-acid fuchsin solution: 90 mL Biebrich scarlet 1% aqueous, 10 mL acid fuchsin, 1% aqueous, 1 mL glacial acetic acid.
   (c) Phosphomolybdic-phosphotungstic acid solution: 25 mL 5% phosphomolybdic acid, 25 mL phosphotungstic acid.

   (d) Aniline blue solution: 2.5 g aniline blue, 2 mL glacial acetic acid, 100 mL distilled water.
   (e) 1% acetic acid solution: 1 mL glacial acetic acid, 99 mL distilled water.
5. Coverslipping
   (a) Mounting media Cytoseal.

2.3. Upright Microscope with Motorized Stage and Drawing Tablet

1. Motorized stage.
2. Color digital camera.
3. PC workstation.
4. 24-in. LCD flat monitor.
5. Drawing tablet (Wacom).
6. Battery backup/surge protector (Tripp-Lite).
7. Upright microscope (Zeiss, Imager MI).
   (a) 10× objective (used to locate and trace the tissue of interest).

2.4. Tracing Software

1. Stereoinvestigator version 9.04 or Neurolucida (MBF Bioscience (Microbrightfield, Inc.)).
2. Nuerolucida Explorer version 9.04 (MBF Bioscience (Microbrightfield, Inc.)).

2.5. Skeletonization Software

1. IMARIS filament tracer (Bitplane).

3. Methods

Using standard histological techniques with state-of-the-art 3D reconstruction technology, we have produced a method to accurately measure branching morphogenesis and nephrogenesis (from vesicles through immature glomeruli) in the developing kidney.

3.1. Processing Tissue for Paraffin Section

1. Time-mated females are sacrificed and embryos harvested at the desired developmental stage (minimally E13.5 to see extensive ureteric branching and significant nephron development). Embryos are then fixed overnight in 4% paraformaldehyde in PBS. Following this, the embryos are placed into cassettes and kept in 70% ethanol at 4°C until they are ready to be processed. The cassettes are then processed as follows:
   (a) 70% Ethanol for 20 min at room temperature.
   (b) 100% Ethanol for 20 min at room temperature.
   (c) 100% Ethanol for 20 min at room temperature.

(d) 100% Ethanol for 20 min at room temperature.
(e) Xylene for 30 min at room temperature.
(f) Xylene for 30 min at room temperature.
(g) Xylene for 30 min at room temperature.
(h) Paraffin wax for 30 min at room temperature.
(i) Paraffin wax for 30 min at room temperature.
(j) Paraffin wax for 30 min at room temperature.

2. Following processing, the cassettes are transferred to the heated paraffin wax tank of an embedding station. The embryos are removed from the cassettes and placed into metal molds sitting upright. As they are held in place with forceps, hot liquid paraffin is poured over the embryos. The cassette lids are placed onto the top of the molds containing the embryos and more hot wax is added to fill the cassette lids. Once filled, the molds are set on the cold plate to harden.

3.2. Sectioning for 3D Reconstruction

1. Before sectioning can commence, the metal molds should be removed (from the surface to be sectioned) and excess wax around the cassettes should be removed using the Paratrimmer. Using a razor blade, trim the block edges to decrease the cutting surface area. Cut a wedge out of the top left corner of the block to make "ribboning" easier.
2. Using the microtome, section into the block until the urogenital sinus is visible. Remove the block from the microtome "chuck" and chill in ice water for 30–40 min. Cut sections at 4 μm through the entire length of the kidney. Float sections on a warm water bath (set at 45°C) and collect serial sections in the correct order on charged slides. Dry the slides for 30–40 min before placing in an incubator set at 55°C for 1–2 h to adhere the sections to the slide.

3.3. De-paraffinize Slides

Prior to any staining, the slides must first be de-paraffinized and rehydrated (see Note 1).

1. Place slides in metal staining racks.
2. Xylene for 5 min
3. Xylene for 3 min
4. Xylene for 1 min
5. 100% Ethanol for 1 min
6. 100% Ethanol for 1 min
7. 100% Ethanol for 1 min
8. Wash in distilled water for 1 min.

3.4. Hematoxylin and Eosin Staining (See Note 2)

1. Place slides into hematoxylin for 1 min.
2. Rinse in running tap water for 1 min.
3. Place slides into clarifier reagent for 1 min.
4. Rinse in running tap water for 1 min.
5. Place slides into bluing reagent for 1 min.
6. Rinse in running tap water for 1 min.
7. Place slides into 95% ethanol for 20 s.
8. Place slides in eosin for 1 min.
9. Place slides into 100% ethanol for 20 s.
10. Place slides into 100% ethanol for 20 s.
11. Place slides into 100% ethanol for 20 s.
12. Place slides into xylene for 1 min.
13. Place slides into xylene for 3 min.
14. Place slides into xylene for 5 min.
15. Coverslip sections with Cytoseal and glass coverslip.

3.5. PAS Staining (See Note 3) (Alternative to H&E Staining)

1. Oxidize sections in 0.5% periodic acid solution for 5 min.
2. Rinse in distilled water for 1 min.
3. Place in Schiff reagent for 15 min (sections will become light pink).
4. Wash in lukewarm tap water for 5 min (sections will turn dark purple).
5. Counterstain with Mayer's hematoxylin for 1 min.
6. Wash in tap water for 5 min.
7. Place slides into 100% ethanol for 20 s.
8. Place slides into 100% ethanol for 20 s.
9. Place slides into 100% ethanol for 20 s.
10. Place slides into xylene for 1 min.
11. Place slides into xylene for 3 min.
12. Place slides into xylene for 5 min.
13. Coverslip sections with Cytoseal and glass coverslip.

3.6. Masson's Trichrome Staining (See Note 4) (Alternative to H&E Staining)

1. Stain in Weigert's iron hematoxylin solution for 10 min.
2. Rinse in running tap water for 10 min.
3. Wash in distilled water for 1 min.
4. Stain with Biebrich scarlet-acid fuchsin solution for 10–15 min.
5. Wash in distilled water for 5 min.
6. Differentiate in phosphomolybdic-phosphotungstic acid solution for 10–15 min (until collagen is not red).

7. Transfer sections directly to aniline blue solution for 5–10 min.
8. Rinse briefly in distilled water and differentiate in 1% acetic acid solution for 2–5 min.
9. Wash in distilled water.
10. Place slides into 100% ethanol for 20 s.
11. Place slides into 100% ethanol for 20 s.
12. Place slides into 100% ethanol for 20 s.
13. Place slides into xylene for 1 min.
14. Place slides into xylene for 3 min.
15. Place slides into xylene for 5 min.
16. Coverslip sections with Cytoseal and glass coverslip.

3.7. Tracing the Kidney Tissues/Lineages and Rendering a 3D Image

1. Examine the stained slides to determine where the first kidney rudiment appears (see Note 5).
2. Launch Stereo Investigator. Place the first slide with visible kidney on the motorized stage (Fig. 1) and set the reference point as the middle of the kidney section.
3. Select Tools > Serial Section Manager. Select the icon for "new section." A window will open in which "Evaluation interval," "Section cut thickness," "mounted thickness," and "Starting Z level" are entered. After these data are entered, tracing can commence (Fig. 2).

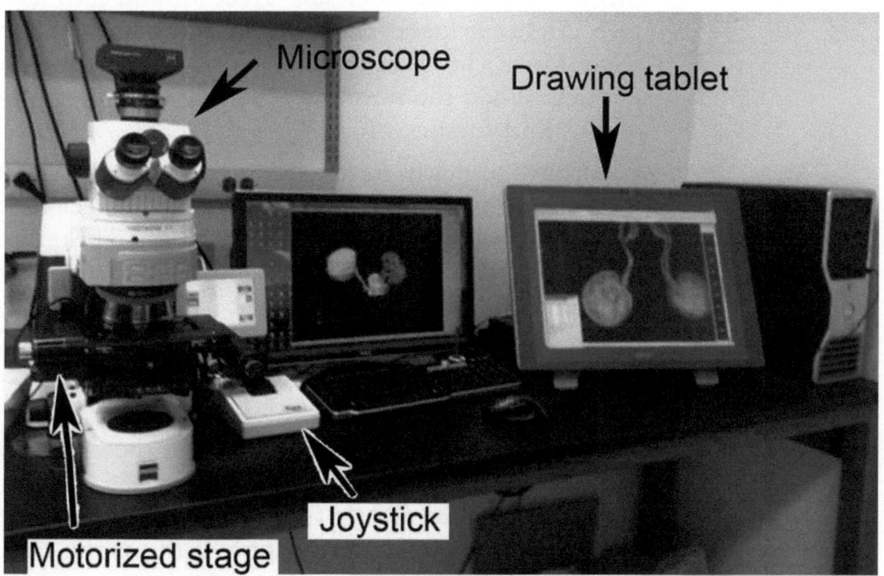

Fig. 1. Microscope setup for 3D reconstruction.

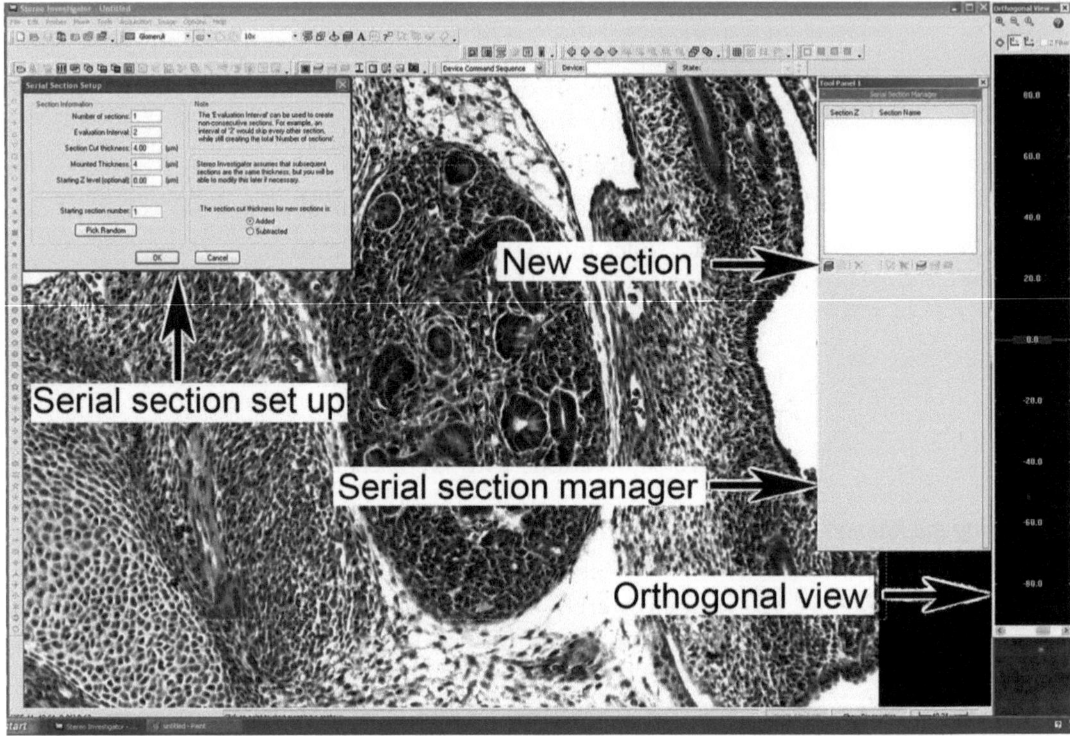

Fig. 2. Software setup for 3D reconstruction.

4. Using the drawing tablet, select the contour to be traced (kidney capsule, ureteric epithelium, etc.) from the drop-down menu in the "Main Toolbar." Trace around each tissue/structure. Right click and select "close contour." Once complete, select Move > Joy Free and move to the next section using the joystick. When the next section is in position, right click and select "End Joystick Mode."
5. Compare the newly traced section with the previously traced section to determine the alignment. To correct for misalignment, select Edit > Select Objects. Right click, and choose Select by Section. Select all contours and click on "Move selected contours" or "Rotate selected contours" to align the newly traced section to the previous section. Once aligned, click on "Create new section" and repeat step 3 until you exhaust the kidney sections (see Note 6).
6. When the entire kidney is traced, select the 3D feature to see the rendering of the entire kidney (Fig. 3e, f). Examine for potential mistakes made in the labeling (e.g., a structure labeled as a vesicle is really a ureteric tip). If this is the case, you can select the inappropriate contour and "change contour type" to the correct contour (see Note 7).

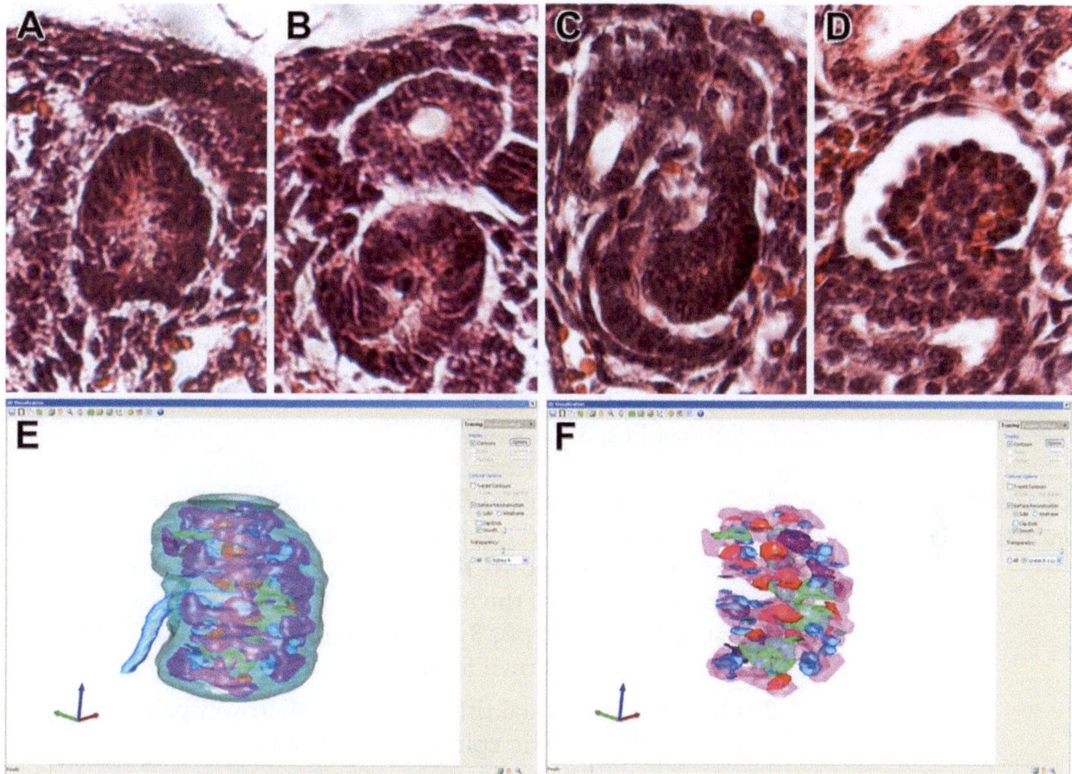

Fig. 3. Segregation of nephron types and 3D reconstruction. (**a–d**) Representative images of the various nephron types: from the earliest renal vesicle (**a**) to comma-shaped bodies (**b**), to S-shaped bodies (**c**) through to a mature nephron (**d**). (**e**, **f**) 3D reconstruction of the developing kidney. (**e**) Reconstruction of the developing kidney, including the outer kidney capsule (*dark green*), the ureter (*light blue*), and ureteric epithelium (*pink*). (**f**) Depiction of the relationship between the ureteric epithelium (*pink*) and the developing nephron types; renal vesicle (*blue*), comma-shaped body (*red*), S-shaped body (*purple*), and glomeruli (*green*).

7. To determine the surface area and the volume of each 3D contour, open up the whole 3D tracing (including all the traced contours) in "Neurolucida Explorer." Under the "analysis" drop-down menu, select the "Marker and region analysis" and select the "3D contour summary" feature. This will then give you the surface area and the volume for the 3D rendering.

3.8. Segregating the Nephrons into the Four Different Developmental Stages

During the initial tracing, it is easiest to label all of the developing nephrons (vesicles through immature glomeruli) the same as "developing glomeruli." However, to determine numbers, volumes, and areas of nephrons at each developmental stage, it is necessary to trace each separately as renal vesicles, comma-shaped bodies, S-shaped bodies, and glomeruli (Fig. 7.3a–d).

1. In order to segregate the various nephron types, it is important to be able to histologically discern them. While comparing the

histologically stained section and the specific level of the 3D image, go through each of the contours and using the "marker" tool label the various structures (1 = renal vesicle, 2 = comma-shaped body, 3 = S-shaped body, 4 = glomeruli).

2. Once the structures are marked, go through and relabel (recolor) each of the nephron contours to match their appropriate developmental stage (Fig. 3f). [You should instead: Select Edit > Select Objects. Left click on the contour you wish to change, right click and select "Change Contour Type," and select the correct contour from the menu.]
3. To determine the volume and area of each developmental nephron type, select "3D contour summary" as in Subheading 3.7.

3.9. Skeletonizing the Ureteric Epithelium

1. Generate tiff images of each layer showing the traced ureteric structures. Record the distance between the first layer containing ureteric tissue to the last layer containing ureteric tissue (i.e., the length of the ureteric tree). Label the layers in sequential order (e.g., 1, 2, 3 … etc.) and save all the tiff images for one kidney in its own folder.
2. Open the individual tiff images in "Microsoft paint" and fill in each of the ureteric epithelium contours.
3. Launch Imaris, select "Open," and then select the folder containing the tiff images of the ureteric tree that you want to skeletonize (simply clicking on one of the images will select them all).
4. Once the images have loaded, invert the image by clicking on the "Image Processing" drop-down menu and then selecting "Contrast change" and "Invert." This process is required to visualize the 3D contours in Imaris.
5. Click on the "Edit" drop-down menu, select "image properties," and change the "X" and "Y" voxel size to "1." Change the "Z" maximum to the distance (in μm) spanning all layers containing ureteric epithelium. Then, in the lower right-hand corner, select the "100%" button to visualize the 3D image in Imaris.
6. Under the "Edit" drop-down menu, select "Show display adjustment." Then, click on the channel to be altered and change the channel color to dark blue and the opacity to 10%. The image is now ready for processing.
7. To begin processing, choose the "Surpass" feature; this is located on the toolbar at the top of the Imaris screen. Choose "Navigate" mode with the pointer (top right-hand corner) to allow the image to be rotated.

8. To begin the skeletonization, select the "Filament tool" ("leaf"-shaped icon on the left-hand side). When the filament tool opens, a four-part guided skeletonization will commence. Use the "Autopath (no loops)" under part 1 of 4 and then click the "blue forward" button on the bottom left (see Note 8).
9. Next (under part 2 of 4), select the largest and the smallest diameter of the ureteric epithelium; typically for E13.5 kidneys, "200 μm" works well as a maximum and "20 μm" works well as a minimum. Make sure that the correct channel is highlighted. Finally, click the "blue forward" button on the bottom left.
10. When part 3 is begun, spheres should appear throughout the ureteric epithelium. The large sphere designates a starting position while the smaller spheres represent an end of a branch. There should only be one starting point located within the ureter (large sphere). If there is more than one large sphere, this needs to be deleted. To delete an unwanted sphere, toggle to select mode (using "esc" key). Subsequently, hold down the "shift" button and move the small formatting box over the large sphere. Click on the large sphere; this should delete the sphere. To change the size of the "select box," use the scroll feature on your mouse.
11. To add terminal tips (small spheres), hold down the "Shift" button and "left" click the mouse. This will place a small blue sphere at the terminal points. If this is not the desired terminal point, then delete it as previously mentioned. Do this for every terminal point that was initially missed by the program. When this is done, click the "blue forward" button in the bottom left. Working with a single 1-pixel line can make connecting or extending point more difficult. Subsequently, to change the thickness of the skeletonized ureteric epithelium, click on the "settings" tab and the option available for the "style" are "line," "cylinder," or "Cone." It is easiest to work with either "Line" or "Cylinder" at a thickness of 3–5. Now, select the button: this is the "double green forward arrow" in the bottom left. This process will take a couple of minutes.
12. When the skeletonization is automatically completed, there are often branches that have not been included or are not extended as much as is required. It is important to as much as possible look at the branch that you want to extend with as little background disturbance as possible. Select on the "draw" feature; this is the third symbol along from the leaf that looks like a fountain pen. Change the Method to "Autodepth." Using the "select" mode, make the box as small as possible and hold down the "shift" key. Click on the mouse to extend the line from as close to the branch that needs to be extended to the terminal tip.

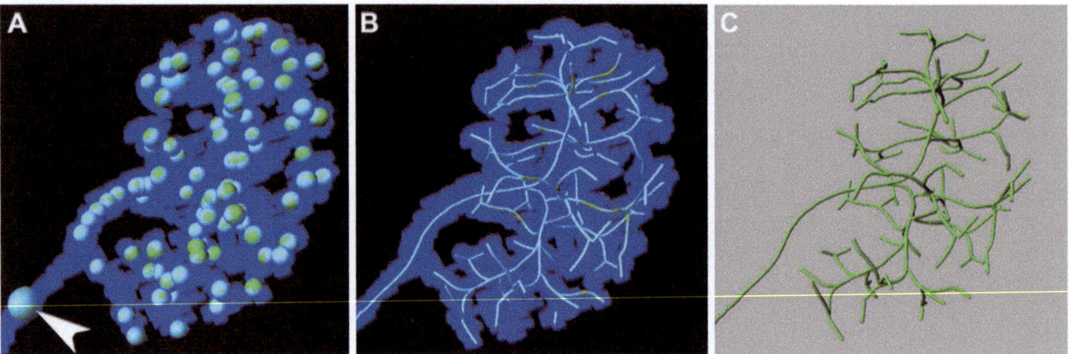

Fig. 4. Skeletonization of ureteric epithelium. (**a–c**) Representative images of the skeletonization process. (**a**) To automate the tracing, spheres are placed inside the ureteric epithelium (*blue*). The large sphere (*arrowhead*) denotes the starting position, while the smaller spheres represent the tract of the skeleton. (**b**) Skeletonization (*green*) within the ureteric epithelium volume (*blue*). (**c**) Skeletonized ureteric epithelium (*green*) with volume subtracted.

13. Once the line has been drawn, it will finally need to be connected to the branch. To connect the line to the branch of interest, select the edit feature "pencil" next to the fountain pen. Then, in the "select" mode, select the branch by moving the box over the branch and clicking on it (the branch will turn yellow). Then, select the extension that was just drawn by holding down "command" and clicking on the end. The branch should also turn yellow. Then, as long as the mouse is in "point" mode, select "Join" under "process selection" (this joins the branches together). Repeat this for every branch that needs to be extended. If you are not satisfied with the placement of a line or the shape that you have drawn, you can try centering and smoothing the line or subsequently you could delete the line and draw it again. When all the lines have been appropriately extended, the ureteric epithelial volume should contain a skeleton (Fig. 4b, c).
14. To run the statistical analysis, click on the sixth button across in the middle on the left-hand side. The statistics button looks like a "red line graph." Then, click on the "detailed" button; this will show you all the analysis that can be done. Each of these data file can then be exported individually (bottom left looks like a "floppy disk") or they can be exported as a whole (bottom left looks like "multiple floppy disks").

4. Notes

1. Before staining, make sure that all the solutions are clean. The various stains can be run through a filter to remove precipitates.

2. For hematoxylin and eosin staining, nuclei will be purple and the cytoplasm will be pink.
3. For PAS staining, the basement membrane will be red, the cytoplasm will be blue, and the nuclei will be purple.
4. For Masson's trichrome staining, collagen will stain blue, the nuclei will be black, and the muscle and cytoplasm will be red.
5. Prior to starting tracing, it is important that all new contours are created for each of the developing kidney structures. It is wise to make the colors of the contours contrast with the section. To create a new contour, go to Options > Display Preferences. Select the Contours tab, and select "Add Contour Type." This can then be changed to desired color (click on the contour and select "Set Color" button or double click on the displayed color square). Define contours for each of your regions: renal vesicle, comma-shaped body, S-shaped body, and glomeruli.
6. When aligning the various section layers, it will become increasingly difficult to visualize the previous section and align it with the current section. To circumvent this, use the "Orthogonal view"; this allows you to set the "z-filter" so that only the last section will be visualized.
7. Due to a software problem, the z-value of a particular layer may change to an inaccurate number. If this is the case, you will need to go through each layer and change the z-value to the appropriate height.
8. For skeletonizing in Imaris, a 3-button mouse must be used. To change the magnification in Imaris, hold down the "command" and "shift" buttons while pressing on the "tertiary" mouse button move forward and backwards to zoom in and out. To Pan and center the image, hold down either "command" or "shift," and clicking on the "tertiary" mouse key move from side to side. To scroll between "Navigate" and "select" pointer, press "esc" button on keyboard.

References

1. Saxen L, Sariola H (1987) Early organogenesis of the kidney. Pediatr Nephrol 1(3):385–392
2. Dressler GR (2006) The cellular basis of kidney development. Annu Rev Cell Dev Biol 22:509–529
3. Costantini F (2006) Renal branching morphogenesis: concepts, questions, and recent advances. Differentiation 74(7):402–421
4. Brenner BM, Garcia DL, Anderson S (1988) Glomeruli and blood pressure. Less of one, more the other? Am J Hypertens 1(4 Pt 1): 335–347
5. Douglas-Denton RN, McNamara BJ, Hoy WE, Hughson MD, Bertram JF (2006) Does nephron number matter in the development of kidney disease? Ethn Dis 16(2 Suppl 2):S2-40–S2-45
6. Clark A, Bertram J (2000) Advances in renal development. Curr Opin Nephrol Hypertens 9(May):247–251

7. Clark AT, Bertram JF (1999) Molecular regulation of nephron endowment. Am J Physiol 276(4 Pt 2):F485–F497
8. Davies JA (1996) Mesenchyme to epithelium transition during development of the mammalian kidney tubule. Acta Anat 156(3):187–201
9. Davies JA, Bard JB (1998) The development of the kidney. Curr Top Dev Biol 39:245–301
10. Cain JE, Nion T, Jeulin D, Bertram JF (2005) Exogenous BMP-4 amplifies asymmetric ureteric branching in the developing mouse kidney in vitro. Kidney Int 67(2):420–431
11. Cebrian C, Borodo K, Charles N, Herzlinger DA (2004) Morphometric index of the developing murine kidney. Dev Dyn 231(3): 601–608
12. Clendenon JL, Byars JM, Hyink DP (2006) Image processing software for 3D light microscopy. Nephron Exp Nephrol 103(2):e50–e54
13. Short KM, Hodson MJ, Smyth IM (2010) Tomographic quantification of branching morphogenesis and renal development. Kidney Int 77(12):1132–1139
14. Sims-Lucas S, Argyropoulos C, Kish K et al (2009) Three-dimensional imaging reveals ureteric and mesenchymal defects in Fgfr2-mutant kidneys. J Am Soc Nephrol 20(12): 2525–2533
15. Sims-Lucas S, Cusack B, Eswarakumar VP et al (2011) Independent roles of Fgfr2 and Frs2{alpha} in ureteric epithelium. Development 138(7):1275–1280

Chapter 8

Three-Dimensional Imaging of Fetal Mouse Kidneys

Deborah Hyink

Abstract

Three-dimensional imaging is a valuable tool for analyzing kidney growth and development. This technique provides information about spatial relationships between the branching ureteric bud, nephrons, and other structures within the kidney. Availability of user-friendly volume-rendering software now puts this technique within the capability of most laboratories with access to a confocal microscope. This paper describes how to prepare samples and acquire images and three-dimensional volume-rendered images.

Key words: Kidney development, Three-dimensional imaging, Volume rendering, Confocal microscopy

1. Introduction

The mammalian kidney is highly patterned with a stereotypic arrangement of nephrons, collecting ducts, and blood vessels. In the past, studies to examine the spatial relationships between renal structures involved painstaking reconstructions from serial sections (1, 2). The software, when available, was not user friendly and required programming skills to achieve good results.

Several changes now permit most laboratories to use three-dimensional imaging techniques. First, the production of bright, endogenous, fluorescently labeled mouse models enables examination of whole fetal kidneys by confocal microscopy (3, 4). Second, RAM has dramatically increased in modern computers, and most computers have video cards capable of generating three-dimensional images. Finally, user-friendly volume-rendering software is available, and is often included with the microscope acquisition suite. This software assembles the optical sections into three-dimensional images. In this paper, I describe how to prepare and acquire images suitable for volume rendering from whole or sectioned fetal kidneys.

Odyssé Michos (ed.), *Kidney Development: Methods and Protocols*, Methods in Molecular Biology, vol. 886,
DOI 10.1007/978-1-61779-851-1_8, © Springer Science+Business Media, LLC 2012

2. Materials

2.1. Whole Mount Samples

1. Whole, endogenously labeled mouse kidneys from embryonic day 11 (E11) to E18.
2. 4% paraformaldehyde (PFA) in phosphate-buffered saline (PBS), pH 7.2–7.4.
3. Rocking shaker.
4. Disposable transfer pipettes.
5. Dumont fine forceps.
6. 24-multi-well plate.

2.2. Labeling

1. Permeabilization/labeling solution (PBS+): PBS with 1% Triton X-100 and 5% bovine serum albumin (BSA).
2. Fluorescently conjugated primary antibody or lectin.

2.3. Clearing/Mounting

1. FocusClear clearing agent (CelExplorer Labs, Co. Taiwan) (see Note 1).
2. MountClear mounting agent (CelExplorer Labs, Co. Taiwan) (see Note 1).
3. CoverWell silicone spacers, 0.5–1.0 mm deep, 20 mm in diameter (Life Technologies).
4. Standard microscope slides.
5. 22-mm^2 cover glass (#1).
6. Pipetman and 200-μL pipette tips.
7. Clear nail polish.

2.4. Image Acquisition

1. Confocal microscope equipped with long working distance glycerol immersion objectives.

2.5. Volume Rendering

1. FIJI volume-rendering software. Free download from http://fiji.sc/wiki/index.php/Fiji.

3. Methods

Carry out all procedures at room temperature (RT) unless otherwise noted. When adding liquids to samples, run the liquid down the side of the well rather than applying directly on top of sample.

3.1. Whole Mount Samples

1. Place whole E11–E13 kidneys into wells of a 24-multi-well plate containing 0.5 mL 4% PFA. Place plate onto a rocker for 15 min. Rocker should be set so that the samples are always

covered by liquid and no liquid spills out of the wells. See Note 2 for labeling later stage kidneys and Note 3 for use of other fixatives.

2. Use disposable pipette to remove fixative. Rinse twice in PBS, 5 min each.
3. Permeabilize kidneys in PBS+. Add 1 mL PBS+ to each well, and then rock for 1 h at RT.
4. Remove PBS+. If no additional labeling is required, proceed to clearing and mounting.

3.2. Labeling

1. Add 0.5 mL of PBS+ containing fluorescently conjugated primary antibody or lectin to wells containing kidneys. See Note 4 for creating fluorescently conjugated antibodies and Note 5 for labeling later-staged kidneys.
2. Incubate for 4 h at RT on a rocker.
3. Remove labeling solution. Wash three times with PBS, 5 min each, at RT.

3.3. Clearing and Mounting

1. Add enough FocusClear to cover kidney in a 24-multi-well plate. Place plate on a rocker and rock until kidneys are translucent (see Note 6).
2. While kidneys are clearing, place clean, dry silicone gasket onto a microscope slide (see Note 7).
3. Gently warm MountClear to 55°C for 30 min prior to use. Swirl to mix.
4. When kidneys are clear, gently transfer into the center of the gasket on the slide. Fill the space in the gasket with warm MountClear (Fig. 1, see Notes 7 and 8).

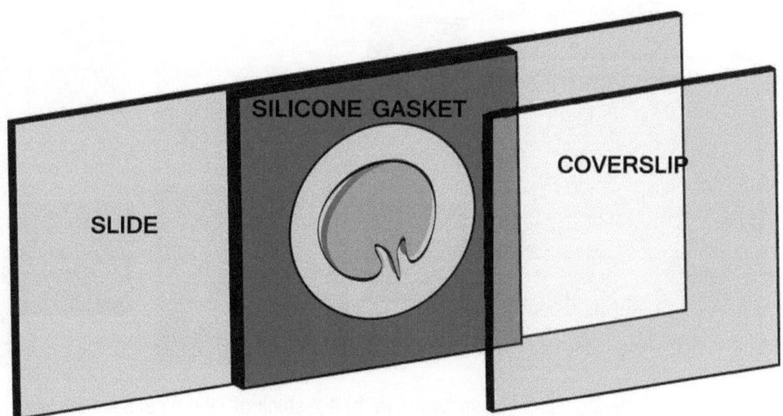

Fig. 1. Imaging chamber for 3D imaging of fetal kidneys. A clean silicone spacer is placed onto a microscopy slide. The labeled and cleared sample is placed in the middle of the imaging well, then the chamber is filled with MountClear, and coverslipped.

5. Cover with a clean coverslip. There should be no air bubbles. Press gently on the coverslip, remove excess MountClear with a Kim-Wipe, and then seal coverslip with clear nail polish. Allow nail polish to dry.

3.4. Imaging

1. Use a long working distance glycerol immersion lens to image the kidneys (see Notes 9 and 10).
2. Set the upper and lower limits for image collection using the image stack function on your confocal microscope. There should be several optical sections above and below the desired image to permit reconstruction.
3. Use the section thickness recommended by the microscopy software. As a rule, the section depth should be no more than two times the *xy* pixel size.
4. If imaging in multiple channels, acquire each channel sequentially to prevent bleed through (see Note 11).
5. Save the image stacks.

3.5. Reconstruction

1. Open the image stacks with FIJI (File, Open). See Note 12 for other options.
2. Once the stack is open, click on the 3D viewer plugin (Plugins, 3D viewer) (Fig. 2a, b).
3. To adjust transparency, click the Edit tab in the 3D viewer plugin. Select attributes, and then transfer function. In the open window, select the alpha channel and adjust the transparency (Fig. 2c–f). You can also adjust the intensity of red, green, and blue channels as needed (Fig. 2g–i).

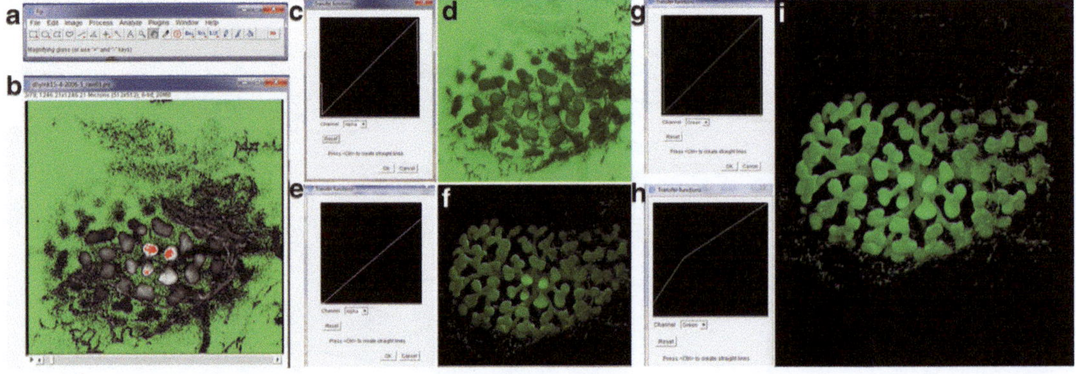

Fig. 2. Volume rendering using FIJI software. (**a**, **b**) A z-stack of 79 optical sections was opened in FIJI. This stack was collected from an endogenously labeled E14 HoxB7-GFP kidney. Initially, the image stack was difficult to view (**d**), so the opacity was adjusted by adjusting the alpha channel (**c** screenshot of control panel before and after, **e**). Panel (**f**) shows the adjusted, volume-rendered image. The intensity of the green channel was adjusted to generate a brighter, more saturated image (**g**–**i**).

4. To add a second channel, click File in the 3D viewer plugin, add Content, and then select from file or from open image. You can adjust the transparency and color before or after import.
5. To capture an image, select View, and then Take Snapshot in the 3D viewer window.

4. Notes

1. FocusClear and MountClear (refractive index (RI) = 1.43) yield better clearing for whole mount fetal kidney imaging than other commonly used clearing/mounting agents, such as 75% glycerol (RI = 1.44 or Vectashield, RI = 1.457).
2. To label whole E14–E18 kidneys, increase fixation time to 30 min and permeabilization time to 2–4 h. The endogenous label must be bright to image structures in the center of the kidney.
3. FocusClear and MountClear are more effective in PFA-fixed kidneys than in kidneys fixed in methanol.
4. AlexaFluor conjugates from Life Technologies work well in 3D imaging. If the desired antibody is not available preconjugated, Zenon Labeling kits (Life Technologies) provide a rapid method to generate conjugates. AlexaFluor 568 (red) and 647 (far-red) work well with EGFP, YFP, and CFP endogenous labels.
5. Antibodies and lectins may not penetrate to the center of later-staged kidneys. If labeling is only seen in the outer cortex, better results may be obtained by labeling 40–60-μm-thick frozen sections. Sections can be floated onto PBS in individual wells of a 24-well cluster and labeled as described in Subheading 3.2. Figure 3 shows an example of volume rendering from a double-labeled thick section.
6. Very small or delicate specimens can be cleared directly on the slide. Set up the imaging chamber, add a 50-μL drop of FocusClear to the center on the chamber, and then add sample. Remove most of the FocusClear prior to using a P20 pipette that has a small pipette tip. Add MountClear and continue.
7. The coverwell imaging chambers are available in several thicknesses. Select a chamber, which will accommodate your specimen without compression. If necessary, silicone spacers may be stacked. Before use, peel off the plastic coverslip and wash with dishwashing liquid to remove the adhesive. Rinse and dry thoroughly before use. Silicone spacers may be reused many times.
8. MountClear becomes firm as it sets. To speed setting, place slide on a flat ice pack for 2–3 min.

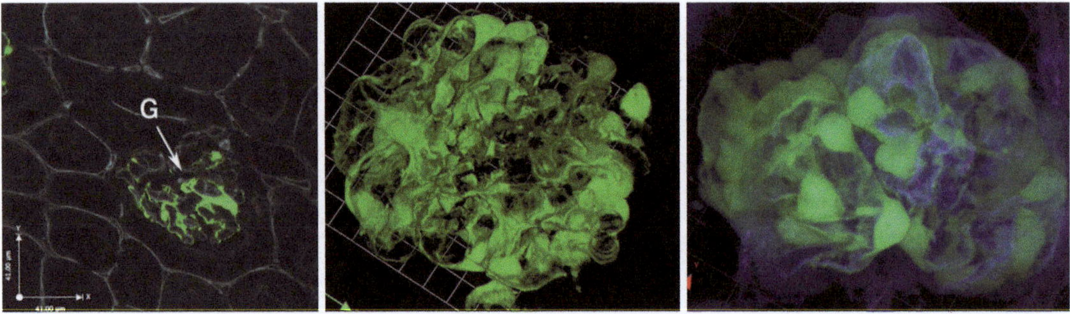

Fig. 3. Volume rendering of whole glomeruli from adult kidneys. 60-μm-thick frozen sections of EGFP-endogenously labeled kidneys were permeabilized and labeled with anti-laminin-Alexa 647. The *panel on the left* shows a single optical section with brightly labeled podocytes in the glomerulus (G). Peritubular capillaries were outlined by anti-laminin. The *middle panel* shows a single glomerulus volume rendered with Volocity software. The *rightmost panel* shows the podocytes covering the capillary loops labeled with anti-laminin. The endogenously labeled podocytes were generated by crossing podocin-cre mice (5) with Z E/G reporter mice (6).

9. Light bends when it crosses boundaries between materials with different refractive indices. RI mismatch causes several problems, which will interfere with high-quality, accurate 3D volume rendering. These problems include spherical aberration, which distorts the 3D image, and alterations of the angle of light, which returns to the objective, thereby decreasing the numerical aperture (NA), which decreases resolution. To acquire the optimal images for reconstruction, the objective, immersion liquid, and mounting media should have the same RI. See the Tutorial at Nikon's MicroscopyU for an in-depth description of RI and NA: http://www.microscopyu.com/tutorials/java/objectives/immersion/index.html.

10. Microscope objectives are manufactured with a wide range of options. Long working distance objectives usually have L, LL, LD, or LWD on the side of the objective. Modern objectives usually state the working distance on the barrel. In most cases, whole mount kidneys can be imaged using a 20× glycerol/multi-immersion lens with a working distance of 350 μm.

11. Bleed through of fluorescent signals can introduce artifacts in 3D imaging. Controls labeled with a single fluorophore should be examined to determine if the signal can be detected in other channels. If so, the emission filters may be adjusted to capture the peak emission for each fluorophore, or a different combination of fluorophores may be selected.

12. 3D volume rendering software options:

    For purchase:

    Volocity: http://www.perkinelmer.com/pages/020/cellular-imaging/products/volocityvisualization.xhtml

    Axiovision: http://www.zeiss.com/micro

Amira: http://www.amira.com/

Imaris: http://www.bitplane.com/

Free:

Voxx: http://www.nephrology.iupui.edu/imaging/voxx/index.html

ImageSurfer: http://imagesurfer.cs.unc.edu/ (leica, zeiss, iplab)

Fiji: http://fiji.sc/wiki/index.php/Fiji

ImageJ distribution with Java3D and analysis plugins

References

1. Hyink DP, Tucker DC, St John PL et al (1996) Endogenous origin of glomerular endothelial and mesangial cells in grafts of embryonic kidneys. Am J Physiol 270(5 Pt 2):F886–F899
2. Zhai XY, Birn H, Jensen KB et al (2003) Digital three-dimensional reconstruction and ultrastructure of the mouse proximal tubule. J Am Soc Nephrol 14(3):611–619
3. Sims-Lucas S, Argyropoulos C, Kish K et al (2009) Three-dimensional imaging reveals ureteric and mesenchymal defects in Fgfr2-mutant kidneys. J Am Soc Nephrol 20(12): 2525–2533
4. Srinivas S, Goldberg MR, Watanabe T et al (1999) Expression of green fluorescent protein in the ureteric bud of transgenic mice: a new tool for the analysis of ureteric bud morphogenesis. Dev Genet 24(3–4):241–251
5. Moeller MJ, Sanden SK, Soofi A, Wiggins RC, Holzman LB (2003) Podocyte-specific expression of cre recombinase in transgenic mice. Genesis 35(1):39–42
6. Novak A, Guo C, Yang W, Nagy A, Lobe CG (2000) Z/EG, a double reporter mouse line that expresses enhanced green fluorescent protein upon Cre-mediated excision. Genesis 28(3–4):147–155

Chapter 9

Analysis of Native Kidney Structures in Three Dimensions

Kieran M. Short and Ian M. Smyth

Abstract

Optical Projection Tomography (OPT) is an imaging technique, which has proven to be ideally suited to the observation and quantification of kidney development in rodents. Unlike confocal microscopy systems, OPT is capable of imaging the organ in toto across a long window of embryonic development at sufficient resolution to capture relative changes in branching dynamics, pelvis development, and nephrogenesis. Here, we describe how to image kidneys by OPT, and initial steps to quantify kidney development from this data.

Key words: OPT, Branching, Kidney, Morphogenesis

1. Introduction

Kidney development is a highly complex process. At a molecular level, significant progress is being made to determine the molecular signaling events required for metanephros formation and development (1, 2). Analysis of the molecular coordination of cellular growth, movement, and differentiation in older embryonic kidneys is complicated by the organ's rapidly increasing size and thickness (3). While optimized confocal microscopy (4) and 2-photon confocal microscopy (5) methods can image outer layers of thick samples to ~100–200 μm, these technologies struggle to capture the entire fluorescence signal from stained older embryonic kidneys, which can grow up to 800 μm thick by late gestation. Embryonic kidneys at age E14 onwards quickly grow and thicken in size (3), and it is these thicker organs which undergo complex, rapid changes in cortical development.

Optical Projection Tomography (OPT) is a new way to image these events in full thickness tissue. This tomographic method (as opposed to medical X-ray CT tomography) relies on the passage of light waves through a sample, with changes in density or

Odyssé Michos (ed.), *Kidney Development: Methods and Protocols*, Methods in Molecular Biology, vol. 886, DOI 10.1007/978-1-61779-851-1_9, © Springer Science+Business Media, LLC 2012

absorption being captured as an interference pattern (6). By imaging the object through multiple angles, tomographic reconstruction mathematics can be used to generate a volumetric dataset describing these internal components. In order for OPT to work, agents are used to clear biological tissue which allows the passage of light through otherwise opaque matter. While clearing reduces visible-light opacity, the tissue structure remains intact and when illuminated the tissue and any markers (fluorescent or colorific) will become illuminated. Antibodies and probes are often used to mark the localization and distribution of proteins and genes within the developing fetus and, if carefully selected, can be specific to particular tissues within an organ. In the process of OPT, when a tissue is stained with markers that respond to particular fluorescent excitation wavelengths, it can be imaged and a 3D dataset of the position and localization of these proteins/genes within the tissue can be identified.

Like all tomographic technologies, software tools are required to make best use of the data acquired. While OPT's ability to rapidly provide qualitative visual feedback is an immediate attraction of the technology, its power lies in the ability to quantify the acquired data. One advance in the study of embryonic kidney development and patterning is the application of OPT and software tools used to image and quantify renal organogenesis. We were able to stain and quantify multiple stages of embryonic kidney development, and using software, we have quantified various measures of kidney development at these stages (3). Methods used to perform this analysis are described within this chapter.

This protocol describes the staining, OPT imaging, and analysis of embryonic mouse kidneys from embryonic day E11.5 to E15.5. We describe in detail the techniques, instrumentation, and software used to quantify and analyze kidney morphometrics, with particular focus on the ureteric tree and developing renal pelvis.

2. Materials

OPT imaging is particularly sensitive to dust contamination, so it is highly recommended to work in a clean environment and use 0.45 μm filtered solutions where possible.

2.1. Dissection and Washing

1. Phosphate-buffered saline (PBS): 0.137 M NaCl, 1.7 mM KCl, 1.4 mM KH_2PO_4, 10 mM Na_2HPO_4, filtered.
2. 4% Formaldehyde fixative: 4% (w/v) in PBS. Make up fresh or store frozen aliquots at −20°C, filtered.
3. Tris-buffered saline (TBS): 50 mM Tris–HCl, pH 7.5, 150 mM NaCl, filtered.
4. TBS-Tx: TBS supplemented with 0.1% Triton X-100.

2.2. Kidney Preparation and Staining

1. Blocking solution: TBS–0.1% Triton X-100, 1% bovine serum albumin, 10% donkey or goat serum (dependent on the species of secondary antibody to be used), 0.02% sodium azide.
2. Primary antibody of choice diluted in blocking solution.
3. Proteinase K for mild digestion of late-stage kidney capsule. A fresh 25 μg/mL Proteinase K solution is made up in TBS-Tx. If using Proteinase K, 100 mM of phenylmethyl sulfonyl fluoride (PMSF) is recommended to neutralize Proteinase K at the end of digestion.
4. Fine Forceps, 200 μL pipette with 200 μL filter tips, 2 mL round-bottom tubes, 10 mL Falcon tubes, 50 mL Falcon tubes.

2.3. Embedding

1. 1% Low melting point agarose made up in ddH_2O.
2. 50 mL syringe with 0.45 μm filter.
3. Pasteur pipettes.
4. 6-multi-well plate, 30 mm tissue culture tray.
5. Scalpel blade.
6. Glass plate (e.g., from Mini protein apparatus).
7. Low lint tissue.
8. Super glue/cyanoacrylate adhesive.
9. OPT sample mounts and forceps and stub tweezers to handle the mounts.
10. Glass vials (recommended Sigma 27181, 40 mL, 29 mm wide × 82 mm high, clear glass) to hold mounted samples in solution.
11. Methanol for dehydration. Concentrations used are 100%, and dilutions of methanol blended with distilled water (v/v) at 95, 75, and 50%.
12. Nitrile gloves for working with Benzyl Alcohol/Benzyl Benzoate (BABB) (as BABB is latex permeable).
13. BABB (a mixture of 1 part Benzyl Alcohol to 2 parts Benzyl Benzoate).

3. Methods

Carry out all procedures at room temperature unless otherwise specified.

3.1. Dissection and Fixation

1. Dissect kidneys from mouse embryos between stage E11.5 and E15.5, with E0.5 being counted as the day that the vaginal plug is identified. Alternatively, whole urogenital tracts can be

dissected and fixed as a complete "unit." There are advantages to individually dissecting kidneys (see Note 1).

2. If dissecting kidneys individually, remove as much surrounding tissue as possible. This permits precise whole kidney organ imaging by auto-fluorescence.
3. Fix in round-bottom Eppendorf tubes at 4°C. Regularly (approximately every 2–3 min) "flick" the tubes in order to keep the kidneys well washed in fixative. If kidneys stick to the side of the tube, release them with a flush of PFA/PBS from a P200 pipette. This is important to minimize uneven fixation.
4. Fixation times (see Note 2 for further information):
   (a) Fix E11.5 kidneys for 5 min in 4% PFA/PBS.
   (b) Fix E12.5 kidneys for 7 min in 4% PFA/PBS.
   (c) Fix E13.5 kidneys for 10 min in 4% PFA/PBS.
   (d) Fix E14.5 kidneys for 12 min in 4% PFA/PBS.
   (e) Fix E15.5 kidneys for 15 min in 4% PFA/PBS.
5. Wash the kidneys three times in ice-cold PBS for 2 min each to remove as much fixative as possible.
6. Wash the kidneys in TBS for 20 min.
7. Wash the kidneys in TBS-Tx for 20 min.
8. Optional for late-stage kidneys:
   (a) In E15.5 and older kidneys, if evidence of capsule can be seen, enzymatic removal may help penetration of antibodies into the whole mount tissue because a PFA-fixed capsule can act as a strong barrier to diffusion and penetration of antibodies (see Subheading 3.2). Great care must be taken not to over-digest the tissue, as it will destroy the tips of the ureteric tree.
   (b) A fresh 25 μg/mL Proteinase K solution in 1× TBS-Tx should be made, and kidneys incubated for 15 min, rocking at room temperature.
   (c) Immediately move samples to ice, inactivate Proteinase K by adding 5 mM (final) PMSF, and rock for 10 min at 4°C to ensure complete inactivation of Proteinase K.
   (d) Finish by washing out inactivated Proteinase K and PMSF with three washes with TBS-Tx for 5 min each.

3.2. Blocking and Antibody Staining

1. Block the samples overnight (see Note 3) at 4°C in TBS-Tx supplemented with 1% BSA and 10% serum. Serum selected should match the species of the secondary antibody to be used.
2. Incubate samples overnight at 4°C in primary antibody (see Note 4 and 5) diluted in blocking solution.

3. Wash out unbound primary antibody with four 15 min washes in 50 mL TBS-Tx, rocking at room temperature, followed by an overnight wash at 4°C, rocking.
4. Incubate samples overnight at 4°C in secondary antibody (see Note 6) diluted in TBS-Tx supplemented with 1% BSA to limit nonspecific binding due to hydrophobic adherence.
5. Wash out unbound secondary antibody with four 15-min washes in 50 mL TBS-Tx, rocking at room temperature, followed by an overnight wash at 4°C, rocking.
6. Wash samples twice in 20 mL TBS to remove the remaining Triton X-100 detergent, 15 min room temperature, rocking.
7. Optional:
   (a) When using Alexa Fluor and Dylight-conjugated secondary antibodies, the stability of the fluorescence is such that samples do not need to be embedded and scanned immediately. If desired, stained kidneys can be post-fixed with 4% PFA/PBS (to fix antibody position), and then stored in PBS supplemented with 0.02% sodium azide (to inhibit microbial growth). This allows the kidneys to remain in storage at 4°C for up to 6 weeks, and also permits transportation at room temperature for up to 4 days.
8. It is advisable to check the surface of the specimens for any lint fibers, plastic burrs from tubes and plates, and other foreign bodies that might have become "stuck." These may fluoresce and cause issues upon reconstruction of the data after OPT scanning. If a problem, physically "clean" the kidneys after washing.
   (a) Use a filtered P200 pipette tip, which has been cut off with scissors to make the tip opening large enough to fit your specimen. Carefully flame the cut tip very lightly to "round" the edges to avoid cutting or shearing of the specimen, and use this to move the kidney between the tube and a dish.
   (b) Under a dissection microscope, use fine forceps to carefully remove any objects that are stuck to the surface of the specimen.
   (c) Make an "eyelash brush" by plucking a single human eyelash and gluing it onto the tip of a rod or pipette tip. Use this to gently "brush" lint and fibers off the kidney. The advantage of this method is that the eyelash will not pierce the specimen like metal forceps can.

3.3. Embedding and OPT Mounting

1. Make up a molten 1% low melting point agarose solution in distilled water. Filter using a 0.45 μm cartridge filter and a 50 mL syringe into a 6-multi-well tissue culture plate. Fill each well to the top of the well (requiring approximately 18 mL per well).

   (a) This can be kept molten in a 37°C incubator until ready to embed, if desired.

2. Make up two glass specimen-positioning hooks.

   (a) Take a glass Pasteur pipette, and flame the end until it becomes bulbous with a 1–2 mm thick end. Let the solid bulb drop to one side to make a "golf club"-like tip.

3. Measure the temperature of the agarose with a clean stick thermometer. When the temperature of the molten agarose has reduced to 29–30°C, pipette the kidneys into the wells using a P200 pipette (see Subheading 3.2, step 8), minimizing carry-over of solution into the agarose.

4. Swirl the specimen around in the agarose to equilibrate the kidney with the mounting medium. As the temperature continues to cool, it will start to gel. At 27°C, this process accelerates. During this time, the samples will start to remain suspended in the agarose.

   (a) Orient the sample in the gelling agarose using the glass positioning hooks into a position that is equidistant from the base of the well and the surface of the agarose (Fig. 1a, b).

   (b) Position the sample to one side of the well so that there is a minimum of 20 mm space between the sample and the opposite side of the well (Fig. 1b).

5. Once the sample is fully supported by the gel matrix, leave it to set further for 5 min, and then place at 4°C to completely set the agarose. This process takes approximately 15 min for 1% low-melting-point agarose chilling down from 26°C.

6. Extract the agarose plug from the casting plate (Fig. 1c). Take a scalpel blade, and on the opposing side of the well, slide the blade between the well and the agarose gel until it goes to the bottom of the well. With a gentle continuous motion, while keeping the handle end of the blade pressed against the sidewall of the well, angle the blade in towards the agarose and tilt up, and push out the agarose "plug" from the well onto a glass plate.

   (a) You will dig some of the agarose up, but minimal damage is done, and any damage is well away from the specimen.

7. You should now have a flat cylindrical plug of set agarose with a kidney sample in it. Trim the agarose so that a rectangular block is made with base of approximately 12 mm square, with the embedded kidney 3–4 mm from one end and 15 mm to the other (Fig. 1d).

8. With a clean OPT mount ready, apply a small amount of cyanoacrylate adhesive (Super glue) to the top of the mount (Fig. 1e).

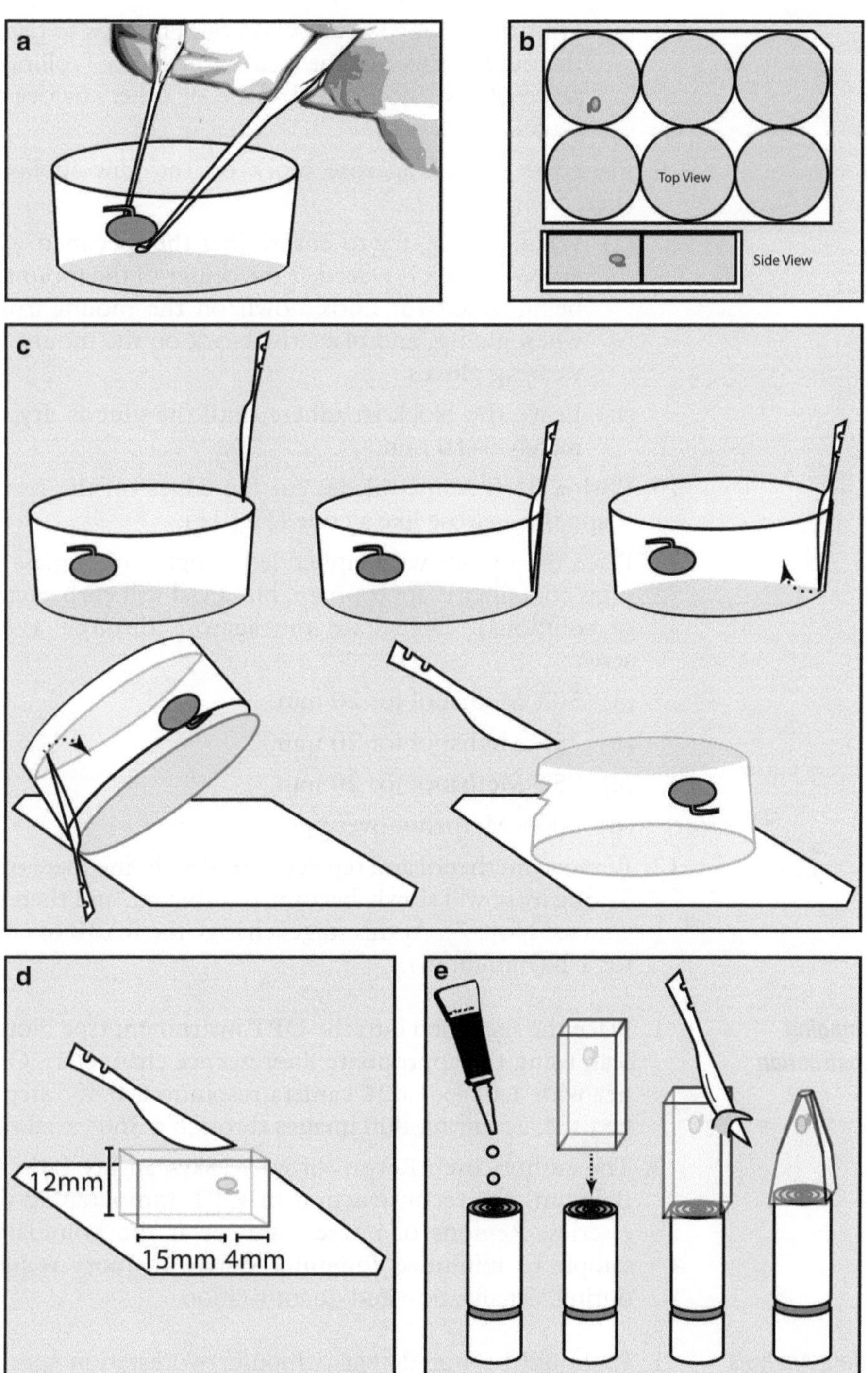

Fig. 1. Embedding and mounting a specimen for OPT imaging. The sample is first placed in a dish of molten agarose, and oriented and positioned with glass hooks (**a**). The sample is held in a position equidistant from the base and surface of the agarose to one side of the dish (**b**). Once set, the agarose plug is extracted from the dish (**c**). The agarose around the sample is trimmed with a scalpel blade to form a rectangular shape, the kidney centered at one end (**d**). Finally, the agarose is glued to a metal mount, and trimmed to a near-conical shape (**e**).

   (a) Hint: In order to get a solid bond, it helps to partially dry the outer surface of the agarose first. Try "rolling" it on a piece of low/no-lint kim-wipe or other, before the next stage.

9. Place the shaped agarose block on the glue-applied mount (Fig. 1e).
   (a) When gluing, try to ensure that the specimen within the agarose block is placed at the center of the mount that it is being glued to. Look down on the mount from above when gluing, and place the block on the mount by hand, wearing gloves.
   (b) Leave the block to adhere until the glue is dry, approximately 5–10 min.
10. With a fresh scalpel blade, cut the edges off the rectangle to shape the agarose like a cone (Fig. 1e).
11. Place the mount with embedded sample into a glass vial (any glass container is appropriate, but a vial will curb excessive use of solutions). Dehydrate the agarose through a methanol series:
    (a) 50% Methanol for 20 min.
    (b) 75% Methanol for 20 min.
    (c) 95% Methanol for 20 min.
    (d) 100% Methanol overnight.
12. Remove methanol and replace with BABB, incubate overnight. The agarose will slowly become translucent, and then transparent (see Note 7). At this stage, change the BABB one final time for 1 h (minimum).

3.4. OPT Imaging and Reconstruction

1. Place the specimen into the OPT instrument (see Note 8), and scan using the appropriate fluorescence channel(s). On a scanner with 1,024 × 1,024 camera resolution, 0.45° steps should be used, acquiring 800 images through a 360° axial rotation.
2. The authors use nRecon software (Skyscan Pty Ltd., Kontich, Belgium) for reconstruction of OPT tomographic data to a *z*-series. Regions of interest are set at the boundary of the sample to minimize computer system memory requirements during visualization and quantification.

3.5. OPT Data Analysis

1. It should be noted that computer workstation specifications need to be sufficient to handle the load of OPT datasets. A system with 4 Gb of RAM is recommended, with a discrete graphics accelerator with a minimum of 1 Gb of onboard RAM. A 64-bit operating system is recommended because it is helpful with handling large datasets with sizeable memory requirements.

2. Qualitative analysis: Due to the inherent nature of the tomographic reconstruction, the OPT dataset has identical distances in *x*, *y*, and *z* planes (i.e., the thickness of any *z* slice is the same as that of a single unit in the *x* or *y* planes). Volumes can be visualized qualitatively with volumetric rendering software. The capability of the software is the only limit to the quality and manipulation of the volume. Some software permits rendering of both external and internal structures.
3. Quantitative analysis: OPT instrumentation is capable of registering a real-world distance to "voxel" (a voxel is a pixel in 3D space) distance ratio. With this figure, it is possible to perform quantitative analysis on data.
   (a) On Bioptonics OPT instruments, measurements have been calibrated for the instrument such that each voxel is of a known dimension, and this is calculated for every zoom position on the instrument. Using this, regions within the dataset can be quantitatively measured for distance, volume, and angle.
4. Software packages which have been successfully used for the visualization and quantification of OPT data include the following.
   (a) Drishti (Windows 32/64 bit, Linux, Mac OSX) offers basic tools to make distance and angle measurements, but its main strength is its ability to visualize volumes in spectacular detail and clarity (Fig. 2). Drishti also has key framing capability for the creation of complex animations, and can output images at any resolution. Please visit: http://anusf.anu.edu.au/Vizlab/drishti/ for more information. This free software is undergoing continual development and new features are constantly added.
   (b) Fiji (Windows 32/64 bit, Linux 32/64 bit, Mac OSX): Fiji is a version of ImageJ, which comes provided with many useful 3D plug-ins. Its strength lies in the stack manipulation tools that come prepackaged which can be useful for segmentation (using the Level Sets plugin), re-slicing, and measurement of 3D data (Fig. 3). Z-data is loaded in as an "Image Sequence," and this is used for the basis of further processing and analysis. This software is also free and undergoing continuous development. Please visit http://pacific.mpi-cbg.de/wiki/index.php/Fiji for more information.
   (c) Osirix (Mac OSX) is capable of rendering and measuring OPT datasets in 3D also, and has some very good segmentation tools (including a 3D "magic wand"). Please visit http://www.osirix-viewer.com/ for more information. The 32bit version is free, and the 64bit version requires a paid license.

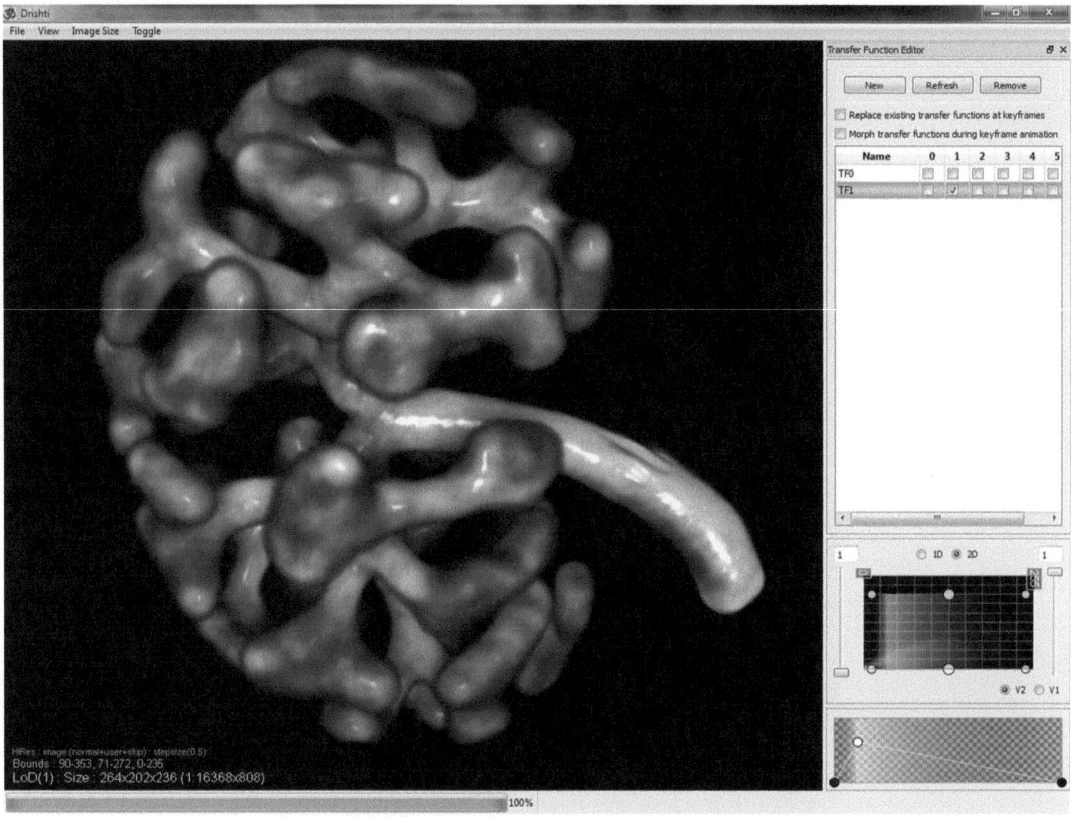

Fig. 2. Drishti. Here showing a representation of an ~E12.5 kidney; Drishti excels at rendering OPT kidney data. This figure also shows some of the Drishti working environment.

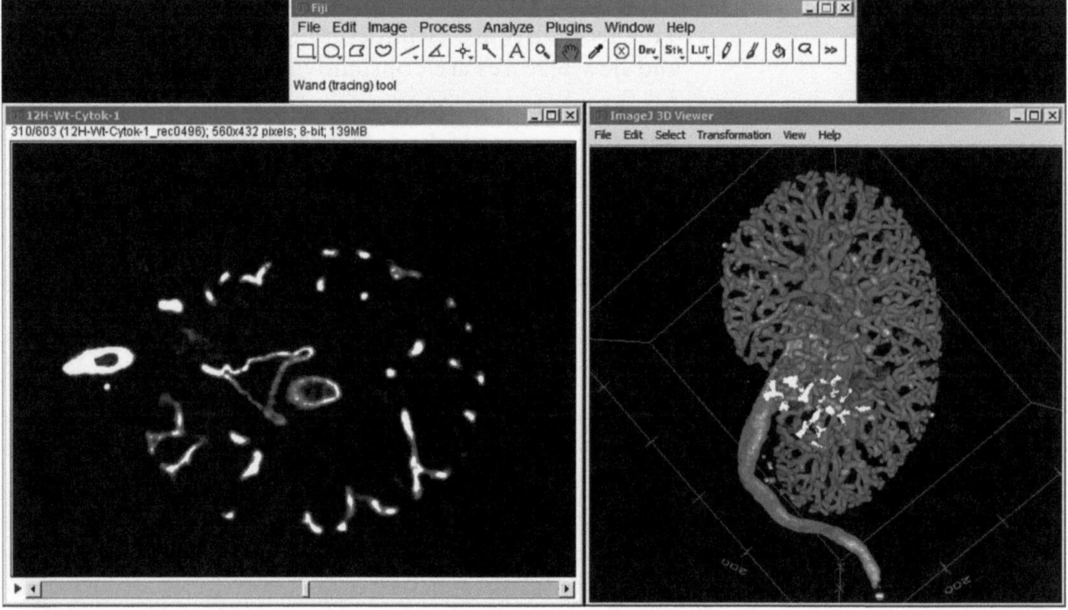

Fig. 3. Fiji is an implementation of ImageJ with many useful stack manipulation tools. Fiji also has simple volume viewers, and has the capability of re-slicing and segmenting datasets.

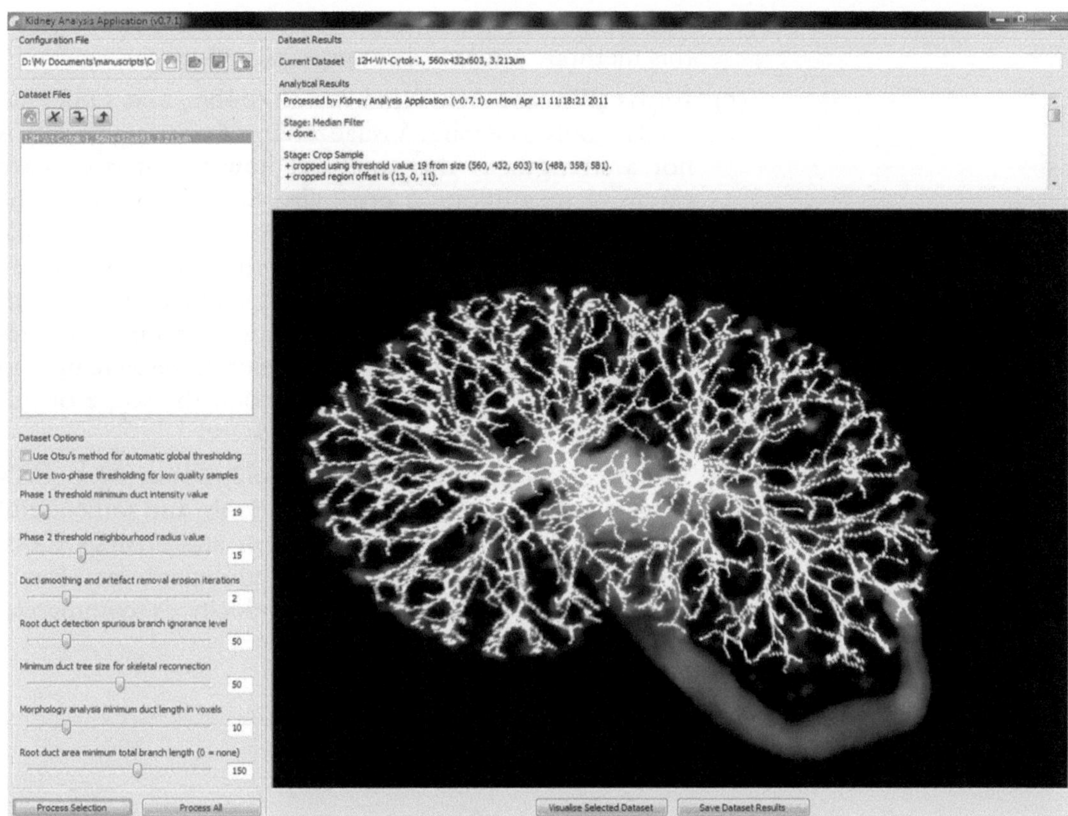

Fig. 4. Kidney analysis application (KAP). KAP was written to skeletonize and quantify scanned ureteric trees from OPT data; here showing the working area with an E15.5 kidney skeletonized.

(d) Kidney Analysis Application (KAP) (Windows 32bit): Kidney branching quantitation software has been developed for use with OPT data (3). It is designed to directly work on data from Bioptonics 3001 OPT scanners, but also able to work on other data such as confocal stacks. The software directly loads z-stack bitmap file format data from Skyscan nRecon, and skeletonizes and analyzes OPT scans of stained ureteric trees. KAP automatically identifies the ureteric tree and excludes the ureter from subsequent analysis (Fig. 4). It reports the number of tips, branches, total tree length, and tip to last branch endpoint distance. This software is free and available upon request.

(e) Amira (Visage Imaging, Windows 32/64bit, Mac OSX, Linux 64bit) has visualization and extensive volume quantification capabilities. The skeletonization tools are optimized for neuronal and vascular datasets, which are able to skeletonize young kidneys from E12.5 to E13.5; testing with Amira v5.3 indicates that the algorithms perform poorly on older kidneys. Amira has many other quantification capabilities, which are beyond the scope of this method. Amira is a commercial software.

(f) Imaris (Bitplane AG, Windows 32/64bit, Mac OSX) has similar tools to Amira. Visualization of volumetric data is not a strength of this software; however, it does have extensive quantification capability. Similar to Amira, the focus of the "Filament Editor" is for dendritic/neuronal datasets, and these typically perform poorly on kidney OPT data (tested with Imaris 7.2.1). The entire breadth of other quantification features these software packages offer is vast, and their implementation in visualizing and quantification of kidney data is beyond the scope of this method. Imaris is a commercial software.

(g) Volocity (Perkin Elmer, Windows32/64bit, Mac OSX 32bit) has some useful visualization tools, and some useful shape-based automatic segmentation and analysis tools. This can be useful for looking at "globular" data, but it has no skeletonization system. Volocity is commercial software.

4. Notes

1. Dissection of kidneys independently permits a much faster whole mount staining protocol and avoids potential issues later in the process with segmenting individual kidneys for analysis from whole urogenital systems during tomographic reconstruction. Whole urogenital ridge staining will not be described here, but incubation times would be approximately 50% longer than those used for E15.5 embryonic kidneys.
2. Fixation times are approximate, but over-fixation can cause issues with antibody penetration. Incomplete fixation can result in tissue degradation because the whole mount staining protocol is performed over several days.
3. The timings in these protocols reflect a "fail safe" for all sizes of tissue up to and including the largest kidneys described at E15.5. In reality, the necessary times for incubation of tissues in solutions to reach saturation point is proportional to the tissue size. Therefore, it takes less time for antibodies, sera, washes, etc. to pass through and saturate smaller tissues than it does for larger tissues. So if your tissue sizes are significantly smaller than E15.5 kidneys (e.g., E12.5), you can speed up the protocol by reducing incubation and washing times for antibody binding and washing stages by 30–50%. If overnight incubations are reduced to 6–8 h incubations, perform them at room temperature rather than 4°C.

4. Antibody concentrations must be determined empirically as antibody–epitope interactions vary greatly. In order to aid rapid penetration of antibody, a higher than normal concentration of antibody is used in the primary antibody incubation compared with other methods such as section staining.
5. Antibody choice: Pan Cytokeratin—ureteric tree specific, E-cadherin—ureteric tree plus descending loops, Six2—cap mesenchyme, Cadherin 6—cap mesenchyme.
6. Alexa Fluor® (Invitrogen)- or Dylight® (Thermo Fisher Scientific)-conjugated antibodies are highly recommended. Their resistance to photobleaching is ideal for withstanding the rigors of OPT scanning, where small specimens can be exposed to intense fluorescent light for extended periods of time (up to a 30-min continuous exposure). They also permit the subsequent use of the specimens for histological examination, keeping their fluorescence through paraffin embedding stages.
7. The time taken to clear varies depending on the size of the specimen and the size of the agarose block after mounting and cutting. It is also advised to leave the lid off the scintillation vial ajar to permit the less dense, volatile methanol to evaporate from the surface of the BABB (which is nonvolatile).
8. A Bioptonics 3001 instrument has been used by the authors for visualization and reconstruction. As new technologies and instruments are released and developed constantly, please refer to your manufacturer's instructions for this stage of the protocol as the fine details of imaging modalities can vary accordingly.

References

1. Costantini F, Kopan R (2010) Patterning a complex organ: branching morphogenesis and nephron segmentation in kidney development. Dev Cell 18:698–712
2. Hendry C, Rumballe B, Moritz K et al (2011) Defining and redefining the nephron progenitor population. Pediatr Nephrol. doi:10.1007/s00467-010-1750-4
3. Short KM, Hodson MJ, Smyth IM (2010) Tomographic quantification of branching morphogenesis and renal development. Kidney Int 77:1132–1139
4. Reihani SN, Oddershede LB (2009) Confocal microscopy of thick specimens. J Biomed Opt 14:030513
5. Leray A, Lillis K, Mertz J (2008) Enhanced background rejection in thick tissue with differential-aberration two-photon microscopy. Biophys J 94:1449–1458
6. Sharpe J, Ahlgren U, Perry P et al (2002) Optical projection tomography as a tool for 3D microscopy and gene expression studies. Science 296:541–545

Chapter 10

Estimating Nephron Number in the Developing Kidney Using the Physical Disector/Fractionator Combination

Luise A. Cullen-McEwen, James A. Armitage, Jens R. Nyengaard, and John F. Bertram

Abstract

Design-based stereology is considered the gold-standard method for estimating the total number of glomeruli, and thereby nephrons, in the adult kidney. However, until recently, a design-based method for estimating nephron number in the developing kidney was not available. For such a method to provide accurate and precise estimates, unambiguous identification of developing nephrons is essential. Here, we describe a combined histochemical/stereological technique for estimating total nephron number in the developing mouse and rat kidney. The method can be modified for use in other species.

Key words: Nephron endowment, Nephron number, Kidney development, Stereology, Disector, Metanephros

1. Introduction

Nephrogenesis ends at approximately 36 weeks' gestation in humans and in early postnatal life in rats and mice (1). After this time, no new nephrons can form. Nephron endowment, the number of nephrons present at the conclusion of nephrogenesis, is known to be influenced either directly or indirectly by specific genes (1–3) and a variety of feto-maternal environmental factors (1).

While many studies have reported total nephron number in kidneys following the completion of nephrogenesis and particularly in adult kidneys (1, 4, 5), a design-based method for estimating nephron number in the developing kidney has not been available until recently (6). Such a method is needed to (1) assess the timing and extent of slowed or accelerated nephrogenesis during kidney development following genetic or environmental perturbations and (2) assess the relative impact of prenatal and

Odyssé Michos (ed.), *Kidney Development: Methods and Protocols*, Methods in Molecular Biology, vol. 886,
DOI 10.1007/978-1-61779-851-1_10, © Springer Science+Business Media, LLC 2012

postnatal environments on nephrogenesis in species in which nephrogenesis continues after birth.

The physical disector/fractionator stereological method is considered the gold-standard method for estimating glomerular, and thereby nephron, number in the adult kidney. This is a relatively simple method to use in the adult kidney because glomeruli can be easily and unambiguously identified. However, random sections through the developing metanephros produce an array of microanatomical features with complex shapes and varying sizes, making feature identification somewhat difficult. For this reason, the standard physical disector/fractionator method is not suited to counting developing nephrons. To overcome the difficulty of nephron identification, we have developed a method that utilises histochemical staining with peanut (*Arachis hypogaea*) agglutinin (PNA), a lectin that identifies podocytes in early S-shaped bodies through to mature glomeruli. Once these structures are unambiguously identified, the physical disector/fractionator method is used to accurately and precisely estimate total glomerular number (N_{glom}), and thereby total nephron number. With the physical disector/fractionator method, the physical disector is used to sample PNA-positive structures—these are sampled with equal probability, regardless of their size or shape, a very important consideration for growing nephrons with complex shapes. These PNA-positive structures are then counted in a known fraction of the kidney using a fractionator experimental design. The method for estimating total nephron number in developing mouse and rat kidneys is described in full below.

2. Materials

1. Fine-tipped forceps.
2. Fixative: We use 10% neutral buffered formalin (100 mL formalin, 900 mL tap water, 4 g of sodium dihydrogen phosphate, monohydrate ($NaH_2PO_4 \cdot H_2O$), and 6 g disodium hydrogen phosphate, anhydrous (Na_2HPO_4)).
3. Hand processing components:
   (a) 70% Ethanol.
   (b) 50% Butanol/50% ethanol mix.
   (c) 75% Butanol/25% ethanol mix.
   (d) 100% Butanol.
4. Microtome fitted with steel blades.
5. Digital micrometer with precision of 1 μm, e.g. Mitutoyo.

6. Dewaxing components:
   (a) Xylene.
   (b) 100% Ethanol.
7. Peanut (*A. hypogaea*) agglutinin staining components:
   (a) Phosphate-buffered saline (PBS).
   (b) H_2O_2.
   (c) Methanol.
   (d) Neuraminidase from vibrio cholerea (Sigma-Aldrich) made at 0.1 u/mL with 1% $CaCl_2$ in PBS.
   (e) 2% Bovine serum albumin, 0.3% Triton X-100 in PBS.
   (f) Biotinylated PNA (Sigma-Aldrich) made up at 20 μg/mL diluted in 0.3% Triton X-100 in PBS, with 1 mM $CaCl_2$/$MnCl_2$/$MgCl_2$.
   (g) Elite streptavidin/biotin amplification ABC kit (Vector Laboratories).
   (h) Diaminobenzidine (DAB) (Sigma-Aldrich) made up at 0.5 mg/mL in distilled water.
8. Haematoxylin counterstaining:
   (a) Haematoxylin.
   (b) Tap water.
   (c) Scott's tap water (0.1% ammonia in tap water).
   (d) 100% Ethanol.
   (e) Xylene.
9. DPX mounting medium.
10. 22 × 60-mm glass coverslips.

3. Methods

3.1. Estimating Glomerular Number in Developing Mouse or Rat Kidney

1. Remove kidney with fine-tipped forceps. Take care not to damage the kidney with the forceps, as nicks to the cortex will result in artefacts in tissue sections.
2. Immersion fix the whole kidneys (see Note 1).
3. Transfer kidneys into 70% ethanol (minimum 20 min). Kidneys can be stored at 4°C for up to 2–3 weeks.
4. Process kidneys to paraffin. We hand process kidneys up to and including embryonic day 16 (E16) in the mouse and E17 in the rat. Older/larger specimens are processed using an automated processor.

5. Hand processing: Place kidneys into microcassettes and dehydrate through a series of graded ethanol/butanol solutions:
   (a) 70% Ethanol for 20 min.
   (b) 50%/50% Butanol/ethanol for 15 min.
   (c) 75%/25% Butanol/ethanol for 15 min.
   (d) 100% Butanol for 15 min (repeat twice).
   (e) Drain cassette well to remove as much butanol as possible (see Note 2), and place cassette into 60°C paraffin for 10 min with agitation (see Note 3).
6. Embed tissue:
   (a) Place kidney into embedding mold (see Note 4).
   (b) Fill mold with paraffin and leave to solidify.
7. Sectioning:
   (a) Place chuck into clamp of microtome fitted with a steel knife.
   (b) Exhaustively section the entire kidney at a nominal thickness of 4 μm, collecting every section (see Note 5).
   (c) Float ribbons of sections on warm water bath to flatten paraffin (see Note 6). We collect sections in ribbons aligned as two columns in a similar orientation on Poly-L-Lysine-coated glass slides (see Note 7).
   (d) Record the number of sections cut or if any sections were lost during sectioning (these will need to be accounted for during sampling).
   (e) Place slides in 37°C oven overnight to ensure adequate section adherence. Slides can then be stored for use as required.
8. Calculate the required sample; using the total number of sections (including those sections not collected), calculate a sampling fraction to achieve approximately 10–12 pairs of sections per kidney consisting of n (reference section) and $n+2$ (lookup section). For example, if 200 sections have been cut, select every 20th and 22nd, 250 sections every 25th and 27th, 300 sections every 30th and 32nd, and so on (see Notes 8 and 9). The first section must be chosen at random (with use of a random number table) within the interval selected (i.e. 1 to n) (see Note 10).
9. Select slides with required sections and histochemically stain with *A. hypogaea* PNA (Fig. 1).
   (a) Deparaffinise sections through a series of three xylene washes, and bring sections to water through a series of three 100% alcohol washes.
   (b) Rinse in PBS.

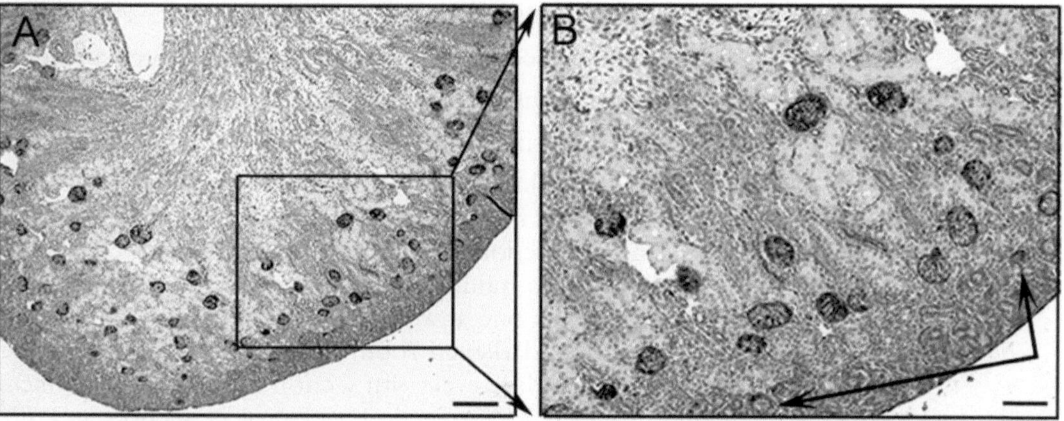

Fig. 1. PNA staining of postnatal day 1 rat kidney. This kidney was sectioned at 5 μm and histochemically stained with PNA, which is visualised with DAB. The glomerular tufts are easily identified (**a**; scale bar represents 150 μm). PNA assists in the unambiguous identification of developing nephrons such as S-shaped bodies shown in the high-magnification view of the same area (*arrow*) (**b**; scale bar represents 50 μm).

(c) Incubate sections for 10 min in 2% H_2O_2 in methanol, 80 μL/slide.

(d) Rinse in PBS for 5 min and repeat.

(e) Incubate for 30 min at 37°C with neuraminidase 0.1 u/mL with 1% $CaCl_2$ in PBS, 80 μL/slide.

(f) Block non-specific binding by incubating with 2% BSA and 0.3% Triton X-100 in PBS for 30 min at room temperature, 80 μL/slide. Do not wash off.

(g) Incubate sections for 2 h with 20 μg/mL biotinylated PNA diluted in 0.3% Triton X-100 in PBS, with 1 mM $CaCl_2$/$MnCl_2$/$MgCl_2$, 80 μL/slide.

(h) Wash with PBS for 5 min and repeat.

(i) Incubate sections with avidin/biotin complex (ABC). We use 10 μL of A and 10 μL of B per 1 mL of 2% BSA and 0.3% Triton X-100 in PBS to make ABC. ABC should be mixed for 20 min prior to use to ensure adequate complex binding. Add 80 μL/slide.

(j) Develop the stain with DAB and 0.01% H_2O_2 in PBS, 80 μL/slide (see Note 11).

(k) End reaction by placing slides in distilled water.

(l) Counterstain sections with haematoxylin for 20 s.

(m) Wash sections under running tap water for 1–2 min (until the water runs clear).

(n) Briefly place sections in Scott's tap water for 1–2 s to turn sections blue.

(o) Wash sections in tap water.

(p) Dehydrate sections in three washes of 100% ethanol.

(q) Clear sections in three washes of xylene.

(r) Coverslip using DPX mounting medium.

10. Count glomeruli using the physical disector principle in which identical regions in the section pairs must be examined. When using paraffin sections, section alignment is often challenging (see Note 6). To minimise difficulty in alignment, we project the section pairs one at a time at approximately 150× onto a table in a semi-darkened room using a microscope modified for projection. Place every *n*th section (reference) on a microscope modified for projection and project section at a final magnification of approximately 150× onto a piece of white paper.

11. If the entire section is projected within the field of view, outline the periphery of the section on the paper. If the entire section is not projected within the field of view, trace the area within the field and move the stage and paper to complete the outline.

12. Identify developing glomeruli and fully developed glomeruli that are PNA positive (Fig. 2a) and mark them on the paper. We outline the circular shape of each PNA-positive structure (Fig. 2) (see Note 12). For those sections that are not completely projected within the field of view, this step is done in stages moving from one side to the other using already marked glomeruli as reference points.

13. Remove the *n*th section and place the *n*th + 2 section (lookup) on the projection microscope. Use glomeruli present in the *n*th section that are also present in the *n*th + 2 section as reference points to line up the *n*th + 2 section with the outline of the *n*th section (Fig. 2c). In the case of those sections not completely projected within the field of view, line up one side.

14. Identify those glomeruli that were present in the *n*th section that are no longer present in the *n*th + 2 section and mark these disappearing glomeruli. We mark these disappearing glomeruli by filling the original circle drawn on the *n*th section (Fig. 2d). Glomeruli present in the *n*th section that are still present in the *n*th + 2 section are not counted and remain as open circles (see Note 12). For those sections that are not completely projected within the field of view, this step is done in stages moving from one side to the other using already marked glomeruli as reference points.

15. Identify those glomeruli present in the *n*th + 2 section that were not present in the *n*th section and mark these appearing glomeruli. We mark appearing glomeruli as closed circles in an

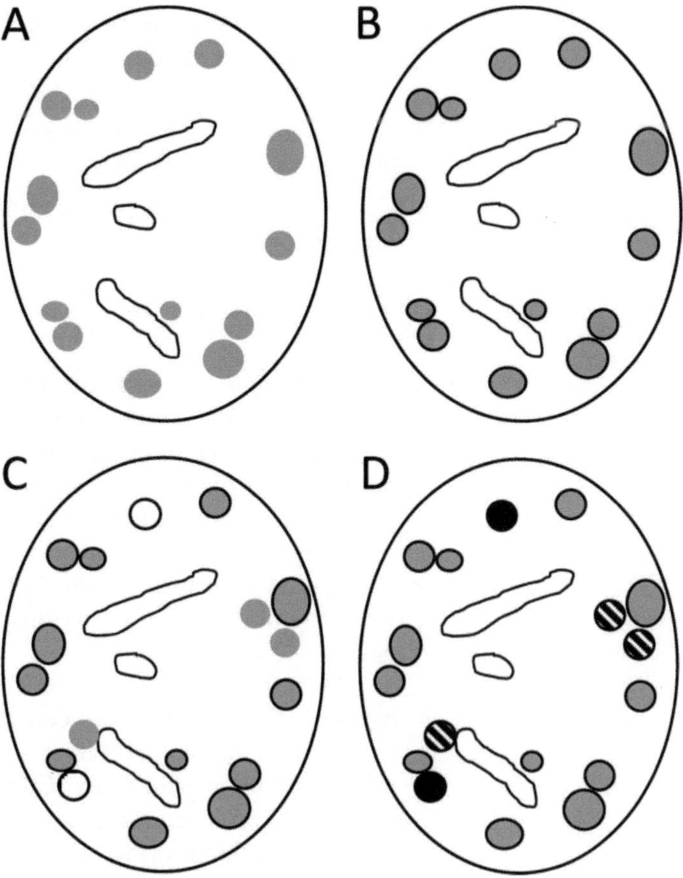

Fig. 2. Counting glomeruli in PNA-stained paraffin sections using the physical disector/fractionator combination. Every *n*th section (reference) is projected at a final magnification of approximately 150× onto white paper and the outline of the kidney and any key landmarks are traced (**a**). PNA-positive glomeruli are clearly distinguished and are then outlined (**b**). The *n*th + 2 section (lookup) is then projected onto the tracing of the *n*th section. Using glomeruli present in the *n*th section that are also present in the *n*th + 2 section as reference points, the *n*th + 2 section is aligned with the outline of the *n*th section (**c**). Those glomeruli that were present in the *n*th section that are no longer present in the *n*th + 2 section are marked (disappearing glomeruli) (**d**—*black circles*). Those glomeruli present in both the reference and lookup sections are not counted and remain as *open circles*. Those glomeruli present in the *n*th + 2 section that were not present in the *n*th section are identified and marked (appearing glomeruli) (**d**—*hatched circles*). This process is repeated for each of the 10–12 complete pairs of sections per kidney. In the example shown, two glomeruli (*black* in **d**) were present in the reference section but not the lookup section, and three glomeruli (*hatched* in **d**) were present in the lookup section but not the reference section. Therefore, Q^{-} for this pair of sections is 5.

alternate colour (Fig. 2d) (see Note 12). For those sections that are not completely projected within the field of view, this step is done in stages moving from one side to the other using already marked glomeruli as reference points.

16. Repeat this process for each complete pair of sections. To estimate the total number of glomeruli in a kidney, we count glomeruli in 10–12 section pairs.
17. Sum the total number of disappearing and appearing glomeruli in all of the section pairs.
18. Calculate the total nephron number (N_{glom}) using the following equation:

$$N_{glom} = \frac{1}{SSF} \times \frac{1}{2} \times \frac{1}{2} \times Q^{-},$$

where N_{glom} is the total number of PNA-positive developing nephrons in the kidney and 1/SSF is the reciprocal of the section-sampling fraction (the number of sections advanced between section pairs).

The first ½ accounts for the fact that the disector pair of sections consisted of the n and the $n+2$ sections.
The last ½ accounts for the fact that PNA-positive structures were counted in both directions between the two sections of a pair.

Q^{-} is the total number of PNA-positive structures appearing and disappearing between the reference and lookup sections for the kidney. For an acceptably low coefficient of error, Q^{-} should be greater than 100 per kidney (6). However, care must be taken when sampling smaller kidneys (such as younger than E19 rat kidneys) to ensure that glomeruli are not sampled twice (see Note 8).

The above protocol needs to be adjusted for small kidneys when only a small number of sections is available, i.e. <200 (see Note 13). We have found, for example, that the E15 mouse kidney contains approximately 70 PNA-positive nephrons in total (7).

4. Notes

1. Embryonic kidney tissue should not be left in fixative for extended periods of time. We fix for up to 1 h in fresh 4% paraformaldehyde. The tissue is then transferred to 70% alcohol.
2. Inadequate removal of butanol will result in poor embedding and tissue falling out of the paraffin block at the microtome. With hand processing, ensure adequate agitation to remove all butanol.
3. Do not leave embryonic kidney tissue in liquid paraffin for extended periods of time. High paraffin temperatures will harden the tissue and make sectioning difficult.

4. When embedding kidneys in paraffin, ensure that there is a thin layer of paraffin on the base of the mold before embedding tissue. As all sections are required to be collected, a thin layer of paraffin ensures that you will get a full block face prior to collecting the first tissue sections.
5. Collection of every section from embryonic/newborn kidneys is a precautionary measure. If some sections in the first sample are lost or damaged, then a second sample is available.
6. Unlike resin sections, paraffin sections are highly susceptible to dimensional changes that occur during sectioning, expansion on the water bath, and mounting. For this reason, we do not cool blocks prior to sectioning, because the block will warm back to room temperature gradually and section dimensions will change. For a similar reason, the temperature of the water bath and the length of time sections are left on the water bath is kept constant in order to minimise the variability in section dimensions. Dimensional changes will affect section alignment, which in turn will slow nephron counting.
7. The use of coated slides is essential to prevent sections from falling off the slides during the staining procedure. We use Poly-L-Lysine-coated slides, but other alternatives ideal for immunohistochemistry (such as Superfrost Plus slides) can be used.
8. For embryonic rat kidneys, we have found that the section-sampling fraction should be a minimum of every 20th section, which provides a distance (20×4 µm = 80 µm) greater than the diameter of the longest arm of an S-shaped body to avoid the same structure being counted twice. Such double counting invalidates this technique. For postnatal kidneys, we use a section-sampling fraction of 30–40 sections. We recommend that a pilot study be conducted prior to a study with new samples/strains to assess the minimal permissible distance between section pairs. To do this, measure the diameter (how many 4-µm sections from one end of a glomerulus to the other) for approximately 50 glomeruli. The section-sampling fraction should not be less than this distance. At the same time, the distance between the reference and lookup sections of a pair should not be greater than the smallest dimension of a feature of interest. For this reason, we use a distance of 8 µm (2×4 µm) between the two sections of a pair. This ensures that no feature can completely exist between the two sections and, therefore, not be seen in either section.
9. Serial sectioning of small kidneys from early embryonic ages (such as E15 mouse kidneys) will result in less than 200 sections. Sampling at the minimal distance of every 20th section will not result in enough section pairs to achieve a precise estimate of nephron number. Therefore, with these young

kidneys, all sections are collected and every nephron in the kidney is counted. This is therefore not an estimate, but rather a complete count of every nephron present in the kidney.

10. In the event that some of the sampled sections are damaged or lost, sections either side of the damaged/lost sections can be used instead. That is, if the section-sampling fraction is every 30th and 32nd and the 120th section is damaged or lost, then the 119th and 121st or the 121st and 123rd can be used to replace that pair. Caution should be taken to avoid going further than two sections either side of the section between the section pairs (i.e. in the case above, the section between the original section pair is the 121st, so sections lesser than the 119th and greater than the 123rd should not be selected to replace damaged or lost sections to minimise changes in the sampling fraction). If sections up to two either side are also damaged/lost, then an alternative random start should be selected resulting in an alternative selection of sections to use.
11. DAB develops the reaction turning the product brown. Sections should be developed under a light microscope, where the researcher can watch the reaction product develop and thereby end the reaction at the appropriate time. Overdeveloping can result in background staining, while under-developing will result in faint staining. Both circumstances will make identification of PNA-positive structures difficult.
12. Sections and PNA-positive structures are outlined at lower magnification for simplicity reasons of fitting tracings onto paper. However, to assist in adequate identification of PNA-positive structures, higher magnification can be used to identify structures with pale staining or those structures with only a few stained cells, such as lower limbs of S-shaped bodies or the very edge of a glomerulus. If identification of features is difficult, adjacent sections can also be used to confirm accurate identification.
13. To obtain nephron number in small kidneys from which there are less than 200 sections (see Note 9), begin by projecting and drawing the outline of the largest section. Circle all PNA-positive structures. Working towards the pole of the kidney one direction at a time, project the next consecutive section and add additional glomeruli not already marked and enclose glomeruli that have disappeared. Continue this process to the pole of the kidney. Return back to the original section and repeat in the other direction until all glomeruli have been marked. The second half of the kidney is often completed on another sheet of paper and the original glomeruli are marked to ensure that they are not counted twice. Sum all PNA-positive structures counted.

References

1. Moritz K, Wintour-Coghlan M, Black MJ et al (2008) Factors influencing mammalian kidney development: implications for health in adult life. Adv Anat Embryol Cell Biol 196: 1–78
2. McMahon AP, Aronow BJ, Davidson DR et al (2008) GUDMAP: the genitourinary developmental molecular anatomy project. J Am Soc Nephrol 19:667–671
3. Walker KA, Bertram JF (2011) Kidney development: core curriculum 2011. Am J Kidney Dis 57(6):948–958
4. Hoy WE, Ingelfinger JR, Hallan S et al (2010) The early development of the kidney and implications for adult health. J Dev Orig Health Dis 1:216–233
5. Puelles VG, Hoy WE, Hughson MD et al (2011) Glomerular number and size variability and risk for kidney disease. Curr Opin Nephrol Hypertens 20:7–15
6. Cullen-McEwen L, Armitage J, Nyengaard J et al (2011) A design-based method for estimating glomerular number in the developing kidney. Am J Physiol Renal 300(6):F1448–F1453
7. Walker KA, Sims-Lucas S, Caruana G et al (2011) Betaglycan is required for the establishment of nephron endowment in the mouse. PLoS One 6:e18723

Chapter 11

An Immunofluorescence Method to Analyze the Proliferation Status of Individual Nephron Segments in the *Xenopus* Pronephric Kidney

Daniel Romaker, Bo Zhang, and Oliver Wessely

Abstract

Organ development requires the coordination of proliferation and differentiation of various cell types. This is particularly challenging in the kidney, where up to 26 different cell types with highly specialized functions are present. Moreover, even though the nephron initially develops from a common progenitor pool, the individual nephron segments are ultimately quite different in respect to cell numbers. This suggests that some cells in the nephron have a higher proliferative index (i.e., cell cycle length) than others. Here, we describe two different immunofluorescence-based approaches to accurately quantify such growth rates in the pronephric kidney of *Xenopus laevis*. Rapidly dividing cells were identified with the mitosis marker phospho-Histone H3, while slowly cycling cells were labeled using the thymidine analogue EdU. In addition, individual nephron segments were marked using cell type-specific antibodies. To accurately assess the number of positively stained cells, embryos were then serially sectioned and analyzed by immunofluorescence microscopy. Growth rates were established by counting the mitosis or S-phase events in relation to the overall cells present in the nephron segment of interest. This experimental design is very reproducible and can easily be modified to fit other animal models and organ systems.

Key words: Cell cycle, Kidney, Metanephros, Mitosis, Pronephros, *Xenopus*

1. Introduction

The mechanism determining the final organ or total body size is an intriguing, yet still poorly understood, question. A multitude of pathways balancing both proliferation and apoptosis has to be tightly monitored to ensure proper size control (1). The core pathways governing proper organ size control were initially identified in the fruit fly *Drosophila melanogaster*. Genetic screens for mutations resulting in tissue overgrowth demonstrated that proteins

Odyssé Michos (ed.), *Kidney Development: Methods and Protocols*, Methods in Molecular Biology, vol. 886, DOI 10.1007/978-1-61779-851-1_11, © Springer Science+Business Media, LLC 2012

involved in two signaling cascades, Insulin/Tsc/TOR and Hippo, were central players (2). These studies were subsequently extended to many vertebrate systems. Importantly, it has become evident that size control mechanisms not only balance proliferation and apoptosis, but also integrate many intrinsic cellular mechanisms like control of mRNA translation, macromolecular synthesis or autophagy, and extrinsic and environmental clues, such as nutrient availability (3, 4).

In humans, an imbalance in size control mechanisms can result in clinical conditions. One example is Autosomal Dominant Polycystic Kidney Diseases (ADPKD). This genetically inherited illness of the kidney is characterized by a cyst-forming tubule epithelium, which constantly expands radially (5). This expansion compresses the renal parenchyma and gradually compromises renal function, leading to end-stage renal failure at later stages of life.

The mammalian metanephric kidney is a complex organ consisting of up to several million functional units, the nephrons, and up to 26 different cell types (3, 6). In respect to size control, it is a rather exceptional organ; not only is its initial size tightly controlled during development, but it is also readily adaptable to partial kidney loss by compensatory growth/hypertrophy (7, 8). However, the intrinsic mechanism and extrinsic clues controlling these processes are still unclear; e.g., it is unknown whether the kidney per se is growing in a linear fashion or if there are distinct growth phases in different nephron segments. This lack of understanding is—in part—due to the fact that the individual nephrons of the metanephric kidney develop asynchronously. As a consequence, nephrons of different differentiation statuses are present at the same time and growth of individual nephrons is difficult to assess.

Here, we provide an alternative approach towards this question, namely, the use of the simpler pronephros. In contrast to the metanephros, the pronephric kidney is composed of only two bilateral nephrons (9). It has been successfully used to study early and late events in kidney development and has provided results that are easily translated to the metanephric kidney (10–12). Among organisms with functional pronephric kidneys, the African clawed frog *Xenopus laevis* is a powerful model organism. The female frog can lay large amounts of eggs, which develop into embryos with a functional kidney after 2 days. Importantly, the developmental timing is highly dependable and precisely documented (13). This allows the collection of embryos from multiple females at precise developmental stages and performing analyses that are highly reproducible and statistically significant.

One prerequisite to addressing the growth characteristics of different nephron segments is their visualization. Different nephron segments are functionally highly specialized and many proteins—in particular glucose, solute, or salt transporters—are specific to individual segments. This segment specificity of individual markers is conserved to the more primitive pronephros as was initially shown in *Xenopus* (14, 15) and subsequently confirmed in zebrafish (16). A simple tool to visualize these subdivisions in *Xenopus* are the two monoclonal antibodies 3G8 and 4A6 that label the proximal tubules or the distal tubules and the pronephric duct, respectively (17). To monitor the cell cycle status of rapidly dividing cells antibodies such as phospho-Histone H3 have been instrumental (18). Conversely, incubating tissues with the thymidine analogue Bromodeoxyuridine (BrdU) or 5-ethynyl-2′-deoxyuridine (EdU) is commonly used to label slow cycling cells (19, 20). These analogues are incorporated into the DNA during chromosomal replication and the number of labeled cells is directly proportional to the length of the cell cycle and the exposure time to BrdU/EdU (21).

Combining these nephron segment- and cell cycle-specific detection systems provides an unprecedented accuracy in the determination of the different proliferation statuses present in the developing nephron. This method (Fig. 1) will provide the baseline for future studies on the underlying molecular mechanisms. In addition, even though we described the technique for the *Xenopus* pronephros, it is extendable to other tissues or organisms. Finally, the method is not restricted to the detection systems described here, but can easily serve as a blueprint for experimental designs using other antibodies or labeling techniques.

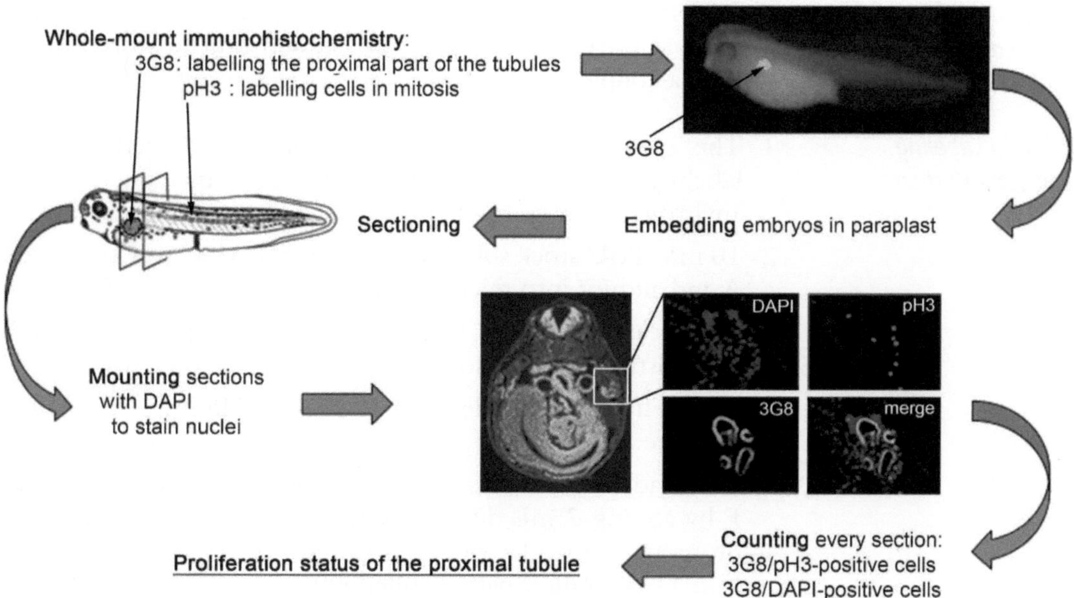

Fig. 1. Experimental workflow using the 3G8 and Phospho-Histone H3.

2. Materials

2.1. Immunohistochemistry

1. DENT'S fixative: 10 mL dimethyl sulfoxide (DMSO), 40 mL methanol.
2. 10× PBS: 80 g NaCl, 2 g KCl, 14.4 g Na_2PO_4, 2.4 g KH_2PO_4, 800 mL distilled water. Mix and adjust pH to 7.4 with NaOH. Adjust to 1 L with millipore water. Autoclave and store at room temperature (RT).
3. PBSw: Prepare 1× PBS using 10× PBS and millipore water, filter with 0.45-μm bottle-top filter and add Tween-20 to a final concentration of 0.1%.
4. Prehybridization buffer: 10% goat serum (heat-inactivated at 56°C for 1 h), 3% (w/v) bovine serum albumin (BSA, Fraction V) in PBSw. Filter using a 0.45-μm syringe filter (see Note 1).
5. Methanol series: Prepare methanol dilutions (25, 50, 75, and 100%) by diluting methanol in 1× PBSw.
6. Ethanol series: Prepare ethanol dilutions (25, 50, 75, and 100%) by diluting ethanol in 1× PBSw.
7. Monoclonal antibodies: The pronephros-specific antibodies 3G8 and 4A6 can be obtained from the European Xenopus Resource Centre at the University of Portsmouth and the pan-kidney α-Na/K-ATPase antibody from the Developmental Studies Hybridoma Bank.

2.2. Embryo Embedding and Sectioning

1. Paraplast: Pellets are placed in a funnel lined with filter paper and melted into a glass bottle overnight using a convection oven at 68°C. Melted paraplast should not be stored longer than a couple of days.

2.3. EdU Labeling and Visualization

1. The components for the EdU (5-ethynyl-2′-deoxyuridine) labeling are part of the Click-iT® EdU imaging kit from Invitrogen, but components can also be obtained individually.
2. 10 mM EdU stock solution: Add 2 mL DMSO to Component A and aliquot into microcentrifuge tubes. Store at −80°C.
3. EdU reaction buffer: Dilute component D to a 1× solution with distilled water and store at 4°C.
4. Alexa Fluor® 594 azide: Add 70 μL of DMSO to Component B. Store at −80°C.
5. Buffer additive: 10× stock solution is prepared from Component F by adding 2 mL distilled water to the vial and mixed well. Store at −80°C. 1× working solution is prepared fresh every time by diluting it with distilled water.

6. EdU working solution: 2.2 mL EdU reaction buffer, 100 μL $CuSO_4$, 6 μL Alexa Fluor® 594 azide, and 250 μL buffer additive. The components have to be added in the indicated order. The solution has to be made freshly each time and cannot be stored. The solution is sufficient for five slides and the amount needs to be adjusted according to the number of slides.
7. 1× PBS: Dilute 10× PBS with distilled water.
8. PBS–BSA: Dissolve 3% (w/v) BSA (Fraction V) in 1× PBS. Mix thoroughly and keep at RT.
9. 4% Paraformaldehyde (PFA): Dissolve 4 g of PFA in 100 mL of 1× PBS by heating to 65°C, vortex frequently, and filter using a 0.45-μm syringe filter.

3. Methods

All procedures are performed at room temperature unless otherwise indicated. For the removal of solutions from vials containing embryos, we recommend using a vacuum aspiration device consisting of a vacuum Erlenmeyer flask attached on one side to a vacuum source and on the other side to a rubber tubing capped by a yellow tip. This allows easy aspiration of most of the liquid without disrupting the embryos.

3.1. Whole Mount Immunohistochemistry

1. *Xenopus* embryos are obtained using standard methods (22) and cultured until the desired stages (23).
2. Embryos are transferred to 3.7-mL glass vials using transfer pipets, which are then filled to the rim with DENT's Fixative (see Note 2).
3. Vials are placed onto a tube rotator and embryos are fixed at 4°C overnight or 4 h at RT.
4. Dent's Fixative is removed; embryos are washed in 100% methanol for 5 min and replaced again with 100% methanol. Fixed embryos can be stored for prolonged periods at –20°C.
5. Rehydrate fixed embryos through methanol series (100, 75, 50, and 25%) to PBSw by removing the fluid and replacing it with the next dilution. Incubate each step at RT for 5 min on a test tube rocker.
6. Incubate embryos in PBSw twice for 1 h each at RT on a test tube rocker.
7. Aspirate PBSw and exchange with 1 mL of freshly prepared prehybridization buffer and incubate at 4°C on a test tube rocker for 2 h.

8. At the same time, prepare a primary antibody master mix by diluting the 3G8 (1:100) and phospho-Histone H3 (Ser10, pH3, 1:500) antibodies in the appropriate amount of prehybridization buffer (you will need a minimum of 1 mL per vial). Pre-incubate the master mix for 2 h at 4°C on a test tube rocker.
9. Aspirate prehybridization buffer and replace with a minimum of 1 mL of primary antibody master mix.
10. Incubate at 4°C on a test tube rocker overnight.
11. Aspirate solution and exchange with 3.5 mL PBSw and incubate at RT for 1 h on a test tube rocker.
12. Repeat step 11 three times.
13. Aspirate PBSw and exchange with 1 mL of freshly prepared prehybridization buffer per vial and incubate at 4°C on a test tube rocker for 2 h.
14. At the same time, prepare a secondary antibody master mix by diluting Alexa Fluor® 488 anti-mouse (1:1,000, detects 3G8) and Alexa Fluor® 594 anti-rabbit (1:1,000, detects pH3) in the appropriate amount of prehybridization buffer (you will need a minimum of 1 mL per vial). Pre-incubate the master mix in the dark for 2 h at 4°C on a test tube rocker (see Note 3).
15. Aspirate prehybridization buffer and replace with a minimum of 1 mL of secondary antibody master mix.
16. Incubate in the dark on a test tube rocker at 4°C overnight (see Note 3).
17. Aspirate solution and exchange with 3.5 mL PBSw and incubate in the dark at RT for 1 h on a test tube rocker.
18. Repeat step 17 four times.
19. Dehydrate embryos through methanol series (25, 50, 75, and 100%) by removing the fluid and replacing it with the next dilution. Incubate each step at RT for 5 min on a test tube rocker.
20. Store embryos in 100% methanol or proceed directly to the next section.

3.2. Embryo Embedding and Sectioning

1. Transfer the number of embryos to be sectioned into a glass vial filled with 3.5 mL 100% isopropanol and incubate at RT for 15 min (see Note 4).
2. Aspirate solution and exchange with 3.5 mL 100% isopropanol. Incubate at 68°C for 15 min using a convection heating oven (see Note 5).
3. Decant solution into a waste container and exchange with 3.5 mL of a premade mixture of isopropanol/paraplast (1:1). Incubate at 68°C for 30 min.

4. Decant solution into a waste container and exchange with 3.5 mL liquid paraplast. Incubate for 1 h at 68°C.
5. Repeat step 4.
6. Repeat step 4, but incubate only for 30 min.
7. In parallel, prepare embedding molds (one per embryo) by filling them with liquid paraplast to the top. Incubate the molds for approximately 30 min at 68°C.
8. Transfer the embryos into the molds filled with liquid paraplast using a pre-warmed transfer pipet.
9. Move one mold at a time to RT. Adjust the position of the embryo so that the head is orientated towards the bottom of the mold and the tail to the top using a straightened paper clip.
10. Let the paraplast solidify overnight at RT without moving the molds (see Note 3).
11. Section the embryos at 25-μm thickness with a rotary microtome (see Note 6).
12. Cover pre-cleaned Superfrost microscope slides with H_2O on a slide warmer adjusted to 45°C. Assemble sections consecutively on the slide and put as many sections as possible on a single slide.
13. Incubate slides on the slide warmer overnight to assure that the sections stretch out and completely attach to the glass surface.
14. Remove slides from the slide warmer, transfer them to Coplin jars, and dewax them in xylene two times, 5 min each (see Note 7).
15. Rehydrate sections into PBSw using a series of ethanol (100, 75, 50, and 25%) by transferring the slides from one Coplin jar to the one with the next dilution. Incubate each step at RT for 5 min.
16. Wash sections three times with PBSw in Coplin jars.
17. Wash sections once with Millipore water in Coplin jars.
18. Mount the sections using a water-based embedding media containing DAPI (e.g., ProLong® Gold Antifade Reagent) using a cover glass and try to avoid any air bubbles.
19. Dry sections at least overnight (see Notes 3 and 8).
20. Analyze the sections with a fluorescence microscope.
21. Identify 3G8-positive proximal tubules on the sections and count all the pH3-positive as well as DAPI-positive cells in this area (see Note 9).

3.3. EdU Labeling and Visualization

1. *Xenopus* embryos are obtained using standard methods (22) and cultured until the desired stages (23).
2. Thaw 10 mM EdU stock solution at RT (see Note 10).
3. Anesthetize *Xenopus* embryos with 250 mg/L Tricaine methane sulfonate (MS222) solution.
4. Inject *Xenopus* embryos with approximately 8 nL of the EdU stock solution into the ventral region at the level of the pronephric tubules using a standard microinjection setup (see Note 11) (22).
5. Return embryos to 0.1× Barth and monitor them until they regained consciousness.
6. Transfer embryos to a new plate containing 0.1× Barth and culture for 12 h (see Note 12).
7. Transfer embryos to 3.7-mL glass vials containing 4% PFA using a transfer pipet (see Note 2).
8. Vials are placed onto a tube rotator and embryos are fixed at 4°C overnight or 4 h at RT.
9. 4% PFA is removed and embryos are dehydrated through methanol series (25, 50, 75, and 100%) by removing the fluid and replacing it with the next dilution. Fixed embryos can be stored for prolonged periods at –20°C.
10. Embryos are embedded and sectioned as described above (Subheading 3.2, steps 1–15).
11. Permeabilize and refix slides in 4% PFA for 15 min at RT using a Coplin jar.
12. Wash the slides in PBS–BSA twice for 5 min each using a Coplin jar.
13. Wash slides in PBSw for 20 min using a Coplin jar.
14. Prepare the EdU working solution. The slides are laid flat into a moist chamber and 500 μL of the EdU working solution is added onto each slide. It is important that the sections never dry out during the procedure, since this will result in background staining. A cover glass is gently put on the solution to ensure that the solution completely covers the slide and does not evaporate. Incubate for 30 min in the dark (see Note 3).
15. Remove EdU working solution (including the cover glass). Wash the slides in PBS–BSA for 5 min using Coplin jars.
16. Wash the slides three times in PBS for 5 min each in Coplin jars.
17. Transfer slides back into the moist chamber, add 500 μL of freshly prepared prehybridization buffer to each slide, and use a cover slide to prevent evaporation. Incubate in the dark at 4°C for 2 h.
18. At the same time, prepare a primary antibody master mix by diluting anti-α-Na/K-ATPase antibody (1:50, see Note 13) in

the appropriate amount of prehybridization buffer (you will need 500 μL per slide). Pre-incubate the master mix for 2 h at 4°C on a test tube rocker.

19. Aspirate prehybridization buffer, replace with 500 μL of primary antibody master mix, and use a cover slide to prevent evaporation.
20. Incubate in the dark at 4°C overnight.
21. Wash the slides briefly in PBSw using Coplin jars.
22. Wash the slides five times for 1 h each in PBSw using Coplin jars.
23. Transfer slides into a moist chamber, cover each slide with 500 μL of freshly prepared prehybridization buffer, and use a cover slide to prevent evaporation. Incubate in the dark at 4°C for 2 h.
24. At the same time, prepare a secondary antibody master mix by diluting Alexa Fluor® 488 anti-mouse (1:1,000, see Notes 3 and 14) in the appropriate amount of prehybridization buffer (you will need 500 μL per slide). Pre-incubate the master mix for 2 h in the dark at 4°C on a test tube rocker.
25. Aspirate prehybridization buffer, replace with 500 μL of secondary antibody master mix, and use a cover slide to prevent evaporation.
26. Incubate in the dark at 4°C overnight.
27. Wash the slides briefly in PBSw using Coplin jars.
28. Wash the slides in the dark five times for 1 h each in PBSw using Coplin jars.
29. Wash slides briefly with distilled water.
30. Mount the sections using a water-based embedding media containing DAPI (e.g., ProLong® Gold Antifade Reagent) using a cover glass and try to avoid air bubbles.
31. Dry sections at least overnight (see Note 8).
32. Analyze the sections with a fluorescence microscope.
33. Identify α-Na/K-ATPase-positive pronephric tubules on the sections (green) and count all the EdU-positive (red) as well as DAPI-positive cells (blue) in this area.

4. Notes

1. We normally prepare the buffer fresh; it can be frozen, but when thawed do not reheat above 37°C, since precipitate will form.

2. Embryos fixed in Dent's or 4% PFA are delicate. Thus, the use of glass vials (e.g., 15 × 45-mm screw thread vials with rubber-lined cap) is recommended. In addition, it is important to completely fill the vials with fixative to prevent embryos from touching the air/fixative interface.
3. Since the secondary antibodies and the EdU working solution contain fluorophores and are therefore light sensitive, we regularly cover the tubes, molds, and sections with aluminum foil to minimize photo bleaching.
4. We normally process as many as five embryos in one glass vial. This number is, however, dependent on the experience of the user and can be adjusted at will. The number should be based on the time needed to process the embryos and transfer them into the molds without premature solidification of the paraplast.
5. All tools used for the embedding (pipets, droppers, and paper clips) need to be kept at 68°C to allow easy handling of the paraplast solutions.
6. To maximize the number of sections that one can put on a single slide, the paraplast block is cut as close as possible to the embedded embryo. For the subsequent analysis, it is important to recover all sections and place them on the slide consecutively. Thus, we do not recommend using a heated water bath to spread the sections. The thickness of 25 μm for the sections has been established empirically. It reflects the size of the cells in the pronephros at the stages analyzed and assures that each section is approximately one cell layer deep. The thickness of sections from different stages, organs, or organisms needs to be adjusted accordingly.
7. The freshness of the xylene is important. While it is possible to reuse it for several times, one has to verify proper dewaxing by visual inspection.
8. Care should be taken to analyze sections after 24 h, since the mounting media has not yet dried completely. Shearing of the coverslip can result in disrupting the tissue integrity and prevent proper subsequent analysis.
9. 3G8 labels the apical membrane of the proximal tubules. The only cells that are counted are those sharing this apical domain. Interstitial cells are neglected.
10. We prefer EdU to the other frequently used Thymidine analogue BrdU, since the methodology to visualize BrdU requires harsh treatments to denature the chromosomal DNA and increase accessibility for the anti-BrdU antibody. Due to the decreasing cell size of the developing embryos, the timing of the treatments for the BrdU staining needs to be adjusted for each individual embryonic stage. In addition, the denaturation

step destroys the epitopes used for immunofluorescence making the double-staining protocol more difficult.

11. In our experience, injection of the EdU into the *Xenopus* embryo is essential for the sensitivity and reproducibility of the assay. Adding the EdU stock solution directly to the culture medium did not reliably work even at higher concentrations of EdU. This seems to be a penetration problem of embryos at stages 38 and higher, since in "bathed" embryos EdU staining was primarily restricted to the epidermis.
12. A 12-h chase is sufficient to allow one mitosis event in the pronephric duct. In other tissues, the timing of the EdU chase may need to be adjusted according to the respective cell cycle length.
13. α-Na/K-ATPase labels epithelial structures, including the entire pronephros. The 4A6 antibody can be used if one only wants to label the pronephric duct and distal tubules.
14. The Click-iT® EdU imaging kit from Invitrogen can be obtained with different fluorescence labels. The protocol here uses the Alexa Fluor® 594 azide, but any other fluorophore combination can be used.

Acknowledgments

We would like to thank U. Tran and V. Kumar for critically reviewing the manuscript. D.R. is a recipient of a DFG postdoctoral fellowship (RO4124/1-1). This work was supported by NIH/NIDDK (7RO1DK080745-03) to O.W.

References

1. Stanger BZ (2008) The biology of organ size determination. Diabetes Obes Metab 10(Suppl 4):16–22
2. Neufeld TP (2003) Body building: regulation of shape and size by PI3K/TOR signaling during development. Mech Dev 120:1283–1296
3. Nyengaard JR, Bendtsen TF (1992) Glomerular number and size in relation to age, kidney weight, and body surface in normal man. Anat Rec 232:194–201
4. Meijer AJ, Codogno P (2008) Nutrient sensing: TOR's ragtime. Nat Cell Biol 10: 881–883
5. Grantham JJ, Cook LT, Wetzel LH, Cadnapaphornchai MA, Bae KT (2010) Evidence of extraordinary growth in the progressive enlargement of renal cysts. Clin J Am Soc Nephrol 5:889–896
6. Al-Awqati Q, Oliver JA (2002) Stem cells in the kidney. Kidney Int 61:387–395
7. Satriano J (2007) Kidney growth, hypertrophy and the unifying mechanism of diabetic complications. Amino Acids 33:331–339
8. Sinuani I, Beberashvili I, Averbukh Z et al (2010) Mesangial cells initiate compensatory tubular cell hypertrophy. Am J Nephrol 31:326–331
9. Wessely O, Tran U (2011) Xenopus pronephros development—past, present, and future. Pediatr Nephrol 26:1545–1551

10. Simons M, Gloy J, Ganner A et al (2005) Inversin, the gene product mutated in nephronophthisis type II, functions as a molecular switch between Wnt signaling pathways. Nat Genet 37:537–543
11. Tran U, Zakin L, Schweickert A et al (2010) The RNA-binding protein bicaudal C regulates polycystin 2 in the kidney by antagonizing miR-17 activity. Development 137: 1107–1116
12. White JT, Zhang B, Cerqueira DM, Tran U, Wessely O (2010) Notch signaling, wtl and foxc2 are key regulators of the podocyte gene regulatory network in Xenopus. Development 137:1863–1873
13. Moody SA (1987) Fates of the blastomeres of the 16-cell stage Xenopus embryo. Dev Biol 119:560–578
14. Zhou X, Vize PD (2004) Proximo-distal specialization of epithelial transport processes within the Xenopus pronephric kidney tubules. Dev Biol 271:322–338
15. Raciti D, Reggiani L, Geffers L et al (2008) Organization of the pronephric kidney revealed by large-scale gene expression mapping. Genome Biol 9:R84
16. Wingert RA, Selleck R, Yu J et al (2007) The cdx genes and retinoic acid control the positioning and segmentation of the zebrafish pronephros. PLoS Genet 3:1922–1938
17. Vize PD, Jones EA, Pfister R (1995) Development of the Xenopus pronephric system. Dev Biol 171:531–540
18. Hendzel MJ, Wei Y, Mancini MA et al (1997) Mitosis-specific phosphorylation of histone H3 initiates primarily within pericentromeric heterochromatin during G2 and spreads in an ordered fashion coincident with mitotic chromosome condensation. Chromosoma 106:348–360
19. Salic A, Mitchison TJ (2008) A chemical method for fast and sensitive detection of DNA synthesis in vivo. Proc Natl Acad Sci USA 105:2415–2420
20. Gratzner HG (1982) Monoclonal antibody to 5-bromo- and 5-iododeoxyuridine: a new reagent for detection of DNA replication. Science 218:474–475
21. Vogetseder A, Palan T, Bacic D, Kaissling B, Le Hir M (2007) Proximal tubular epithelial cells are generated by division of differentiated cells in the healthy kidney. Am J Physiol Cell Physiol 292:C807–C813
22. Sive HL, Grainger RM, Harland RM (2000) Early development of *Xenopus laevis*: a laboratory manual. Cold Spring Harbor Laboratory Press, Cold Spring Harbor, NY
23. Nieuwkoop PD, Faber J (1994) Normal table of *Xenopus laevis*. Garland Publishing, Inc, New York

Part III

Renal Primary Cell Cultures and Cell Lines

Chapter 12

Dissociation of Embryonic Kidney Followed by Re-aggregation as a Method for Chimeric Analysis

Jamie A. Davies, Mathieu Unbekandt, Jessica Ineson, Michael Lusis, and Melissa H. Little

Abstract

This chapter presents three methods for re-constructing mouse foetal kidney tissue from simple suspensions of cells. These techniques are very useful for a number of purposes: (1) they allow the production of fine-grained chimaeras in which cell autonomy of mutations can be tested, (2) they provide an environment that allows the renal differentiation potential of stem cells to be assessed, and (3) they are an excellent system in which to study the mechanisms of self-organization. Each of the methods described here begins with disaggregation of embryonic mouse kidneys, followed by re-aggregation and culture; the main differences are in the culture methods, each of which has advantages for particular purposes.

Key words: Tissue engineering, Metanephros, Chimaera, Self-organization, Mosaic, Organ culture

1. Introduction

The ability to construct "embryonic kidney tissue" by re-aggregation of initially dissociated renogenic cells adds a powerful weapon to the armoury of kidney culture techniques. As well as uncovering basic processes of anatomical self-organization, the system allows experimenters to make fine-grained chimaeras that place "test" cells in the context of developing kidney tissue. This provides a convenient way to assess the abilities of these cells to differentiate into various renal cell types or their abilities to interfere with or promote the differentiation and morphogenesis of the host tissue. Formation of an embryonic kidney tissue from simple suspensions of cells is also a promising technique for stem cell-based tissue-engineering techniques in regenerative medicine, but these applications are beyond the scope of this article.

Odyssé Michos (ed.), *Kidney Development: Methods and Protocols*, Methods in Molecular Biology, vol. 886, DOI 10.1007/978-1-61779-851-1_12, © Springer Science+Business Media, LLC 2012

Here, we present two broadly similar methods for disaggregating embryonic mouse kidneys to obtain renogenic cells and then re-aggregating them to form organotypic tissue, with or without the addition of other cells to make chimaeras. One method was developed in Edinburgh, and the other in Brisbane; both were published in 2010 (1, 2) and highlighted by editorials in their respective journals (3, 4). The methods each begin with enzymatic dissociation of kidneys, followed by random re-aggregation of cells using centrifugation. They then use conventional organ culture of the resulting aggregate to allow renal structures to re-form. Both have been used for published studies on the fates of exogenous cells in chimeric re-aggregates (2, 5). The Edinburgh method uses a temporary drug treatment to promote cell survival, while the Brisbane method uses a feeder layer of *Wnt*-secreting support cells.

Simple re-aggregations of the type described above result in the re-formation of ureteric bud epithelia and the induction of nephron epithelia from mesenchyme, followed by eventual connection of the nephrons to the ureteric bud tubules in the usual manner. At high magnification, there is little apparent difference between the tissues and those of an embryonic kidney that developed *in vivo*, but on low-power examination there is one very obvious difference: a normal embryonic kidney is arranged around a single, branched ureteric bud/collecting duct tree that leads back to a single ureter, whereas in the re-aggregates many small, disconnected ureteric bud "tree-lets" form. This difference prevents the development of the normal cortico-medullary axis of the kidney, and would be a major handicap to clinical use since the drainage purpose of the collecting ducts is defeated and the urine-concentrating function of cortico-medullary organization is also missing. A very recent development of the Edinburgh method, which uses two sequential rounds of disaggregation and re-aggregation, results in a re-aggregate that is arranged around one single ureteric bud (6); either the bud or the mesenchyme can be chimeric in this system, and they can even be chimaeras with different exogenous cells.

2. Materials

Observe good sterile technique when preparing and handling all instruments, solutions, and hardware. Ensure that your supply of enzymes does not have sodium azide as a preservative.

2.1. The Edinburgh Method

1. Dissecting medium: Eagle's Minimum Essential Medium.
2. Kidney culture medium (KCM): Dissecting medium with 1× penicillin/streptomycin and 10% fetal calf serum (FCS).
3. Trypsin-EDTA 10× made up at 1× in phosphate-buffered saline (PBS).

4. Glycyl-H1152 dihydrochloride (Tocris, Bristol, UK), made up to 1.25 μM in KCM.
5. Optional for tracking test cells: Green CMFDA CellTracker dye (Molecular Probes, Invitrogen).
6. Optional for "standard immunostaining": Methanol stored at –20°C, mouse anti-calbindin-D28K (Ab9481, Abcam, Cambridge MA, USA), rabbit anti-laminin (L9393, Sigma), goat FITC anti-mouse (F0257, Sigma), and goat TRITC anti-rabbit (T5268, Sigma).
7. 5 μm polycarbonate filter, Millipore.
8. Stainless steel culture grids. (These are for supporting the culture filters at the liquid/gas interface. Make them from fine stainless steel mesh: cut the mesh into triangles about 1.5 cm per side, and bend the corners down to make legs about 3-mm high—the height is not critical, but having them very high wastes medium.) We find it useful to force a pointed scissor blade into the mesh and to turn it to make small "holes" about 3 mm across, across which pieces of filter will later be placed.
9. Microcentrifuge.
10. Tubes.
11. 3.5-mm Petri dishes.
12. Cell strainer—40 μm.
13. Haemocytometer.
14. Optional—Fluorescence microscope (this is our favoured method for visualizing marked cells and immuno-stained antigens, but other methods such as sectioning and enzymatic staining are alternatives).
15. A good dissecting microscope. The difference that quality makes to the ability of an experimenter to place samples accurately on the culture filters cannot be over-emphasized. We use the Zeiss Stemi-2000 series; other excellent microscopes are available.

2.2. The Brisbane Method

1. Confluent *Wnt4*-expressing NIH3T3 cells (available from Andreas Kispert).
2. 100 μg/mL mouse collagen IV solution (BD Biosciences, 354233) and 0.65 N HCl.
3. 0.4 μm polycarbonate filters (LabQuip Technologies, K04CP01300).
4. Dissecting medium: Dulbecco's modified Eagle's medium (DMEM), High Glucose.
5. Scalpel blades.

6. Microscopes: Dissecting microscope for harvesting embryonic kidneys; standard light microscope for checking paraffin sections; fluorescence microscope for visualizing immunofluorescence of resulting sectioned samples.
7. Accutase (Millipore, SCR005).
8. PBS.
9. Gilson P1000 and P200 pipettes.
10. Optional: DiI or GFP-labelled test cells for analysis of renal potential. These may include cell lines, freshly isolated tissue, or FACS-sorted cell populations.
11. Shaking water bath.
12. Culture medium: DMEM supplemented with 100 u/mL penicillin, 100 g/mL streptomycin, 2 nM/Ll-glutamine, and 10% FCS.
13. Standard tissue culture incubator at 37°C, 5% CO_2.
14. Stainless steel culture grids. (These are for supporting the culture filters at the liquid/gas interface. Make them from fine stainless steel mesh: cut the mesh into triangles about 1.5 cm per side, and bend the corners down to make legs about 3-mm high—the height is not critical, but having them very high wastes medium).
15. Plastic ware: 1.5-mL microcentrifuge tubes, 15-mL Falcon tubes, 4-well dishes, and 60-mm tissue culture dishes for dissection of kidneys.
16. Cell strainer—70 or 100 μm.
17. Haemocytometer for quantitation of cells prior to re-aggregation.
18. Benchtop centrifuge for pelleting re-aggregations in 15-mL tubes.
19. Standard glass microscope slides.
20. Microtome for cutting sections.

2.3. Optional for "Standard Immunostaining"

1. 4% Paraformaldehyde stored at −20°C.
2. Alcohol series (70, 80, 90, and 100%).
3. Xylene.
4. Paraffin wax and microtome for paraffin embedding and sectioning.
5. Antibodies: Mouse anti-calbindin D28K (Abcam, Ab9481), mouse anti-Six2 (Sapphire Biosciences, H00010736), mouse anti-Aquaporin1 (Millipore, #AB2219), rabbit anti-Pax2 (Zymed Laboratories, #71-6000), mouse anti-WT1 (DakoCytomation, #6F-H2m3561), rabbit anti-pan-laminin (Sigma, L9393), rabbit anti-GFP (Sapphire Bioscience,

#ab13970), Alexa Fluor 488 anti-rabbit (Invitrogen, A10254), Alexa Fluor 594 anti-mouse (Invitrogen, A10256).

3. Methods

Both methods begin with kidney rudiments isolated from E11.5–E12.5 mouse embryos. Given the specialized natures of this volume, it is assumed that any reader is capable of performing this dissection, and a proper description of the process would require a chapter in itself. Such a chapter can be found in a previous volume of this journal (7).

3.1. The Basic Edinburgh Method

See Subheading 3.2 for a refinement that results in a re-aggregate arranged around a single re-aggregated ureteric bud.

This method involves significant micro-manipulation of tissues, in open air, in media that are intended to be buffered against 5% CO_2: pay close attention to the colour of the pH indicator in the medium while you work, and change medium if it begins to look significantly more alkaline than equivalent medium in a 5% CO_2 incubator. This is important—pH drift is bad for the cells (but so, alas, are all of the non-CO_2 buffers we have tried in an attempt to obviate the problem).

1. Isolate at least 10 fresh E11.5 metanephric rudiments in dissecting medium.
2. Using a fine (pulled) Pasteur pipette, transfer the rudiments to a 3.5-mm Petri dish containing trypsin-EDTA solution and incubate them for 4 min at 37°C, 5% CO_2.
3. Using a glass Pasteur pipette, transfer the kidneys to a 3.5-mm Petri dish containing KCM. The precise volume does not matter much, but the presence of serum in the KCM is important for quenching (competing for) the trypsin-EDTA. Incubate the rudiments in this for 10 min at 37°C.
4. This incubation is a good time to prepare culture filters for later use. Immerse a 5-μm polycarbonate filter in KCM and cut it into squares about 5 mm per side using a scalpel (rounded blades are less inclined to tear the filter). If necessary, small notches can be cut into filters as an identification code for samples, one notch being the filter for sample 1, two notches being for sample 2, etc. Cut one filter fragment into a triangle shape for the control kidney. Place filter grids in fresh 3-cm Petri dishes, and fill these dishes with KCM with H-1152 until the surface of the grids is just wet but the meniscus away from the grid still bends a little lower than the grid surface (excess KCM with H-1152 can be pipetted away to achieve this state of

affairs). Place the pieces of filter on top of the grid (across the holes in the mesh if you made them). Several pieces of filter can be put on one grid. Place the whole dish in the 37°C, 5% CO_2 incubator until it is needed (see Note 3).

5. Place the organs in a 0.5-mL Eppendorf tube containing 200 μL of KCM. Dissociate the organs by trituration—that is, pipetting them up and down through a yellow Gilson tip adjusted to 100 μL. This step may need practice—too much violence results in shear stresses lethal to the cells, while too little fails to separate cells into a single-celled suspension (see Note 1).
6. Filter the resulting suspension through the cell strainer. Stain a sample of it with Trypan Blue and apply the stained cells to a haemocytometer both to check that (a) the cells are in a single-celled suspension and (b) that they are alive (our results show an average of about 90% of cells being alive, see Note 2) and (c) to measure their concentration.
7. Divide the cell suspension in the main, unstained sample into aliquots of 8×10^4 cells, placing each aliquot in a 500-μL microcentrifuge tube. Complete with KCM medium to obtain a solution of 150–200 μL per tube.
8. Optional: Add test cells to the suspensions. If these cells do not carry an intrinsic marker, e.g. GFP, they can first be stained with CellTracker according to the manufacturer's directions (a typical labelling procedure uses CellTracker at 4 μM, but we recommend that a pilot experiment be performed to determine the maximum concentration of CellTracker compatible with viability of the cell type in question: in our experience, this varies with both cell type and batch of CellTracker). The number of cells to be added must be determined by trial and error, typically by running a series of parallel experiments in which the test cells form increasing proportions of the final mix. When mixing labelled E11.5 kidney cells, we can use any proportion. In our experiments in which human amniotic fluid cells (hAFSCs) were incorporated into kidney re-aggregates, we found that the optimum ratio, for the best possible incorporation, was 10% of the final mix to be of hAFSC origin (5).
9. Centrifuge each suspension of cells for 2 min at $800 \times g$ to make a pellet (see Notes 4 and 5).
10. Use a yellow pipette tip, on a pipette, to aspirate a little medium and then expel it, very gently, at each pellet to persuade the pellet to break free of the tube.
11. Remove the Petri dish containing the filters in the grid, prepared earlier at stage 4, from the incubator and place it at the stage of the dissecting microscope. Collect the pellets from their microcentrifuge tube with a glass Pasteur pipette and

release them gently on to a square filter (one re-aggregate, one filter). Each will be just visible as a brownish "stain". Beware the risk of releasing so much medium that the re-aggregate is washed over the side of the filter.

12. Place the dish with all of its occupied filters in the incubator, taking great care to treat it gently (and warning other incubator users of the need not to slam doors, etc.). Incubate for 24 h.
13. Remove the dish from the incubator, remove the grid with filters, and place it in a new Petri dish. Quickly fill with fresh pre-warmed KCM with no H-1152 (continued presence of H-1152 prevents nephrons forming properly (1)). Return to the incubator for as long as desired (3 days is typical).
14. Optional—Fix in 4% formaldehyde (made freshly from paraformaldehyde) in PBS for 30 min, wash in PBS, and immerse in methanol for 10 min. The formaldehyde fix is necessary if CellTracker has been used because fixation directly in methanol results in its loss. Methanol is needed for antibody access to the cytoplasm. If Cell tracker has not been used, fixation can be directly in ice-cold methanol. Use forceps to transfer filters to a bijou tube with PBS, and incubate them for at least 30 min at room temperature. Replace the PBS with a solution of primary antibody (each at 1/100, for the antibodies mentioned in Subheading 2) and leave it overnight at 4°C. Wash in PBS during the next day, and incubate in secondary antibodies overnight at 4°C. Wash again in PBS, mount, and observe.

3.2. The Revised Edinburgh Method

For making a re-aggregate arranged around a single re-aggregated ureteric bud.

This method consists essentially of two sequential rounds of the basic method, with some micro-dissection in between. It is significantly more labour intensive than the basic method, so should be used only when having a single ureteric bud is important.

1. Begin by setting up a conventional disaggregation and re-aggregation culture using the method described in Subheading 3.1 above. (Optional: If chimeric ureteric buds are required, add labelled test cells as appropriate.) Culture for 1 day in KCM with H-1152 and 3–4 days in plain KCM. This culture will contribute only the ureteric bud to the final experiment, and is referred to henceforth as the "UB-donor culture".
2. Prepare a new culture dish for the final culture (step 4 of Subheading 3.1); plain KCM can be used for this.
3. Isolate a fresh batch of E11.5 kidneys. Under a dissecting microscope, use 25-gauge needles to pull the mesenchyme away from the ureteric bud without using enzymes.

4. Place the mesenchymes only in a Petri dish containing 0.5× Trypsin-EDTA for 2 min at 37°C in the incubator.
5. Place the mesenchymes in a Petri dish containing KCM and leave them for 10 min at 37°C in the incubator.
6. Place the mesenchymes in a 0.5-mL Eppendorf tube containing 200 μL of KCM and triturate them using a yellow tip, the pipette being adjusted to 100 μL, until they are a single-cell suspension (filter them and verify their viability and that they are a suspension of single cells by the method of stage 6 in Subheading 3.1). If it is critical to know that the final experiment is not contaminated by any ureteric bud cells carried over with this mesenchyme, keep a sample of the suspension and either immunostain it for a ureteric bud marker such as calbindin-D28K or use RT-PCR.
7. Optional: If the mesenchymal component of the final re-aggregate needs to be chimeric, add test cells to the suspension of mesenchymal cells now.
8. Pellet the mesenchyme cells and recover the pellet using steps 9 and 10 of Subheading 3.1; use about 10^5 cells per re-aggregate.
9. Recover the UB donor culture from the incubator, gently scrape it off its filter in KCM using a 25-gauge needle, and under a dissecting microscope, cut out "ureteric buds". (These can be distinguished from developing nephrons by their large diameter and branched shape. The easiest to cut out are those that are only just branched.) It is almost unavoidable that a few mesenchymal cells will come with the bud.
10. At the dissecting microscope, place one of these recovered "ureteric buds" on each filter of the Petri dish prepared in step 2. These are almost invisibly small when on a filter, so it helps to place them exactly in the middle of a hole in the underlying metal grid.
11. Pipette one re-aggregate of fresh mesenchyme, prepared in step 6, on top of the ureteric bud.
12. Incubate for as long as required (3–4 days typical), and fix and stain as in step 14 of Subheading 3.1 (Fig. 1).

3.3. The Brisbane Method

1. 24 h prior to setting up the re-aggregate, seed 5×10^4 *Wnt4*-expressing NIH3T3 cells in 50-μL droplet of culture medium onto a 0.4-μm polycarbonate filter (one filter per re-aggregate). Float seeded filters in 1 mL culture medium in a 4-well dish. Incubate at 37°C, 5% CO_2.
2. Dilute 100 μL concentrated collagen IV in 600 μL 0.65 N HCl. Pipette 100 μL diluted collagen IV onto a 0.4-μm

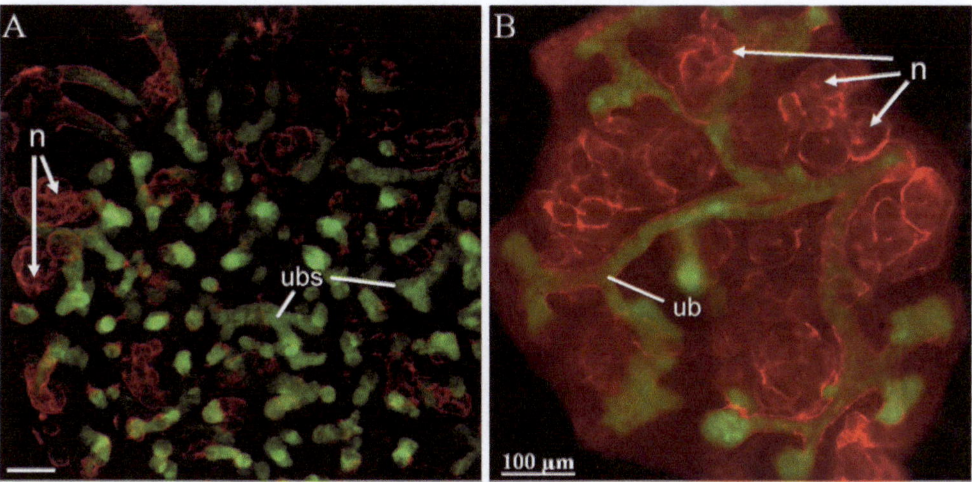

Fig. 1. (**A**) A re-aggregate produced by the basic Edinburgh method (Subheading 3.1) cultured for a total of 7 days and stained with anti-calbindin (*green*) and anti-laminin (*red*). Nephrons ("n") and numerous small "ureteric buds", some of which are branched, are visible ("ubs"). (**B**) A re-aggregate produced by the refined Edinburgh method (Subheading 3.2) and stained with anti-calbindin (*green*) and anti-laminin (*red*). Note how the arrangement of the tissues is much more like that of a normal embryonic kidney, with nephrons ("n") arranged around a single-branched ureteric bud ("ub"). Scale bar = 100 μm.

polycarbonate filter (one filter per re-aggregate). Incubate at room temperature for 1 h before washing in 1× PBS.

3. Harvest embryonic kidneys in dissection media, and allow three to four kidneys per re-aggregate.
4. Collect kidneys into a pile, remove all media, and roughly mince kidneys using a sterile scalpel blade.
5. Collect minced kidneys into 1 mL pre-warmed (37°C) Accutase. Digest in shaking water bath at 37°C for 15 min, manually pipetting fragments every 5 min to aid digestion.
6. Centrifuge kidneys at 300 rpm ($15 \times g$), 5 min.
7. Resuspend pellet in 500 μL pre-warmed (37°C) culture medium, manually dissociating with a P1000 pipette to single-cell suspension.
8. Pass cells through a 100-μm cell strainer to remove any remaining cellular clumps.
9. Count cells using haemocytometer (see Note 2).
10. If including labelled test cells in re-aggregate, harvest cells into culture medium and obtain cell count using haemocytometer.
11. Into a 15-mL tube, aliquot embryonic cells and the appropriate portion of test cells to give a final cell number of 4×10^5 cells in 600–700 μL culture medium. We usually would not add more than 10% test cells to a re-aggregation.

12. Centrifuge at 2,000 rpm (650 × *g*), 2 min.
13. Culture dish set-up: Into an organ culture dish, layer one piece of triangular mesh, one filter with feeder cells (feeder cells facing upwards), and one collagen IV-coated filter (collagen layer upwards). Add enough culture medium to just reach the level of the filters without making them too wet.
14. Using a P1000 pipette, carefully blow the re-aggregate off the side of the 15-mL tube and draw up into the pipette.
15. Carefully pipette the re-aggregate onto the top collagen IV filter. Let rest for 2–3 min and then top up the medium level so that the re-aggregate is at a media–air interface.
16. Culture for 4 days at 37°C, 5% CO_2.
17. Keeping re-aggregate on the collagen IV filter but discarding the filter seeded with feeder cells, fix in 4% paraformaldehyde for 10 min on ice, and then wash in 1× PBS for 5 min, twice.
18. Process re-aggregate into paraffin wax as described previously (8). Briefly pass tissue through an ascending ethanol series (15 min in each of 70, 80, 80, 90, 90, and 100% ethanol) followed by 2 × 20 min in xylene, and wax for 30 min at 60°C, 15 min at 60°C, twice.
19. Trim filter into square shape with 1–2-mm clearance around pellet using scalpel blade.
20. To embed, position filter/pellet on the smallest edge with pellet on the side such that pellet will be cut on sagittal plane.
21. Using microtome, cut into 7-μm sections using the remaining filter as a guide. Regular checking on a standard light microscope is necessary to determine the progress of sectioning.
22. After sectioning, sections can be stained and morphology assessed using standard histochemistry (haematoxylin and eosin or other stain) or assessed for contribution of test cells into re-aggregation via standard immunofluorescence with the desired antibodies. Our preferred options when using GFP-labelled test cells is anti-GFP with a marker of ureteric epithelium (calbindin D28K or Pax2; note that Pax2 also marks the cap mesenchyme and developing tubules), cap mesenchyme (Six2 or WT1; note that WT1 also marks early tubules and developing podocytes), basement membrane (pan-laminin; collagen IV), or a specific tubule marker (Aqp1 for proximal tubules) (Fig. 2).

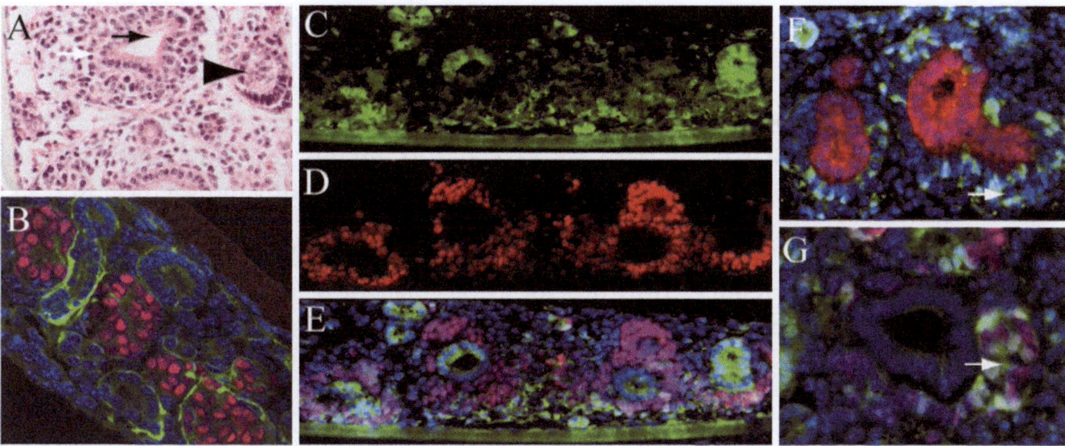

Fig. 2. Section analyses of chimeric re-aggregations. (**A**) Histological section of embryonic kidney re-aggregation showing evidence for a ureteric tip (*black arrow*), surrounding cap mesenchyme (*white arrow*) and developing nephron (*arrowhead*). (**B**) Immunofluorescence of embryonic kidney re-aggregation illustrating expression of WT1 (*red*; metanephric mesenchyme and developing nephrons) and pan-laminin (*green*; epithelial basement membranes). (**C–E**) Immunofluorescence of 50:50 re-aggregation between wild-type and GFP+embryonic kidney. GFP; *green*. WT1, *red*. (**F**, **G**) Re-aggregations of 50:50 wild-type embryonic kidney and cells FACS sorted from the embryonic kidneys of Sall1-GFP mice demonstrating the application of the method to test renal potential of an isolated cell population. Sall1GFP+cells (*white arrows*); *green*. (**F**) Calbindin D28K (ureteric epithelium), *red*. (**G**) WT1, *red*.

4. Notes

1. During the dissociation step (step 5 of Subheading 3.1), do not be too gentle. If the kidneys are not pipetted repeatedly and fast enough, they will stick to the pipette tip and the dissociation will be inefficient.
2. Do not leave the cells for too long in suspension. The longer the cells will stay in suspension, the more cell death will be observed.
3. Observe good sterile techniques to avoid culture contamination. Place metal grids and forceps in ethanol when they are not used, and sterilize them by burning the remaining ethanol covering them before use.
4. If cells are left too long in a microcentrifuge tube, they will start to attach to the walls of the tube and the centrifugation step will not be efficient. Mix the cell suspension before centrifugation.
5. After centrifugation, the pellet should have a nice round shape at the bottom of the tube. The line along the walls corresponds to the presence of cellular debris and can mean that the cells were dissociated too strongly or that they were left for a long time in suspension.

Acknowledgements

This work was supported by NC3Rs grant G0700480 and EU Star-t-Rek network FP7 223007 grants to J.A.D. and Australian Stem Cell Centre P067 and National Health and Medical Research Council of Australia ID631362 grants to M.H.L. M.H.L. is a Principal Research Fellow of the NHMRC. We thank Caroline Hendry, Institute for Molecular Bioscience, for assistance with Figures.

References

1. Unbekandt M, Davies JA (2010) Dissociation of embryonic kidneys followed by reaggregation allows the formation of renal tissues. Kidney Int 77:407–416
2. Lusis M, Li J, Ineson J et al (2010) Isolation of clonogenic, long-term self renewing embryonic renal stem cells. Stem Cell Res 5:23–39
3. Schmidt-Ott KM (2010) ROCK inhibition facilitates tissue reconstitution from embryonic kidney cell suspensions. Kidney Int 77: 387–389
4. Abraham J, Keller C (2010) Renal stem cell biology starts to take spherical shape. Commentary on: Lusis et al., Isolation of clonogenic, long-term self renewing embryonic renal stem cells. Stem Cell Res 5:1–3
5. Siegel N, Rosner M, Unbekandt M et al (2010) Contribution of human amniotic fluid stem cells to renal tissue formation depends on mTOR. Hum Mol Genet 19(17):3320–3331
6. Ganeva V, Unbekandt M, Davies JA (2011) An improved kidney dissociation and re aggregation culture system results in nephrons arranged organotypically around a single collecting duct system. Organogenesis 7:83–87
7. Davies JA (2010) The embryonic kidney: isolation, organ culture, immunostaining and RNA interference. Methods Mol Biol 633:57–69
8. Rumballe B, Georgas K, Little MH (2008) High-throughput paraffin section in situ hybridization and dual immunohistochemistry on mouse tissues. CSH Protoc Jul 1

Chapter 13

Analysis of Migration in Primary Ureteric Bud Epithelial Cells

Satu Kuure

Abstract

Kidney development has been widely used as a model system to study molecular control of inductive tissue interactions and mechanisms through which branching organs form. Due to lacking or poor methods, less focus has been in understanding details of cellular events that accomplish example ureteric bud (UB) branching. In order to form a branch point, cells need to proliferate, move in relation to each other, and change their shape as well as adhesive properties. In this chapter, detailed description is given how to set up primary UB epithelial cell cultures and study cell motility in these cells.

Key words: Kidney development, Ureteric bud, Primary epithelial cells, Migration, Scratch assay, Microdissection

1. Introduction

Kidney develops as a result of reciprocal inductive interactions between epithelial cells of Wolffian duct (WD; also called nephric duct)-derived ureteric bud (UB) and metanephric mesenchymal (MM) cells. In mouse, which is a widely used mammalian model organism for studies of organogenesis, UB forms around E10 when MM secretes signals that attract WD cells first to cluster and bulge on the area where MM resides (1, 2). Epithelial branching morphogenesis begins at E11 when an ampulla develops in the tip of the primary UB, which then half a day later gives rise to a T-shape bud (3). Similar bifurcation of the T-shape bud is reiterated throughout the development, as each UB gives rise to two new tips for about 10–11 cycles (4). From its very early bud stage (Fig. 1), UB is divided into subpopulations, the so-called tip and stalk domains, which are characterized by different gene expression patterns and cell proliferation rates (5–9). The majority of new branches are formed at the tips of UB while the stalk region potentially has the capability to branch at least in vitro (10, 11).

Odyssé Michos (ed.), *Kidney Development: Methods and Protocols*, Methods in Molecular Biology, vol. 886, DOI 10.1007/978-1-61779-851-1_13, © Springer Science+Business Media, LLC 2012

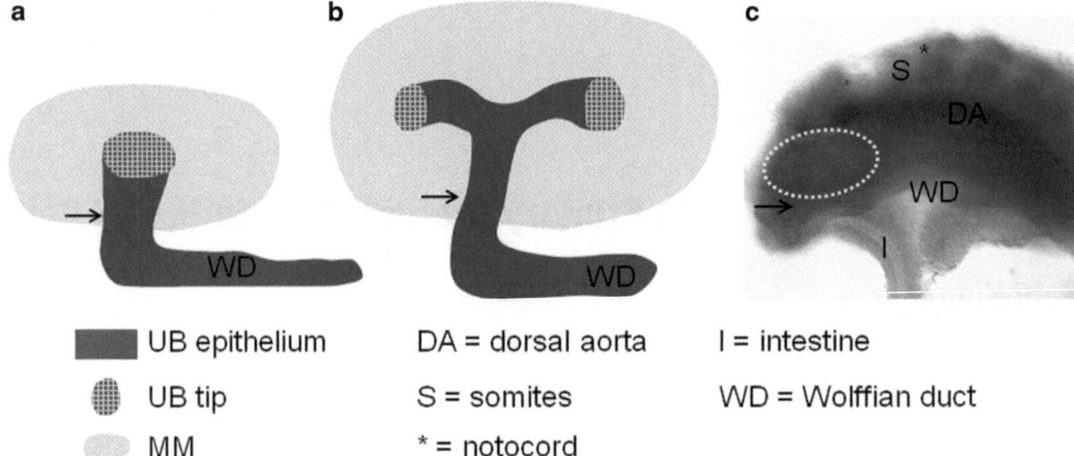

Fig. 1. Schematic illustration of an early ureteric bud (UB) morphology. (**a**) Bud-stage kidney at E10.5 shows that from its very early appearance the UB that has grown out from the Wolffian duct (WD) and invaded the metanephric mesenchyme (MM) is subdivided into tip (*lighter squared area*) and trunk (*arrow*) domains. (**b**) Branching morphogenesis begins by the formation of the so-called T-bud kidney, where UB has branched once to give rise two new tips. Tip–trunk subdomains within the UB epithelium are maintained in intact kidneys as long it grows. (**c**) Kidney primordium as indicated by *white dotted circle* beneath of dorsal aorta (DA), somites, and notochord, all of which run through the anterior–posterior body axis of an embryo.

Simultaneously to branching, the UB signals back to the MM to induce the development of nephrons, the functional units of kidney (1). Nephrogenesis is characterized by mesenchyme-to-epithelium transformation (MET), which takes place in the armpits of T-shape buds. First, MM condenses and then turns into nephron epithelium through a series of morphologically distinct steps (12). Therefore, UB branching is not only important for the growth and determination of organ shape, but it also instructs the final number of nephrons (13). Quite some knowledge on molecular control of UB branching has been accumulating during the past 10 years (14), but the cellular basis for branch point formation is less well understood (15).

The development of primary UB requires localized proliferation (8) and cell movements (2) within the epithelium itself. Proliferation keeps playing an important role when the UB invades the MM and starts its branching morphogenesis (8), but less is known how cell motility affects elongation and branch formation. Currently, genetic labeling of individual UB epithelial cells, or even cell clusters, is very challenging due to technical restrictions, and therefore following cell movements or migration in the living organ is very limited. Generation of chimeric embryos that express a genetic marker under the Hoxb7-promoter (16) only in a few UB cells (the so-called low chimeric embryos) can be used for studying cell movements by time-lapse imaging (11). Alternatively, as explained here, cell cultures obtained from UB epithelium (17) can be used for classical scratch assay to measure cells' motility (18).

The scratch assay is a straightforward and cheap method to study migration of cell populations in vitro (18). The basic idea is that cells in the confluent culture are challenged to move by creation of an artificial gap, the so-called scratch. The cells on the edge of the newly produced gap are activated, and start moving toward the opening to close the scratch. This movement/migration occurs until the edges meet again and the cells are able to establish new cell–cell contacts. Generally, the scratch assay is considered as a technique that requires relatively large amounts of cells due to confluence requirement, but as shown previously, it can be applied on small sample size as well (19).

Assaying UB epithelial cell motility involves setting up the UB cell cultures on fibronectin-coated plates, manual generation of the scratch, careful documentation of the cells' movements in time-lapse manner while they fill the gap produced by the scratch, and quantification of the migration rate. The most challenging and laborious step is to establish primary cell cultures, which involves dissection of early embryonic kidneys out of the abdominal cavity followed by separation of cell lineages from each other (20). Enzymatic treatment either with pancreatin–trypsin or collagenase eases microdissection of UBs free from mesenchymal cells, which can be further facilitated by using a transgenic mouse model to visualize UB lineages by the expression of fluorescent marker in these cells only (21, 22). In the conditions described below, isolated UBs adhere to the fibronectin-coated plastic to form a monolayer in approximately 48 h. UB cells in these cultures do not proliferate but survive approximately 2 weeks (19). Potential MM cell contamination in the cultures is not fundamentally critical for setting up homogenous UB cell cultures as mesenchymal cells die off due to loss of inductive capacity of UB cells in monolayer (23).

In conclusion, the scratch assay on primary UB epithelial cells is a relatively crude but inexpensive method to study the ability of epithelial cells to move. This system is particularly useful for comparing the motility between cells from different origin, e.g., those derived from mutant versus wild-type kidneys (19), but it can also be further developed for other types of applications.

2. Materials

2.1. Reagents and Tools for Dissections

1. E11–E12 mouse embryos.
2. Small scissors and fine forceps (see Note 1).
3. Glass or plastic dishes (100, 60, and 30 mm).
4. Stereomicroscope (for example, Leica MZ7.5 or Olympus SZ x9).

5. Needles (Tungsten needles, 22- or 25-gauge disposable injection needles with syringes).
6. 70% Ethanol (EtOH), diluted in ddH_2O.
7. Dulbecco's PBS (with Ca^{2+} and Mg^{2+}) (see Note 2).
8. DMEM/F12 supplemented with 10% fetal bovine serum (FBS).
9. Collagenase (200 mg/mL stock in phosphate-buffered solution (PBS)).
10. DNase I.

2.2. Cell Culture Reagents

1. PBS, cell culture grade.
2. 0.2% bovine serum albumin (BSA) in PBS.
3. Fibronectin (1 mg/mL stock in PBS).
4. 24-multi-well plates.
5. Culture medium: DMEM/F12 supplemented with 10% FBS, 1× penicillin–streptomycin, and 1× L-glutamine.
6. GDNF (recombinant rat, R&D Systems).
7. HGF (recombinant human, Sigma-Aldrich).
8. FGF2 (recombinant human, Sigma-Aldrich).
9. Drummond Wiretrol 10 μL, capillaries, and delivery plunger.
10. Small pipette tips.
11. Inverted microscope with camera.

3. Methods

As mentioned earlier, the most difficult step in setting up the primary UB cultures is isolation of UBs free of MM from newly dissected kidney rudiments. Embryonic kidneys at E11–E11.5 are relatively small and potentially challenging to identify (Fig. 1). By E12, the organ rudiments become more apparent and therefore their recognition is easier, but at the same time the isolation of UB unfortunately becomes slightly more complicated. Another issue that affects the choice of embryonic stage of the samples is the fact that the early-phase UBs (E11–E11.5) that are at bud or T-bud phase (Fig. 1), respectively, contain fewer cells and accordingly give rise to smaller cultures than the several branches of UBs at the later stages. Therefore, the balance between dissection skills and sample material amount actually dictates the stage of kidneys used for establishing the UB cell cultures. The most important parameter for steady experimental setup is, however, an equal amount of starting material, the ureteric buds, in order to reliably compare migration in different samples.

3.1. Collecting Embryonic Kidneys

1. Euthanize pregnant mouse, spray its belly with 70% EtOH, cut out the uterus with E11–E12.5 embryos, and place it in a 100-mm petri dish containing Dulbecco's PBS.
2. Open the uterus by holding it still with forceps and simultaneously incising with scissors.
3. Tease embryos out and rip them free of extraembryonic tissues with thin forceps.
4. Cut the embryo with needles below the fore limbs, and remove intestine and everything above it (see Notes 3 and 4) to get good access to the developing kidney.
5. Dissect kidneys out from the body by first removing the spinal cord, then turning the embryo to lie on the back, and finally gently removing the remaining body walls. Once the kidneys are separated, dissect away extra-renal tissues as much as possible and place kidneys on ice in Dulbecco's PBS (see Note 5).

3.2. Separation of UB and Setup of Primary UB Epithelial Cell Culture

1. Treat kidneys with 4 mg/mL collagenase by incubating them at 37°C for 15 min (see Note 6).
2. Stop collagenase reaction with 25 u/mL DNase I in DMEM/F12 + 10% FBS and let them rest for 10–15 min at 37°C.
3. Separate UBs free of MM with needles by gently scraping mesenchyme away (see Note 7). Penetrate the mesenchyme with your needles at the stalk region of UB (the portion of UB that is closest to the Wolffian duct), and then remove MM by pushing it away from the epithelium moving toward UB tips. E12 kidneys have more complex UB tree, and therefore it is easier to access UBs from tip direction rather than via stalk (see Notes 8 and 9).
4. Place isolated UBs in the middle of fibronectin-coated plate (see Notes 10 and 11) already containing culture medium supplemented with GDNF (5 ng/mL), FGF2 (25 ng/mL), and HGF (50 ng/mL). All buds should be close to each other in order to form a single monolayer culture.
5. Take the 24-multi-well plate to cell culture incubator paying extra careful attention not to move easily floating UBs all over the well (see Note 12).
6. Let the UBs settle and adhere for 42–48 h during which they form monolayer cultures (Fig. 2 and see Note 13).

3.3. Scratch Assay and Analysis of Results

1. With 10-μL pipette tip edge, make a scratch across the circular epithelial cell culture (see Note 14). Change tip between the wells to avoid cross contamination of cells.
2. Take photographs immediately after creation of the scratch (start point), and then at chosen time points (for example, 3, 8, and 20 h) (see Note 15).

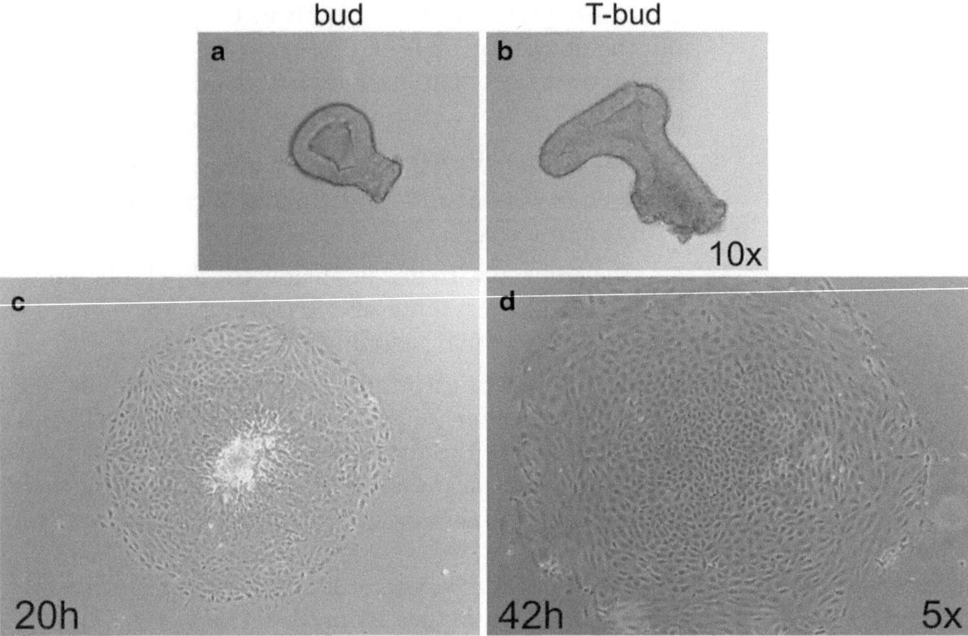

Fig. 2. Establishment of ureteric bud epithelial cell cultures. Morphology of isolated ureteric bud at (**a**) bud (E10.5) and (**b**) early T-bud (E11) stages. When isolated, UBs are placed on fibronectin-coated plates they adhere to the surface and start to form a spherical monolayer culture. (**c**) In 20 h, most of the cells have already formed a monolayer while some still remain in tightly packed, tube-like structures as observed in the middle of the culture (*a bright spot*). (**d**) Circular monolayer of UB epithelial cells is established 42 h after plating of isolated ureteric bud.

3. At the end of the culture, cells can be fixed for antibody staining or other purposes (see Note 16).
4. Analyze the migration in different samples by measuring the gaps at each time point with, for example, ImageJ software (for free downloads, check http://rsbweb.nih.gov/ij/).
5. To give numerical value (in percent) for how much the initial gap has shrunk at certain time point (the so-called gap remaining—value), divide the width at a given time point by the initial gap width and multiply it with hundred. Gap filled—value describes how large proportion of the initial gap is filled in certain time and can be calculated by subtracting gap remaining percentage from 100%.

4. Notes

1. Use always clean, sterile dissection tools to avoid possible microbe contamination.
2. Instead of Dulbecco's PBS, dissections can be also done in CO_2-independent medium.

3. While dissecting the kidneys, keep all other embryos, except the one you are working with, on ice.
4. E11–E12.5 kidneys are located bilaterally on the dorsal midline, ventral to the neural tube and somites, at the level of the hind limbs.
5. If studying kidneys of genetically modified mouse lines, store and treat kidneys pairwise from now on, for example by placing them in 24-multi-well plates.
6. 1–2 mL of collagenase is enough for treating dozens of early kidney rudiments, as it is enough just to cover the samples with collagenase. Pipette collagenase on dry, clean 30-mm dish so that it forms a nice drop. Then, add and remove the kidneys for treatment with the help of a Wiretrol glass capillary. When dealing with kidneys on 24-multi-well plates (see previous note), it is better to add and remove the solution rather than move around the kidneys.
7. Before starting the actual isolation of UBs, it is pivotal to clearly perceive where the UB runs within the MM. The earlier the kidney is, the easier it is to spot the UB epithelium, which appears as a bright bud- or T-bud-shaped tube at E10.5–E11 (Figs. 1 and 2a, b).
8. It is very important that the relative amount or the number of UBs employed in setting up the culture is the same, or as close as possible, between the samples in order to establish comparable cultures for scratch assay.
9. If needed, it is possible to set up the culture with UB tips only, but this generates fewer cells and is therefore recommended only for E11.5 or older kidneys.
10. Fibronectin-coated plates can be purchased and used according to the manufacturer's instructions. Remember to warm up ready-made plates at least 30 min prior to use.
11. Homemade fibronectin coating is cheaper than the commercial plates and easy to do: incubate 10 μg/mL fibronectin on each well of 24-multi-well plates for 1 h at room temperature or alternatively for 30 min at 37°C. Then, wash with 0.2% BSA 3×15 min at 37°C, add culture medium, and the plates are ready to use.
12. Once the UBs are placed on fibronectin, it takes them a few hours to adhere on the surface. Be extra careful when moving the plates right after UB plating because UBs float easily at this point, and if they end up adhering to the edges of the well it is impossible to observe and document their behavior later during the experiment.
13. It is good to observe the UB cultures once per day during the first 48 h to get an idea where on the well they are settling.

If studying UBs from different genetic background, it may also be useful to take pictures in order to get an idea of potential differences in their adhesive properties.

14. Similar scratch width in every UB epithelial cell culture is pivotal for quantification of migration rate. Hold pipette tip at about a 45° angle and press firmly but not too hard while sliding the tip steadily across the culture. It is advisable to make few test scratches on the empty wells before performing the actual experiment to get an idea how the fibronectin-coated surface feels in your hands and to see the width of scratch created.
15. Wild-type UB epithelial cells typically close the gap produced by the scratch in 20–24 h.
16. Instead of, or in addition to, scratch assay, UB epithelial cells can be studied with antibody staining. For this, samples are easier to handle and observe with a microscope if the cultures are established on fibronectin-coated coverslips rather than 24-multi-well plates.

References

1. Saxen L (1987) Organogenesis of the kidney. Cambridge University Press, Cambridge
2. Chi X, Michos O, Shakya R et al (2009) Ret-dependent cell rearrangements in the Wolffian duct epithelium initiate ureteric bud morphogenesis. Dev Cell 17:199–209
3. Airik R, Kispert A (2007) Down the tube of obstructive nephropathies: the importance of tissue interactions during ureter development. Kidney Int 72:1459–1467
4. Cebrian C, Borodo K, Charles N, Herzlinger DA (2004) Morphometric index of the developing murine kidney. Dev Dyn 231:601–608
5. Lin Y, Zhang S, Rehn M et al (2001) Induced repatterning of type XVIII collagen expression in ureter bud from kidney to lung type: association with sonic hedgehog and ectopic surfactant protein C. Development 128:1573–1585
6. Carroll TJ, Park JS, Hayashi S, Majumdar A, McMahon AP (2005) Wnt9b plays a central role in the regulation of mesenchymal to epithelial transitions underlying organogenesis of the Mammalian urogenital system. Dev Cell 9:283–292
7. Kispert A, Vainio S, Shen L, Rowitch DH, McMahon AP (1996) Proteoglycans are required for maintenance of Wnt-11 expression in the ureter tips. Development 122: 3627–3637
8. Michael L, Davies JA (2004) Pattern and regulation of cell proliferation during murine ureteric bud development. J Anat 204:241–255
9. Michael L, Sweeney DE, Davies JA (2007) The lectin Dolichos biflorus agglutinin is a sensitive indicator of branching morphogenetic activity in the developing mouse metanephric collecting duct system. J Anat 210:89–97
10. Sweeney D, Lindstrom N, Davies JA (2008) Developmental plasticity and regenerative capacity in the renal ureteric bud/collecting duct system. Development 135:2505–2510
11. Watanabe T, Costantini F (2004) Real-time analysis of ureteric bud branching morphogenesis in vitro. Dev Biol 271:98–108
12. Quaggin SE, Kreidberg JA (2008) Development of the renal glomerulus: good neighbors and good fences. Development 135:609–620
13. Schedl A (2007) Renal abnormalities and their developmental origin. Nat Rev Genet 8: 791–802
14. Costantini F, Kopan R (2010) Patterning a complex organ: branching morphogenesis and nephron segmentation in kidney development. Dev Cell 18:698–712
15. Nigam SK, Shah MM (2009) How does the ureteric bud branch? J Am Soc Nephrol 20: 1465–1469
16. Kuure S, Chi X, Lu B, Costantini F (2010) The transcription factors Etv4 and Etv5 mediate formation of the ureteric bud tip domain during kidney development. Development 137: 1975–1979
17. Ye P, Habib SL, Ricono JM et al (2004) Fibronectin induces ureteric bud cells branching

and cellular cord and tubule formation. Kidney Int 66:1356–1364

18. Liang CC, Park AY, Guan JL (2007) In vitro scratch assay: a convenient and inexpensive method for analysis of cell migration in vitro. Nat Protoc 2:329–333
19. Kuure S, Cebrian C, Machingo Q et al (2010) Actin depolymerizing factors cofilin1 and destrin are required for ureteric bud branching morphogenesis. PLoS Genet 6:e1001176
20. Saxen L, Lehtonen E (1978) Transfilter induction of kidney tubules as a function of the extent and duration of intercellular contacts. J Embryol Exp Morphol 47:97–109
21. Srinivas S, Goldberg MR, Watanabe T et al (1999) Expression of green fluorescent protein in the ureteric bud of transgenic mice: a new tool for the analysis of ureteric bud morphogenesis. Dev Genet 24:241–251
22. Chi X, Hadjantonakis AK, Wu Z, Hyink D, Costantini F (2009) A transgenic mouse that reveals cell shape and arrangement during ureteric bud branching. Genesis 47: 61–66
23. Barasch J, Pressler L, Connor J, Malik A (1996) A ureteric bud cell line induces nephrogenesis in two steps by two distinct signals. Am J Physiol 271:F50–F61

Chapter 14

Investigating Primary Cilia in Cultured Metanephric Mesenchymal Cells

Lijun Chi and Norman Rosenblum

Abstract

Primary cilia are present in most vertebrate cells. They have complex structures that are required for signal transduction in developing tissues. The embryonic kidney consists of two major cell lineages, ureteric and metanephric mesenchyme. Here, we describe a method to isolate metanephric mesenchyme from ureteric bud, culture metanephric mesenchyme cells, and study primary cilia in cell culture.

Key words: Primary cilia, Kidney, Metanephric mesenchyme, Ureteric epithelium, Primary cell culture, Immunofluorescence

1. Introduction

Primary cilia are present in most vertebrate cells (1, 2). Primary cilia are generated and maintained by the conserved mechanism of intraflagellar transport (IFT), which is essential for signal transduction in many developing tissues (3–5). Genetic studies demonstrated that primary cilia are crucial for Hedgehog (HH) signaling (6), and may be involved in Planar Cell Polarity (PCP) (7, 8). Mutations in genes whose protein products are located in the primary cilium are important in the pathogenesis of autosomal and recessive forms of Polycystic Kidney Diseases (PKD), including Nephronophthesis which can involve the retina, cerebellum, and limbs in addition to the kidney (2, 9, 10). Development of methods for investigating the primary cilium has potential value in the understanding of its structure and function during organogenesis. Here, we developed a technique for visualizing primary cilia in the isolated and cultured metanephric mesenchyme (MM) cells from embryonic day 11.5 (E11.5) mouse kidney, which is the main malformation organ in the cilia protein dysfunction during development. After considering whether the cells have 90% confluence in

Odyssé Michos (ed.), *Kidney Development: Methods and Protocols*, Methods in Molecular Biology, vol. 886, DOI 10.1007/978-1-61779-851-1_14, © Springer Science+Business Media, LLC 2012

the culture dish, we use antibody against acetylated α-tubulin to detect the primary cilia in the MM cells. This model is applied in our laboratory and can be used for further studies of the roles of primary cilia.

2. Materials

2.1. Dissection of Mouse Kidney Tissue

1. Pregnant mouse (E11.5) (see Note 1).
2. Straight dissecting forceps (length 110 mm).
3. Curved forceps (length 120 mm).
4. Straight scissors (length 140 mm).
5. Glass dissection plate (60 mm) (see Note 2).
6. Tissue culture dish (35 mm).
7. Fine needle (30-gauge 1/2).
8. Syringe (1 mL).
9. Syringe filter (0.22 mm).

2.2. Equipment

1. Dissection microscope (e.g., Leica MZ10F).
2. 37°C water bath.
3. Tissue culture incubator 37°C, 5% CO_2.
4. Tissue culture hood.
5. Microscope cover glass.
6. Confocal microscope with proper lasers (e.g., Olympus).

2.3. Cell Culture Dishes

1. Tissue culture dish (35 mm).
2. Cell culture dish (12 well).
3. 2 Chamber tissue culture glass slide (BD Falcon™, 354112).

2.4. Reagents, Solutions, and Antibodies

1. 70% Ethanol.
2. Methanol, precooled at −20°C.
3. 1× PBS, pH 7.4.
4. 25% pancreatin, store at +4°C: 0.25 g pancreatin, 0.17 g NaCl in 20-mL volume with sterile H_2O (see Note 3).
5. Tyrode's solution: 8 g NaCl, 0.2 g KCl, 0.05 g NaH_2PO_4, 1 g glucose, 1 g $NaHCO_3$ in 1 L of sterile H_2O (see Note 4).
6. 2.5% pancreatin–trypsin: 0.450 g trypsin, 2 mL 25% pancreatin, 18 mL Tyrode's solution. Aliquot into 0.5 mL, and store at −20°C (see Note 5).
7. DMEM (high glucose), store at 4°C.

8. Fetal bovine serum (FBS), store at –20°C.
9. Penicillin–streptomycin solution stabilized (P4333, Sigma), store at –20°C.
10. Collagenase B (11088807001, Roche), store at 4°C.
11. 0.25% trypsin-EDTA, store at 4°C.
12. Blocking buffer: 2% BSA (stock: 30% BSA), 5% goat serum, 1% Tween 20 in PBS.
13. Acetylated α-tubulin antibody (1:1,000, Sigma, T6793).
14. Anti-KIF3A antibody (1:100, Sigma, K3513).
15. Alexa Fluor® 488 goat anti-rabbit IgG and Alexa Fluor® 546 goat anti-mouse IgG (1:1,000, Molecular Probes, Invitrogen).
16. DAPI (Sigma, D9564).
17. Vectashield Hard Set mounting medium (VECTOR, H-1400).

3. Methods

To prevent contamination, all solutions, tools, and equipment in contact with kidney tissue and living cells must be sterile. Metanephric kidneys (E11.5) are dissected in PBS. The culture system is demonstrated in Fig. 1.

3.1. Metanephric Mesenchyme Isolation

1. Kidneys are dissected from embryos isolated from pregnant mice at embryonic day 11.5 (Fig. 2d) (11, 12).
2. Transfer and incubate kidneys in 2.5% pancreatin–trypsin in Tyrode's solution for 1 min at room temperature (13) (see Note 6).
3. Remove kidneys and place in DMEM containing 10% FCS to stop the enzyme activation, and maintain them in holding medium from 20 min to 2 h.

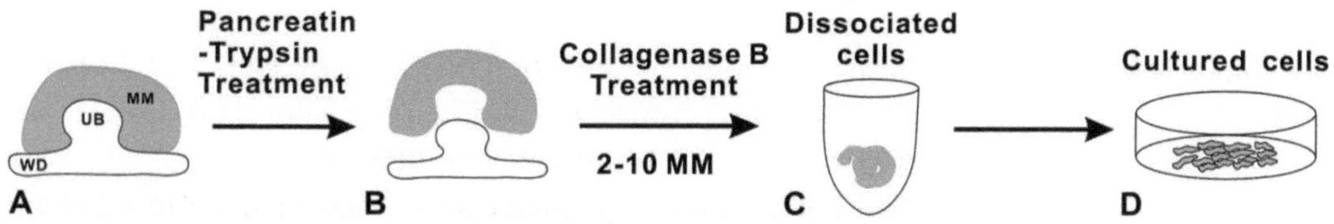

Fig.1. Metanephric mesenchyme cell culture system. (**a**) The ureteric bud (UB) and metanephric mesenchyme (MM) constitute the mouse embryonic kidney at E10.5–E11.0. (**b**) The UB can be separated from the MM by pancreatin–trypsin enzyme treatment. (**c**) Dissociating MM cells in Collagenase B. (**d**) The metanephric mesenchymal cells are cultured in a Petri dish.

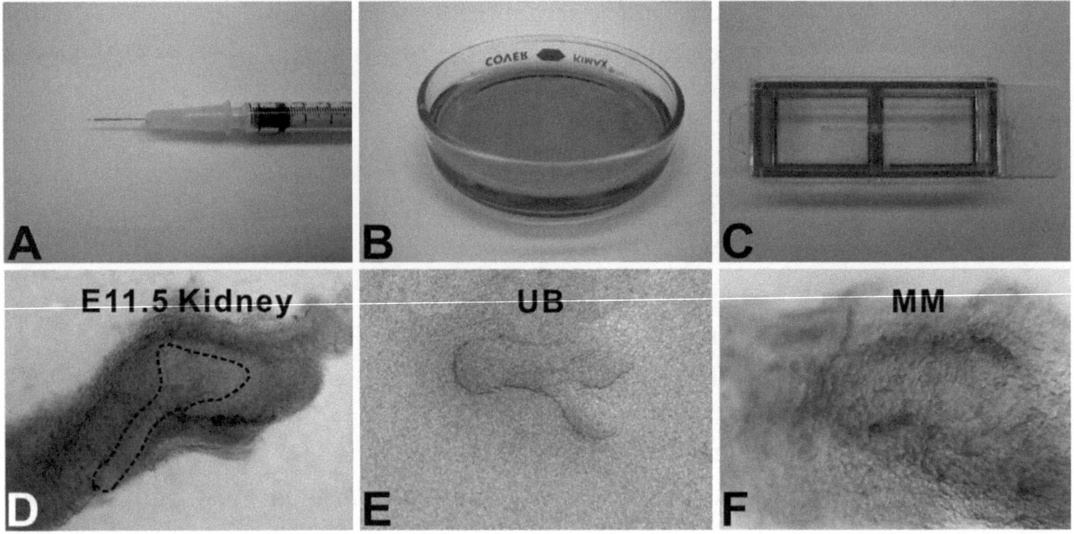

Fig. 2. Dissection tools and kidney. (**a**) Fine needle with syringe. (**b**) Glass plate containing DMEM. (**c**) Two-chamber Cell Culture Glass Slide. (**d**) Kidney at E11.5; *dotted line* indicates the ureteric bud and ureteric stalk. (**e**) Ureteric bud isolated from kidney at E11.5. (**f**) MM separated from kidney at E11.5.

4. Using two sterilized fine needles with syringe (Fig. 2a), gently separate metanephric mesenchyme (Fig. 2f) away from the ureteric bud (Fig. 2e) in DMEM in a glass dissection plate (Fig. 2b).

3.2. Dissociation of MM

1. Collect MMs (e.g., ten) into a 1.5-mL microcentrifugue tube and then dissociate MM cells in Collagenase B (10 mg/mL, in Tyrode's solution) for 10 min at 37°C.
2. Mechanically dissociate cells by gentle aspiration by repeated pipetting.
3. Add 200 μL DMEM + 10% FBS to stop the digestion and centrifuge at <1000 × *g* for 10 min. Add another 200 μL DMEM + 10% FCS and centrifuge for 5 min at <1000 × *g*, and then aspirate supernatant.

3.3. Culture of MM Cells

1. Resuspend cells in 300 μL DMEM with 10% FBS and 0.5% penicillin–streptomycin solution (penicillin 100 U/mL and streptomycin 0.1 mg/mL), and mix gently.
2. Add 100 μL of resuspended cells to each chamber in a 2 chamber Cell Culture Glass Slide (Fig. 2c) and in one well of a 12-multi-well plate. Then, add 400 μL DMEM to each cell aliquot.
3. Incubate cells at 37°C for 2 days (48–72 h) (Fig. 3a, c) before further manipulation.

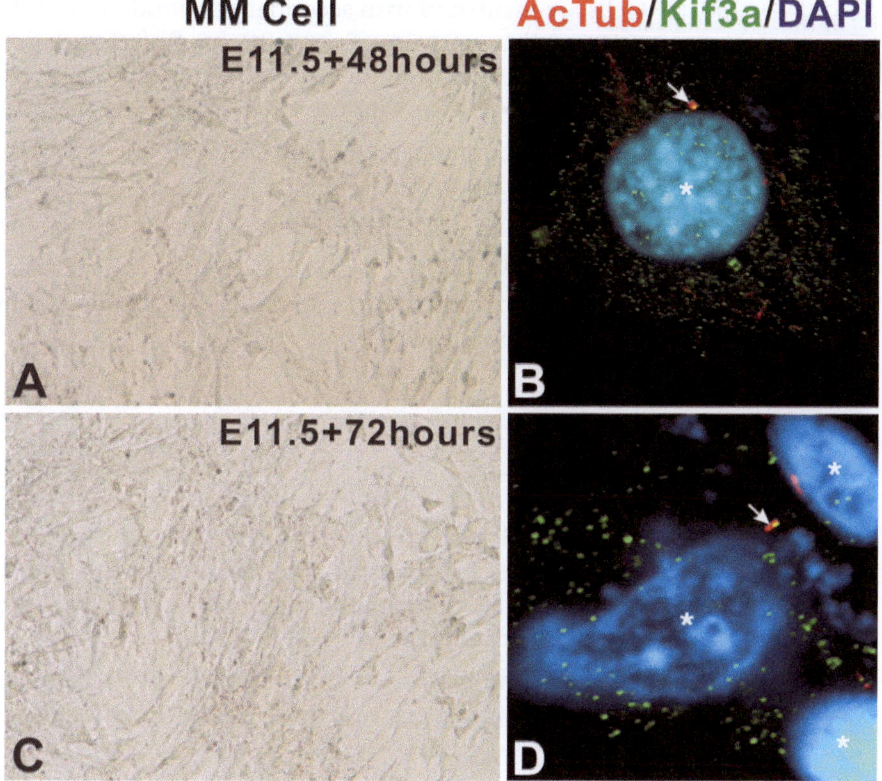

Fig. 3. MM cell culture and imaging of primary cilia. (**a–c**) E11.5 MM cells were cultured for 48 or 72 h and imaged by light microscopy. (**b–d**) KIF3A co-localizes with acetylated tubulin in primary cilia (*arrows*); nuclei are stained with DAPI (*asterisk*).

3.4. Immuno-fluorescence Imaging of Primary Cilia in Culture MM Cells

Following MM cell culture, the cell density needs to be evaluated. The desired cell confluence is 50–60% at 48 h and 70–80% at 72 h (Fig. 3a, c).

Immunofluorescence staining procedure is as follows.

1. MM cells grown on the glass slide are fixed in cold methanol (-20°C) for 10 min at room temperature.
2. After fixation, cells are washed with PBS twice for 10 min per wash. Next, blocking buffer (2% BSA, 5% goat serum, 1% Tween-20 in PBS) is added to cells for 30 min in a humidified chamber at room temperature.
3. Cells are incubated with primary antibodies in 1% BSA, 2.5% goat serum, and 1% Tween-20 in PBS at the following concentrations overnight at 4°C: acetylated α-tubulin (1:1,000), anti-KIF3A (1:100).
4. Cells are washed in 0.2% BSA, 0.5% goat serum, and 0.1% Tween-20 in PBS twice.

5. Cells are incubated with secondary antibodies in 1% BSA, 2.5% goat serum, and 1% Tween-20 in PBS for 1 h at room temperature: Alexa Fluor® 488 goat anti-rabbit IgG and Alexa Fluor® 546 goat anti-mouse IgG (1:500).
6. Cells are counterstained with DAPI (1 μg/mL) to visualize nuclear chromatin.
7. After washing with PBS, glass coverslips are mounted with mounting medium.
8. Images are obtained with a Spinning Disk Confocal Microscope with appropriate lasers (Fig. 3b, d).

4. Notes

1. All protocols and procedures for the humane treatment of live animals must be observed at all times. Consult your local animal facility for guidelines and regulations for the care and use of laboratory animals.
2. All metal and glass tools must be autoclaved. All reagents and solutions must be sterile and aseptic technique should be used.
3. After making the 25% pancreatin, stir the solution for 3–4 h at room temperature and then overnight at 4°C. Next day, centrifuge for 10 min at 5,000 rpm for 10 min, sterile filtrate the supernatant, and aliquot for storage at −20°C.
4. After dissolution of Tyrode's solution, sterile filter with a 0.22 mm Millipore filter and store at room temperature.
5. Dissolve the trypsin by drawing the solution into and out of a pipette. Keep the solution ON ICE to decrease activation of the enzyme. A pH of 7.4 is important because variance of the pH from 7.4 can adversely affect the effectiveness of digestion.
6. The time of treatment in pancreas-trypsin is critical. We found that a treatment time of 1 min in 2.5% pancreas-trypsin at room temperature permits easy separation of the metanephric mesenchyme and ureteric bud.

References

1. Scholey JM, Anderson KV (2006) Intraflagellar transport and cilium-based signaling. Cell 125(3):439–442
2. Gerdes JM, Davis EE, Katsanis N (2009) The vertebrate primary cilium in development, homeostasis, and disease. Cell 137(1):32–45
3. Goetz SC, Anderson KV (2010) The primary cilium: a signalling centre during vertebrate development. Nat Rev Genet 11(5):331–344
4. Lancaster MA, Gleeson JG (2009) The primary cilium as a cellular signaling center: lessons from disease. Curr Opin Genet Dev 19(3):220–229

5. Silverman MA, Leroux MR (2009) Intraflagellar transport and the generation of dynamic, structurally and functionally diverse cilia. Trends Cell Biol 19(7):306–316
6. Huangfu D, Liu A, Rakeman AS et al (2003) Hedgehog signalling in the mouse requires intraflagellar transport proteins. Nature 426(6962):83–87
7. Ross AJ, May-Simera H, Eichers ER et al (2005) Disruption of Bardet-Biedl syndrome ciliary proteins perturbs planar cell polarity in vertebrates. Nat Genet 37(10): 1135–1140
8. Jones C, Roper VC, Foucher I et al (2008) Ciliary proteins link basal body polarization to planar cell polarity regulation. Nat Genet 40(1):69–77
9. Pazour GJ (2004) Intraflagellar transport and cilia-dependent renal disease: the ciliary hypothesis of polycystic kidney disease. J Am Soc Nephrol 15(10):2528–2536
10. Baker K, Beales PL (2009) Making sense of cilia in disease: the human ciliopathies. Am J Med Genet C Semin Med Genet 151C(4):281–295
11. Barak H, Boyle SC (2011) Organ culture and immunostaining of mouse embryonic kidneys. Cold Spring Harb Protoc: pdb prot5558
12. Sakai T, Onodera T (2008) Embryonic organ culture. Curr Protoc Cell Biol Chapter 19:Unit 19 18
13. Kispert A, Vainio S, Shen L, Rowitch DH, McMahon AP (1996) Proteoglycans are required for maintenance of Wnt-11 expression in the ureter tips. Development 122(11):3627–3637

Chapter 15

Making Immortalized Cell Lines from Embryonic Mouse Kidney

Guanping Tai, Peter Hohenstein, and Jamie A. Davies

Abstract

Immortalized cell lines derived from embryonic mouse kidneys are useful tools for exploring signaling pathways, morphogenetic mechanisms, and gene function in renal development: they also provide a means for efficient first-round screening of panels of small molecules intended to combat renal pathologies such as the development of cysts, and such cell line-based screening can allow a valuable reduction in the numbers of animals needed for a given line of research. This chapter presents a simple method for generating cell lines from the "Immortomouse," which carries a temperature-sensitive SV40 antigen, under the control of an interferon-regulated promoter.

Key words: Kidney, Ureteric bud, Metanephric mesenchyme, SV40, Immortomouse, 3Rs

1. Introduction

Transgenic knockout mice, and the various techniques for renal organ culture explained elsewhere in this volume, provide powerful methods for manipulating gene function in the context of a whole developing kidney. They have been largely responsible for our current understanding of renal development (1–6). There are studies, though, for which whole-organ experiments are inappropriate. Biochemical measurement of the protein phosphorylation response to activation of a signaling pathway, for example, is easier when only one cell type is present. For studies like this, it is very helpful to have a cell line that represents the cell type of interest and that can be grown in flasks to very large numbers. Cell lines that represent particular components in the developing kidney also show great promise for high-throughout screens for the ability of small molecules to affect cell behavior. This screening might be for basic research in identifying important signaling proteins or for applied research in identifying drugs able to interfere with pathways

Odyssé Michos (ed.), *Kidney Development: Methods and Protocols*, Methods in Molecular Biology, vol. 886, DOI 10.1007/978-1-61779-851-1_15, © Springer Science+Business Media, LLC 2012

that cause cystic disease, for example. Performing such screens in whole animals would both be very expensive, financially and ethically, and very slow compared to rapid screening in cell culture.

It is difficult to raise cell lines from the kidneys of wild-type mouse embryos, possibly because each cell type requires survival signals from another (7). This problem can be mitigated by immortalizing cells artificially. A straightforward approach to this, and one that is safer than using vectors capable of immortalizing any cell they transfect, is to begin with kidneys of the Immortomouse strain (8). This mouse expresses a temperature-sensitive version of the SV40 large T antigen under the control of an interferon-inducible promoter. Both interferon and temperature can, therefore, be used to modulate SV40-based immortalizing activity. Cells isolated from such a mouse can be grown in culture at 33°C with gamma-interferon (IFN-γ) and sub-cloned into separate lines.

It is important to note that cell lines produced in this way, while showing many of the properties of their parent tissues, are not exactly the same as them because they are selected for genetic and epigenetic changes that facilitate growth in culture. Many of the cell lines we have made, for example, express correct sets of markers and show responses to signals in the manner of their cell type of origin, but they will not reintegrate properly into a disaggregation/reaggregation culture system (9). The limitation is also true for the widely used mouse kidney cell lines M15, mIMCD3, and MDCK. Nonetheless, such cell lines can be excellent models for morphogenesis and cell signaling.

2. Materials

2.1. Hardware

1. CO_2 incubator capable of running at 33°C, and one running at 37°C (see Note 1).
2. Dissection microscope (we use a Zeiss Stemi 2000).
3. Fine forceps.
4. Syringe needles (BD Microlace-3 25-gauge 0.5 × 16 mm) and 1.0-mL disposable syringes for dissection (these needles are good dissecting instruments and are cheap enough to be discarded when blunt).
5. Cloning cylinders, glass.
6. Dow Corning® high-vacuum silicone grease (Z273554-1EA, Sigma).
7. Cell culture dishes.
8. T-25 tissue culture flasks.
9. 6-multi-well cell culture plates.
10. 24-multi-well cell culture plates.

2.2. Animals

1. H-2Kb tsA58 transgenic immortal mice (8).

2.3. Media

1. Coating solution: 2% solution of Matrigel (BD biosciences) in ice-cold 1:1 DMEM/F12 (see Note 2). Make this freshly each day.
2. Dissecting medium: Dulbecco's modified Eagle's medium (DMEM).
3. Separation medium: 2 u/mL Dispase II in dissecting medium. This remains active for about 2 weeks at 4°C.
4. Disaggregation solution: 1× Trypsin-EDTA.
5. Immortalization medium: 1:1 mix of DMEM/F12 with 10% heat-inactivated fetal bovine serum, IFN-γ 100 u/mL (ProSpecBio cyt-358), 1% ITS supplement (Sigma I2521—i.e., a final 1 in 100 dilution of the manufacturer's stock: this supplement contains 1 mg/mL insulin, 0.55 mg/mL human transferrin, and 0.5 μg/mL sodium selenite), 1× glutamine, 1× penicillin/streptomycin (these last three coming from a single stock solution, Invitrogen 10378016), and 1× antioxidants (Sigma A1345).
6. Enriched immortalization medium: Immortalization medium with a total of 200 u/mL IFN-γ, 2% ITS, and 2× antioxidants.
7. ROCK inhibitor medium: Immortalization medium with 10 μM Y-27632 (Sigma Y0503).

3. Methods

3.1. Initial Culture of Cells

1. Prepare culture dishes by placing 5 mL of coating solution in each and leaving them on a flat surface at room temperature for a few hours. Rinse in dissecting medium before use.
2. Isolate metanephric rudiments from mouse embryos by microdissection in dissecting medium. It is assumed that anyone reading this chapter will be familiar with a suitable technique for doing this and it would take up too much space to explain it here. Detailed guidance is available in a previous volume of this journal (10).
3. (*Optional*—see Note 3) Isolate the individual renal tissue of interest. For our work on E11.5 kidneys, we separate metanephric mesenchyme from ureteric bud by incubating kidney rudiments for 5–10 min in room temperature separation medium, and then gently pull the ureteric bud away from the mesenchyme using needles (Fig. 1); rinse in dissecting medium.

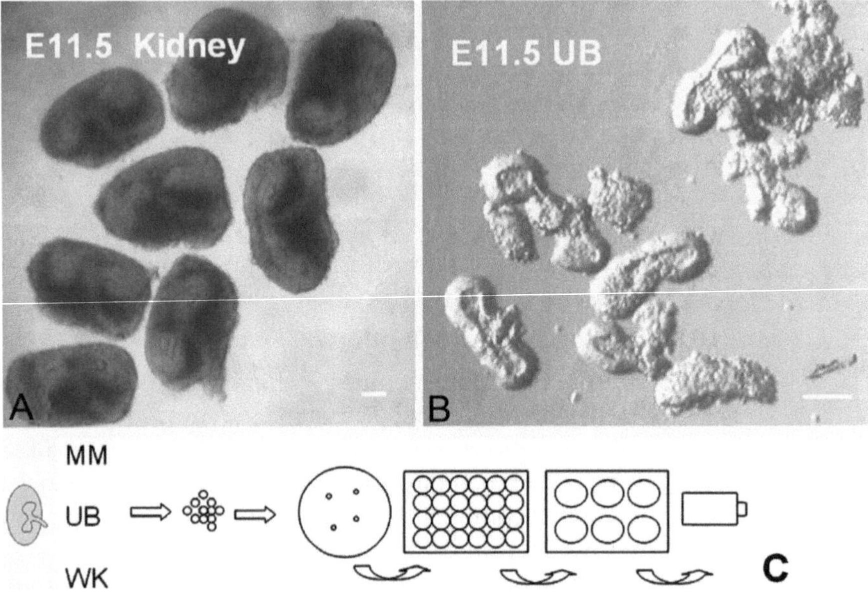

Fig. 1. Microdissection of E11.5 kidney. (**a**) At E11.5, the ureteric bud has made a "T shape" but no nephrons have formed. (**b**) Dispase digestion allows mesenchymes to be pulled away from ureteric buds (the buds being shown here, although there is some mesenchyme at the *top right* of the image). (**c**) A cartoon illustrating the sequence of events described in this chapter; *MM* metanephrogenic mesenchyme, *UB* ureteric bud, *WK* whole kidney. Scale bar = 100 μm.

4. Disaggregate tissues to make a single-celled suspension. This is done by placing three to four E11.5 kidneys, eight to ten isolated ureteric buds, eight to ten isolated mesenchymes, or about one E14.5 kidney crudely chopped into pieces into disaggregation solution for 4–10 min at 37°C. Using a glass pipette, transfer the tissue to an Eppendorf tube containing about 200 μL immortalization medium. Leave it for 5–10 min and then complete its dissociation by trituration (pipetting repeatedly into and out of a yellow Gilson tip). Monitor the cells on a microscope to verify that they are in single-celled suspension.
5. (*Optional*—sort cells by FACS or magnetic beads at this point—see Note 3.)
6. Plate the cell suspension in coated cell culture dishes in 8 mL ROCK inhibitor medium. Leave in a 33°C incubator for 48 h.
7. Replace the medium with immortalization medium (with no ROCK inhibitor). Incubate at 33°C for 72 h.
8. Repeat step 6.

9. Replace medium with enriched immortalization medium and leave for 4–10 days, watching for the appearance of small proliferating clones of cells.

3.2. Cloning

1. When clones of 20–40 cells can be seen, use a marker pen to draw around them (on the underside of the dish—see Note 4). Continue to incubate the dish until the clones each acquire about 150 cells.
2. Place a thin layer of silicone grease in a glass dish and autoclave it: this will result in a thin layer of sterile grease.
3. Press the bottom of the sterile cloning rings firmly on to the silicone grease film so that they acquire a thin coat of it.
4. Place disaggregation solution in an incubator to warm up to 37°C.
5. Rinse the culture dish in sterile PBS, and then place cloning rings firmly over the clones in which you are interested (see Note 5). Add 100 μL warm disaggregation solution and leave at 37°C for 2 min.
6. Add 100 μL immortalization medium to each cloning ring, recover the suspended cells, and centrifuge at 200 × g for 2 min. Discard the supernatant.
7. Resuspend the cells in 1 mL immortalization medium and culture in a 24-multi-well plate for 1–2 weeks at 33°C, changing the medium every 3 days. Inspect the cells, and move to the next step when they reach about 85% confluence.

3.3. Expansion of Clones

1. When the cells have reached about 85% confluence, rinse with 1× PBS and replace this with pre-warmed disaggregation medium for 2 min. Recover and centrifuge cells as in step 6 above. Replate in a 6-multi-well plate in immortalization medium.
2. When 85% confluence is again achieved, passage the cells again, as in step 1, and transfer to a T25 culture flask. For reasons of economy, 50 u/mL IFN-γ can be used.
3. When a culture has been established, it is worth testing whether it will grow without IFN-γ. (Adaptation to cell culture often means that the cells become IFN-γ independent. We detect expression of the SV40 transgene in our cell lines even without it—Fig. 2.)
4. Optional: Test the expression of markers of interest by standard RT-PCR (Fig. 2).

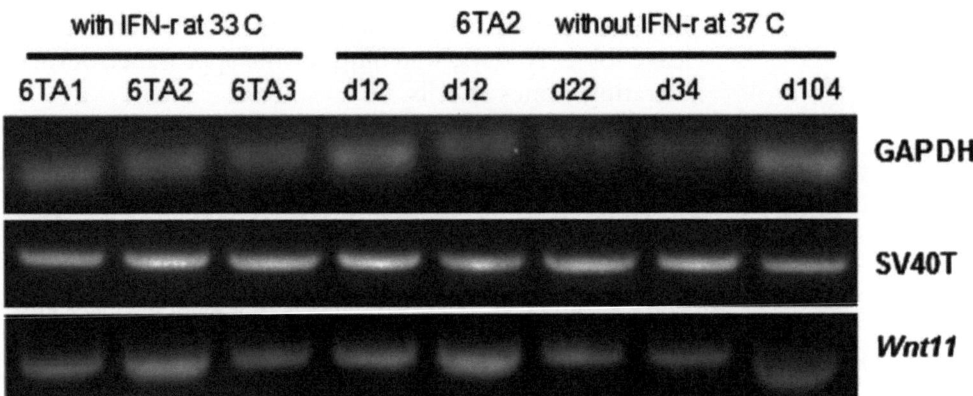

Fig. 2. Expression of SV40T in established lines with and without IFN-γ. The figure shows RT-PCR detection of GAPDH (a control housekeeping gene), Wnt11 (a marker for ureteric bud tips, which we wished our cell lines to represent), and the SV40 large T transgene. The SV40 large T was expressed even without addition of IFN-γ, and at both 33 and 37°C, although coding for a temperature-sensitive protein, it would not be expected to give rise to significant activity at 37°C. The numbers "6TA1," etc. are clone numbers, and the d12, d22, etc. were days of culture since sub-cloning.

4. Notes

1. The 33°C should be in addition to a conventional one at 37°C because some of the enzyme digestions mentioned in this protocol require the higher temperature.
2. It is essential that coating medium be kept ice cold until coating begins (otherwise, it will gel).
3. It is possible to raise cell lines by culturing mixed cells from whole kidney rudiments, making clones and then identifying the cells each clone represents by a study of marker genes ("anchor genes" in the language of Thiagarajan et al. (11), who list many). It may be much more efficient, however, to put effort into separating tissues to isolate only the desired cell type in the first place. When cell lines are being raised from young (<E12) kidneys, mechanical dissection may be all that is needed. Later, the structure of the organ becomes too intricate for this, so FACS or magnetic sorting is needed.
4. Choose only clones that are distant enough from other clones that cloning rings can be put around them alone.
5. Choose no more than eight clones in one dish: dealing with more introduces too much delay in which cells are being manipulated and reduces viability.

Acknowledgments

This work was supported by NC3Rs grant G0700480.

References

1. Costantini F, Kopan R (2010) Patterning a complex organ: branching morphogenesis and nephron segmentation in kidney development. Dev Cell 18:698–712
2. Davies JA, Ladomery M, Hohenstein P et al (2004) Development of an siRNA-based method for repressing specific genes in renal organ culture and its use to show that the Wt1 tumour suppressor is required for nephron differentiation. Hum Mol Genet 13:235–246
3. Kreidberg JA (2010) WT1 and kidney progenitor cells. Organogenesis 6:61–70
4. Jain S (2009) The many faces of RET dysfunction in kidney. Organogenesis 5:177–190
5. Davies JA, Fisher CE (2002) Genes and proteins in renal development. Exp Nephrol 10:102–113
6. Pulkkinen K, Murugan S, Vainio S (2008) Wnt signaling in kidney development and disease. Organogenesis 4:55–59
7. Coles HS, Burne JF, Raff MC (1993) Large-scale normal cell death in the developing rat kidney and its reduction by epidermal growth factor. Development 118:777–784
8. Jat PS, Noble MD, Ataliotis P et al (1991) Direct derivation of conditionally immortal cell lines from an H-2Kb-tsA58 transgenic mouse. Proc Natl Acad Sci USA 88:5096–5100
9. Davies JA, Unbekandt M, Ineson J, Lusis M, Little M (2011) Dissociation of embryonic kidney followed by re-aggregation as a method for chimaeric analysis. Meth Mol Biol 886:135–146
10. Davies JA (2010) The embryonic kidney: isolation, organ culture, immunostaining and RNA interference. Methods Mol Biol 633:57–69
11. Thiagarajan RD, Georgas KM, Rumballe BA et al (2011) Identification of anchor genes during kidney development defines ontological relationships, molecular subcompartments and regulatory pathways. PLoS One 6:e17286

Chapter 16

Engineered Tissues to Quantify Collective Cell Migration During Morphogenesis

Sriram Manivannan, Jason P. Gleghorn, and Celeste M. Nelson

Abstract

Renal development is a complex process involving the dynamic interplay of over 25 different cell types. One distinct step in this process is the formation of the ureteric tree, which develops from the repeated branching of the ureteric bud. During branching of the ureteric bud, cells migrate collectively in unison to form the complex structure of the tree. Here, we present a microlithography-based 3D culture model in which multiple identical kidney epithelial tissues are used to quantify collective cell migration during the process of branching morphogenesis.

Key words: Patterning, Engineered tissue, Persistence time

1. Introduction

The functional units of the kidney are the nephrons, which are connected together by the collecting ducts. These collecting ducts develop from the repeated branching of the ureteric bud, whereas the nephrons develop from the surrounding mesenchymal cells (1). During the initial stages of renal development, the dorsal intermediate mesoderm coalesces to form the Wolffian duct. Through cues from the surrounding mesenchyme, the Wolffian duct buds to form the ureteric bud, which then collectively migrates into the surrounding metanephric mesenchyme (MM) (1, 2). As the ureteric bud elongates, it branches to form the ureteric tree. The cells at the tips of these branches induce the surrounding mesenchyme to undergo mesenchymal-epithelial transition to form the nephrons, which elongate and segment to form the final filtration structure of the kidney (1). Movement of the ureteric bud into the MM,

Odyssé Michos (ed.), *Kidney Development: Methods and Protocols*, Methods in Molecular Biology, vol. 886, DOI 10.1007/978-1-61779-851-1_16, © Springer Science+Business Media, LLC 2012

branching of the ureteric bud, and segmentation of the nephrons all rely on the coordinated migration of cell populations (3). Disrupting any of these processes affects the structure and function of the renal system, and can lead to birth defects, hypertension, or renal failure in the adult (1). Thus, it is vital to understand the role of collective cell migration during renal development.

The process of kidney development can be studied using intact animals, organ explants, or three-dimensional (3D) culture models. Whereas in vivo studies allow for examination of the phenotypic effects of genetic manipulations, live imaging of organs as they are developing is challenging in the intact animal. Organ explants help to overcome these challenges, but organs can be difficult to culture, and their growth ex vivo is often affected by dissection techniques (4). To achieve a greater degree of spatial, temporal, and physical control, simple 3D epithelial cultures have been used. These usually comprise kidney-derived cells embedded in an extracellular matrix (ECM). These models achieve the goal of producing tissues that resemble the in vivo system. However, these culture models rely on self-assembly of the cells, a process that produces tissues that are very heterogeneous in size, shape, and composition, thus making it impossible to directly compare tissues and difficult to quantify results (5).

Microlithography-based techniques can be used to overcome the problem of heterogeneity and create well-controlled, quantifiable arrays of engineered 3D tissues (5, 6). Collagen matrices with cavities of defined geometry are created using microlithographically patterned silicone molds. These cavities are filled with epithelial cells to create multiple micrometer-scale epithelial tubules initially identical in size and shape. The development of these tissues can be followed over time to investigate the control processes and collective motions that define branching morphogenesis.

2. Materials

2.1. Cell Culture

1. Madin-Darby Canine Kidney (MDCK) epithelial cells (ATCC).
2. 0.05% Trypsin-EDTA.
3. Recombinant adenovirus encoding histone 2B (H2B)-mCherry (Vector Biolabs).
4. Minimum Essential Medium (MEM) Eagle, supplemented with 10% fetal bovine serum and 1% glutamine–penicillin–streptomycin.

2.2. 3D Microlithography

1. Poly(dimethyl siloxane) (PDMS, Sylgard 184; Dow Corning).
2. Micropatterned silicon master.

3. Vacuum desiccator.
4. Ethanol.
5. 1× Phosphate-buffered saline (PBS).
6. 1% Bovine serum albumin (BSA) in PBS.
7. Collagen I, rat tail (BD Biosciences).
8. 10× Dulbecco's modified Eagle's medium Nutrient Mixture F-12 (DMEM/F12).
9. 0.1 N NaOH.
10. MEM.
11. Hepatocyte growth factor (HGF; Sigma).
12. Round glass coverslips (15 mm diameter).

2.3. Imaging and Analysis

1. Microscope incubation chamber (e.g., LiveCell; Pathology Devices).
2. Cell-tracking software (e.g., IMARIS; Bitplane).
3. MatLab or other numerical analysis software.

3. Methods

Here, we describe a 3D engineered tissue model used to quantify collective cell migration during morphogenesis of kidney epithelial cells. Collagen matrices with cavities of defined geometry are created using microlithography; epithelial cells, transduced with a fluorescent nuclear marker, are embedded in these cavities to create multiple identical micrometer-scale epithelial tubules. These tubules are imaged using time-lapse confocal microscopy and analyzed using automated cell-tracking software to study collective cell behavior during morphogenesis in a 3D environment.

3.1. Labeling Cells with a Fluorescent Nuclear Marker

1. Twelve to eighteen hours before the start of the experiment, trypsinize a plate of MDCK cells that is approximately 30% confluent (see Note 1).
2. Add recombinant adenovirus encoding H2B-mCherry at >100 MOI to the cell suspension and replate the cells (see Note 2).

3.2. Three-Dimensional Microlithography

1. Prepare the PDMS molds (stamps) and supports by mixing 60 g PDMS (10:1 w/w PDMS polymer: curing agent).
2. Mix the PDMS pre-polymer mixture thoroughly and place in a vacuum desiccator to remove air bubbles.
3. Pour 55 g of the PDMS mixture onto the silicon master and 5 g onto a polystyrene Petri dish.

4. Place the samples in an oven and bake at 60°C for 3 h.
5. Peel the PDMS from the silicon master and cut it into stamps ~10 mm × 8 mm × 2 mm in size.
6. Peel the PDMS from the Petri dish and cut it into supports ~10 mm × 8 mm × 0.4 mm in size.
7. Sterilize the PDMS stamps, supports, and coverslips with ethanol and dry them using a vacuum aspirator.
8. Coat the feature-containing surface of the stamps with ~100 μl of 1% BSA solution. After removing any air bubbles that might be present, incubate at room temperature for 30 min (see Note 3).
9. Prepare neutralized collagen by mixing 800 μl collagen, 100 μl 10× DMEM/F12, 200 μl 0.1 N NaOH, and 60 μl MEM. This volume is sufficient to make eight samples.
10. Remove the BSA from the PDMS stamps using a vacuum aspirator and rinse the stamps twice with ~25 μl of neutralized collagen.
11. Add ~40 μl of neutralized collagen to the stamp. Flip the stamp over onto supports that are placed ~8 mm apart.
12. Incubate at 37°C for 30 min to allow the collagen to gel.
13. Trypsinize the H2B-mCherry-transduced cells to prepare a concentrated suspension and keep on ice.
14. Place ~30 μl of neutralized collagen on top of the 15-mm coverslips and incubate at 37°C for 10 min.
15. Use sterilized tweezers to remove the PDMS stamps gently from the molded collagen gels without distorting the cavities.
16. Add one drop of the cell suspension (~25 μl) to the collagen gel and wait for the cells to settle into the cavities (see Note 4).
17. Once the cavities are full, wash off excess cells by pipetting 400 μl of cold media across the surface of the collagen gel.
18. Repeat the washing step as needed to remove the excess cells.
19. Place the sample at 37°C for 10 min to allow the cells to attach to the collagen.
20. Place the collagen-coated glass coverslip on top of the sample.
21. Add 2 ml of culture media to the sample.
22. Place the sample in a 37°C incubator overnight to allow the formation of MDCK tubules (see Note 5).

Figure 1 summarizes the procedure of creating epithelial tubules and Fig. 2 shows MDCK tubules created using this method.

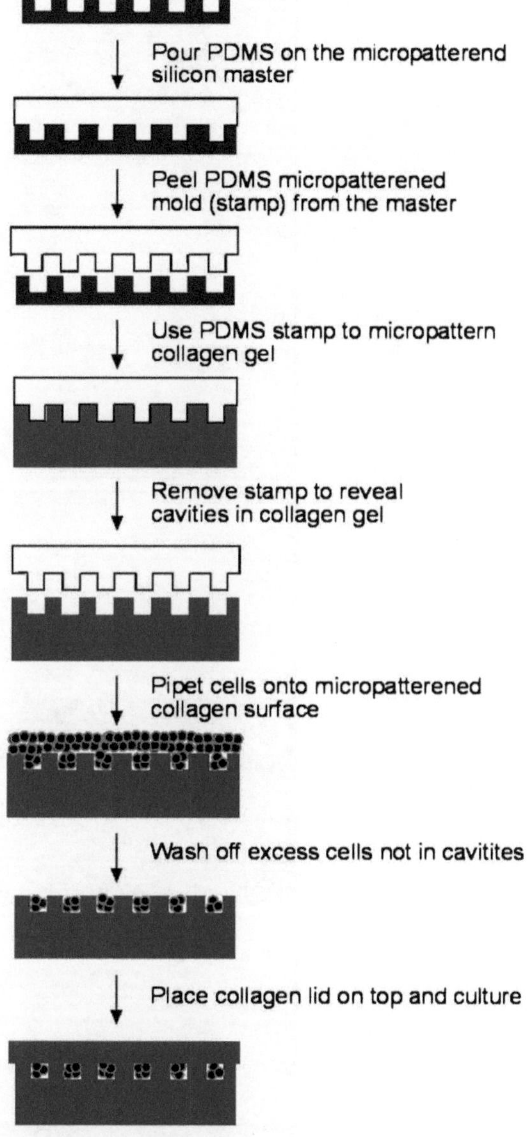

Fig. 1. Schematic of 3D microlithography procedure.

3.3. Imaging and Tracking

1. Equilibrate the microscope incubation chamber to 37°C, 5% CO_2, and ~90% relative humidity.
2. Place the sample inside the incubation chamber and choose the locations to be imaged using the microscope software (see Note 6).
3. Bring each tubule to be imaged in focus and set the Z steps (see Note 7).
4. Image for 12–24 h at 5–10-min intervals (see Note 8).
5. To analyze the images, import the time-lapse image sequence into IMARIS (see Note 9).

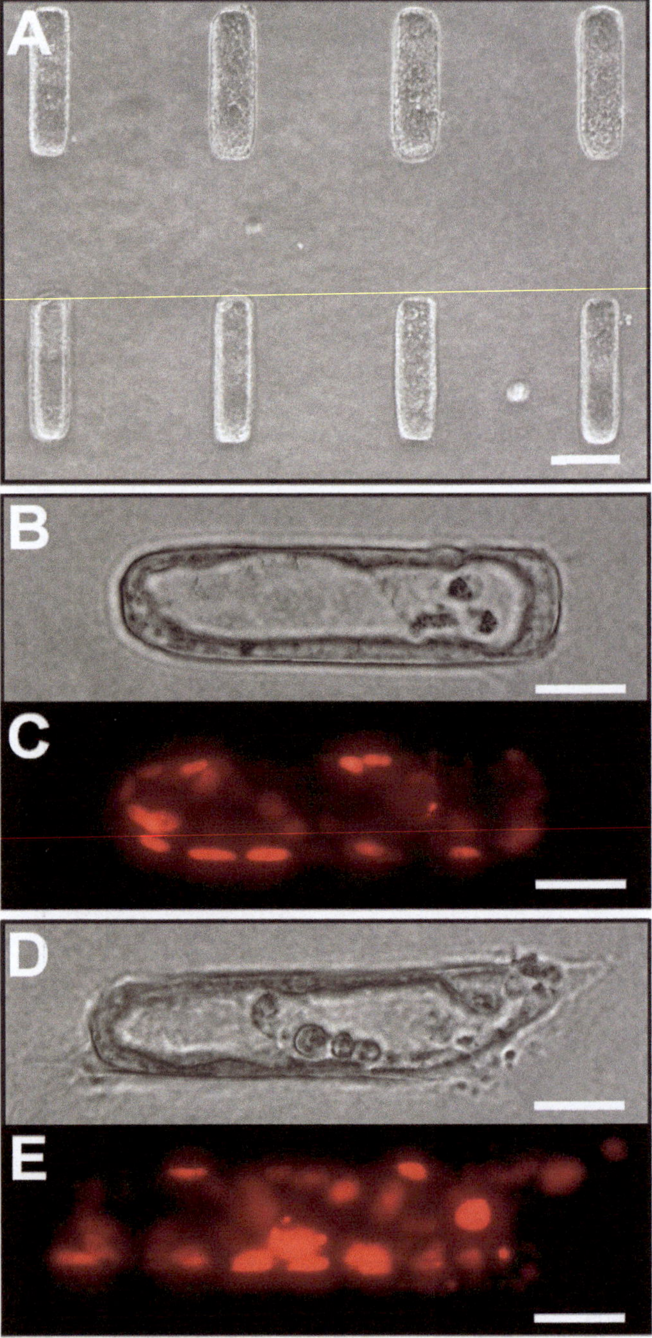

Fig. 2. After overnight incubation, the cells embedded in the collagen gel organize to form a tubule. (**a**, **b**) Phase images and (**c**) fluorescence image of quiescent MDCK tubules expressing H2B-mCherry. (**d**) Phase image and (**e**) fluorescence image of H2B-mCherry-expressing MDCK tubules induced to undergo branching by addition of 10 ng/ml HGF. Scale bars, 100 μm (**a**), 50 μm (**b**–**e**).

6. Use "Image Properties" option found under Edit menu to adjust the voxel (pixel) size and time points (see Note 10).
7. To track the cells, select "Spots" from Surpass menu and follow the Spots wizard.
8. Choose "Track Spots over time" and click next (see Note 11).
9. Under "Spots detection," enter estimated diameter of 10 μm and click next.
10. The spots algorithm will highlight the cells it has identified by placing a grey sphere (spot) on them.
11. Adjust the quality threshold to include any cells the algorithm might have missed (see Note 12).
12. After thresholding, move through the time steps of images and add spots to any cells that might have been missed in auto detection. Similarly, delete any erroneously placed spots.
13. Upon finishing the spots wizard, the software will display the trajectories of the cells (see Note 13).

Figure 3 shows a tubule that was tracked using IMARIS.

3.4. Analysis

Several parameters, including mean speed, displacement, and persistence time, are commonly used to quantify cell movement. The mean speed and displacement denote the rate at which a cell is moving and the distance between its initial and final positions, respectively. The mean speed and displacement, along with other related parameters, can be exported directly from IMARIS. The persistence time is a calculation of the time it takes a cell to change its direction of travel, and thus cells with a longer persistence time change direction less often than those with a shorter persistence time. Persistence time is calculated by fitting the mean-squared displacement (the average distance a cell traveled) and other measured parameters to a persistent random walk model (7–15).

1. Export the tracking results data (including speed, *x*-displacement, *y*-displacement, *z*-displacement, and position for all cells as a function of time, and total displacement and total track length) by clicking "Export all Data" found under statistics in the spots option dialogue.
2. Calculate the mean-squared displacement ($\langle \mathrm{d}^2(t_i) \rangle$) for time interval $t_i = i \times \Delta t$ using the positional information for each cell and the following formula,

$$\langle \mathrm{d}^2(t_i) \rangle = \frac{1}{N-i+1} \sum_{n=0}^{N-i} \left[\left(x(t_{n+i}) - x(t_n)\right)^2 + \left(y(t_{n+i}) - y(t_n)\right)^2 + \left(z(t_{n+i}) - z(t_n)\right)^2 \right],$$

where N = number of observations and $5 \le i \le (N/2)$ (see Note 14).

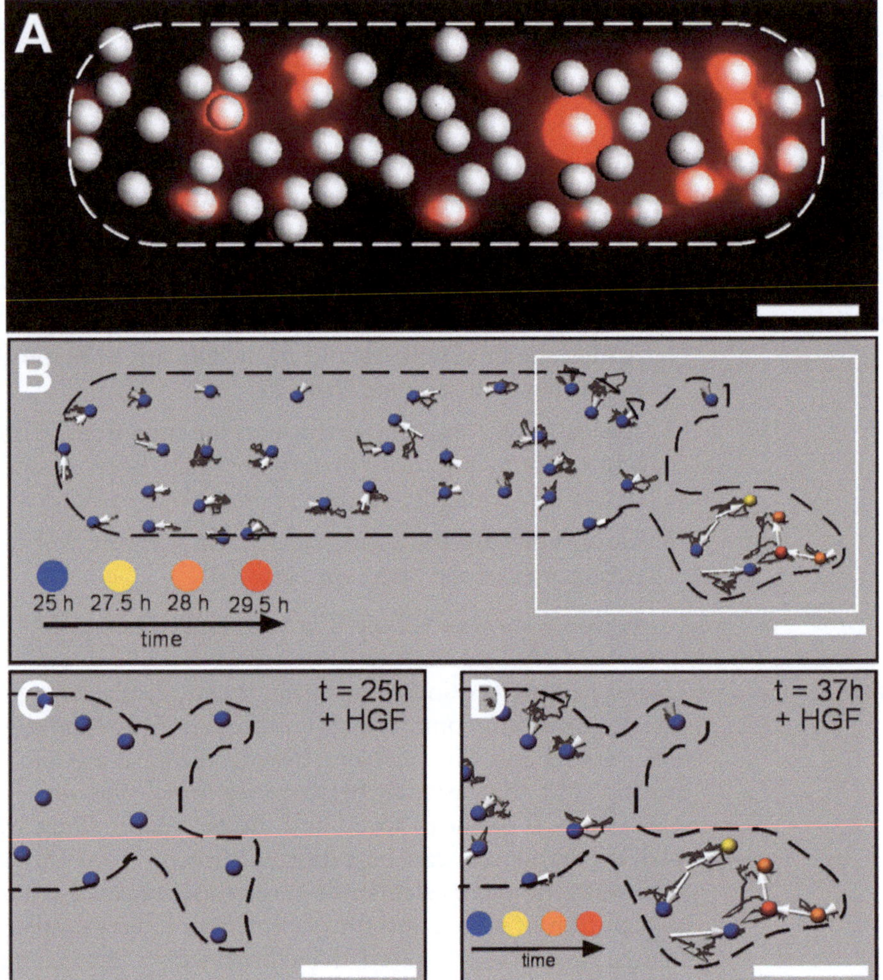

Fig. 3. (**a**) MDCK tubule in the process of branching with the nuclei identified (*white spots*). *Dotted line* denotes boundary of the tubule. (**b**) Nuclei displacement vectors (*white arrows*) and tracks (*black lines*) for cells of an MDCK tubule over 12 h. Fewer nuclei are identified for clarity and *spot colors* denote the age of cells. The branch (*boxed region*) is shown in panels (**c**, **d**). Branch of the tubule at the (**c**) start and (**d**) end of imaging. Scale bars, 30 μm.

3. Calculate persistence by fitting the data to the persistent random walk model using a least squares regression method.

$$\left\langle d^2(t) \right\rangle = 2V^2P\left[t - P\left(1 - \exp\left(-\frac{t}{P}\right)\right)\right],$$

where V = average cell speed and P = persistence time.

For MDCK tubules imaged for 12 h at 10-min intervals starting 24 h after treatment with 10 ng/ml of HGF, we found that the cells moved with a velocity of ~14 μm/h and a persistence time of ~18 min. Over this time period, the branches are just starting to form. To observe robust branching, we recommend imaging and tracking for longer time periods (~24 h) with short intervals.

4. Notes

1. It is difficult to transduce MDCK cells without first suspending them. Transduction becomes even more difficult as their confluence increases and they form a monolayer (16).
2. We found that adding ~700 MOI gives 100% transduction after 15 h for this particular virus; if the transduction is not 100%, increase the amount of virus added.
3. To remove air bubbles, try gently scratching them off using a pipette tip. Incubating the BSA-coated stamps at 4°C overnight will also help to remove bubbles.
4. It takes about 60–90 s for the cells to fill the cavities. Gently shaking the dish will help the cells fall into the cavities.
5. After ~12 h, the MDCK tubules should be fully formed.
6. Pretreating samples with 5–10 ng/ml of HGF increases the motility of the cells (17).
7. Set Z step ~2 μm and image 60 μm above and below zero location.
8. The interval of time between subsequent images should be chosen such that it is much smaller than the persistence time of the cells being imaged.
9. When importing the sequence of images into IMARIS, specify that the images are time steps by clicking on "Setting" in the open file window and selecting T.
10. Voxel size depends on the microscope, camera, and the objective used.
11. Reducing the area of interest using "Segment only a Region of Interest" can increase automated spot detection speed and decrease computational resources.
12. Lowering the quality threshold allows the software to identify faint signals as cells to track, but this also increases noise.
13. To correct for drift during imaging, click "Drift Correction" found under Edit in the spots menu.
14. Mean-squared displacement is not calculated for time intervals shorter than $5 \times \Delta t$ or longer than $(N/2) \times \Delta t$ to minimize errors. These errors may be caused by incorrect choice of Δt at short intervals or by the overlapping interval calculations of MSD at long intervals (11, 18).

Acknowledgments

We thank Nikolce Gjorevski for assistance with the imaging and tracking software. This work was supported in part by grants from the NIH (CA128660 and GM083997), Susan G. Koman for the Cure (FAS0703855), the David and Lucile Packard Foundation, and the Alfred P. Sloan Foundation. C.M.N. holds a Career Award at Scientific Interface from the Burroughs Wellcome Fund.

References

1. Costantini F, Kopan R (2010) Patterning a complex organ: branching morphogenesis and nephron segmentation in kidney development. Dev Cell 18:698–712
2. Pohl M, Stuart RO, Sakurai H, Nigam SK (2000) Branching morphogenesis during kidney development. Annu Rev Physiol 62:595–620
3. Vasilyev A, Liu Y, Mudumana S et al (2009) Collective cell migration drives morphogenesis of the kidney nephron. PLoS Biol 7:e1000009
4. Sakurai H, Nigam SK (1998) In vitro branching tubulogenesis: Implications for developmental and cystic disorders, nephron number, renal repair, and nephron engineering. Kidney Int 54:14–26
5. Nelson CM, Inman JL, Bissell MJ (2008) Three-dimensional lithographically defined organotypic tissue arrays for quantitative analysis of morphogenesis and neoplastic progression. Nat Protoc 3:674–678
6. Nelson CM, VanDuijn MM, Inman JL, Fletcher DA, Bissell MJ (2006) Tissue geometry determines sites of mammary branching morphogenesis in organotypic cultures. Science 314:298–300
7. Zaman M, Matsudaira P, Lauffenburger D (2007) Understanding effects of matrix protease and matrix organization on directional persistence and translational speed in three-dimensional cell migration. Ann Biomed Eng 35:91–100
8. Dickinson RB, Tranquillo RT (1993) Optimal estimation of cell movement indices from the statistical analysis of cell tracking data. AIChE J 39:1995–2010
9. Dikeman DA, Rivera Rosado LA, Horn TA et al (2008) $\alpha 4\beta 1$-Integrin regulates directionally persistent cell migration in response to shear flow stimulation. Am J Physiol Cell Physiol 295:C151–C159
10. Mori H, Gjorevski N, Inman JL, Bissell MJ, Nelson CM (2009) Self-organization of engineered epithelial tubules by differential cellular motility. Proc Natl Acad Sci USA 106:14890–14895
11. Rosello C, Ballet P, Planus E, Tracqui P (2004) Model driven quantification of individual and collective cell migration. Acta Biotheor 52:343–363
12. Parkhurst MR, Saltzman WM (1992) Quantification of human neutrophil motility in three-dimensional collagen gels. Effect of collagen concentration. Biophys J 61:306–315
13. Zaman MH, Trapani LM, Sieminski AL et al (2006) Migration of tumor cells in 3D matrices is governed by matrix stiffness along with cell–matrix adhesion and proteolysis. Proc Natl Acad Sci USA 103:10889–10894
14. Huang S, Brangwynne CP, Parker KK, Ingber DE (2005) Symmetry-breaking in mammalian cell cohort migration during tissue pattern formation: role of random-walk persistence. Cell Motil Cytoskeleton 61:201–213
15. ReinhartKing CA (2008) Endothelial cell adhesion and migration, In: Cheresh DA (ed) Methods in Enzymology. Academic Press, Oxford, pp 45–64
16. Arcasoy SM, Latoche J, Gondor M et al (1997) MUC1 and other sialoglycoconjugates inhibit adenovirus-mediated gene transfer to epithelial cells. Am J Respir Cell Mol Biol 17: 422–435
17. O'Brien LE, Tang K, Kats ES et al (2004) ERK and MMPs sequentially regulate distinct stages of epithelial tubule development. Dev Cell 7:21–32
18. Shreiber DI, Tranquillo RT (2006) Three-dimensional, quantitative in vitro assays of wound healing behavior. In: Celis JE (ed) Cell biology: a laboratory handbook, 3rd edn. Academic Press, Oxford, p 2328

Part IV

Detecting Gene/Protein Expression and Signaling

Chapter 17

Access and Use of the GUDMAP Database of Genitourinary Development

Jamie A. Davies, Melissa H. Little, Bruce Aronow, Jane Armstrong, Jane Brennan, Sue Lloyd-MacGilp, Chris Armit, Simon Harding, Xinjun Piu, Yogmatee Roochun, Bernard Haggarty, Derek Houghton, Duncan Davidson, and Richard Baldock

Abstract

The Genitourinary Development Molecular Atlas Project (GUDMAP) aims to document gene expression across time and space in the developing urogenital system of the mouse, and to provide access to a variety of relevant practical and educational resources. Data come from microarray gene expression profiling (from laser-dissected and FACS-sorted samples) and in situ hybridization at both low (whole-mount) and high (section) resolutions. Data are annotated to a published, high-resolution anatomical ontology and can be accessed using a variety of search interfaces. Here, we explain how to run typical queries on the database, by gene or anatomical location, how to view data, how to perform complex queries, and how to submit data.

Key words: Organogenesis, Renal, Kidney, Metanephros, Mesonephros, Wolffian, Nephric, Ureter, Bladder, Testis, Prostate, Seminal vesicle, Ovary, Oviduct, Uterus, Cervix, Vagina, Vulva, Phallus, Urethra, Penis, Clitoris, Development, Bioinformatics, Atlas

1. Introduction

The Genitourinary Development Molecular Anatomy Project (GUDMAP), begun by an international consortium in 2005, is building a comprehensive and easy-to-use online database of gene expression during mouse urogenital development. Data types already present include microarray analyses of laser-captured and FACS-sorted cells, low-resolution in situ analyses of whole-mounts, high-resolution in situ analyses of sections, and immunohistochemical data. Table 1 summarises the scale and range of the data currently accessible in the database at the time of writing (February 2011).

Odyssé Michos (ed.), *Kidney Development: Methods and Protocols*, Methods in Molecular Biology, vol. 886,
DOI 10.1007/978-1-61779-851-1_17, © Springer Science+Business Media, LLC 2012

Table 1
A summary of the contents of the GUDMAP database at the time of writing (February 2011)

Dataset	Type of data	Stage, tissue type and sex	Number of genes/ entries	Contributing laboratory	Resulting publications
Murine transcription factors	WISH	TS23 UGT M/F	1,500 genes	McMahon	(7)
High resolution analysis of compartment-specific Murine TFs	SISH	TS23 & adult metanephros	772	Little	
Antibody markers of renal structures	IHC	TS23 & adult metanephros	7 genes 14 entries	Little	(8)
Validation of subcompartment enriched genes in the developing kidney	SISH	TS23 metanephros	38 genes/entries	Little	(9)
Validation of renal vesicle enriched genes	SISH	TS23 metanephros	66 genes/60 entries	Little	(10)
Genes expressed by the mesonephric and metanephric tubules	WISH	TS17, TS20 & 21 UGT M/F (WISH)	76 genes/367 entries	Little	(11)
Anchor genes specific to key renal compartments	SISH	TS23 & adult metanephros	200 genes/entries	Little	(12)

Validation of genital tubercle, urethra and bladder enriched genes	WISH	TS21 UGT incl. genital tubercle M/F	43 genes	Little	(13)
Sexually dimorphic genes in the gonad	WISH	TS19, 20, 21, 22, 23 UGT M/F	39 genes/239 entries	Little	
Gene expression across cessation of nephrogenesis	SISH	TS21, P0, P2, P4	212	Little	
Testis-expressed genes	SISH	TS22 testis	1846	Gaido	(14)
Validation of pelvic ganglia genes in the LUT	SISH	TS23 LUT incl. bladder/urethra, genital tubercle	12 genes/24 entries	Southard-Smith, Little	
Spatial and temporal validation of urothelium-specific bladder genes	SISH	TS23 & TS27 (P2) bladder	44 genes/92 entries	Mendelsohn, Little	
Validation of temporal and spatial profiling of layer-specific bladder genes	SISH	TS23 & TS27 (P2) bladder	33 genes/70 entries	Lessard, Little	
TFs in the bladder	WISH	(In process)	(In process)	Mendelsohn	

Expression data are annotated according to a high-resolution, hierarchical ontology (1). This ontology is compatible with, and effectively forms an extension of, the ontology of the eMouse Atlas Project, EMAP (2). Submissions (see Subheading 3.6) contain extensive metadata to describe how, when and by whom they were obtained. Each item is assigned a unique identifier and is subject to careful quality control and curation by a full-time editorial office, and then entered into the online database. Each type of data follows appropriate international conventions: for example, array data conform to the MIAME standard (3), also used by databases such as the Gene Expression Omnibus (GEO (4)), and in situ data conform to the MISFISHE standard (5). Interfaces in the database allow extensive inter-operability with other databases and bioinformatic tools. As well as containing expression data, the GUDMAP site is also a resource for phenotype–gene associations, disease associations, tutorials on urogenital development, and lists of transgenic mouse lines made for, and made available by, the project.

The interface of the GUDMAP site provides many different ways of querying the database and performing both simple and complex searches. There are far too many possible ways of using the database than can be explained in this short chapter. The rest of this text therefore presents instructions for a few common searches, ranging from the basic to the more complex, to give the reader sufficient experience to perform other types of search. It also indicates how data may be submitted.

2. Materials

Computer with a compatible web browser. The system is tested regularly on a number of browsers and operating systems (see Note 1), but we recommend Mozilla Firefox v3.5.3 or later. This can be obtained from http://www.mozilla.com/en-US/firefox/

3. Methods

The methods described here, and the screen-shots used to illustrate them, are correct for the database as it was at the time of writing (February 2011). From time to time, interfaces and search facilities may be developed in response to users' feedback and details may change; an up-to-date tutorial can always be found from the "help" tab on the home page.

For all searches, begin by directing your browser to http://www.gudmap.org—it may be useful to save a bookmark to this site (see Note 2).

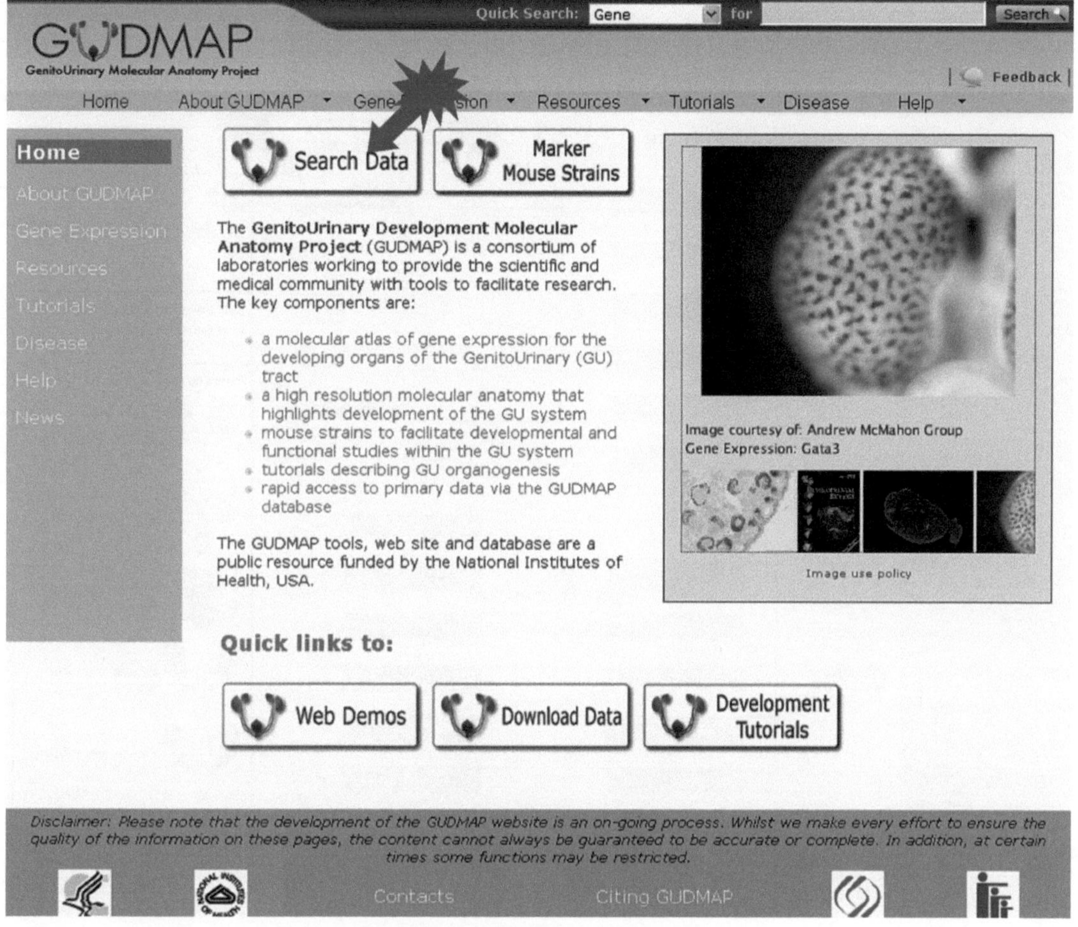

Fig. 1. The GUDMAP home page (the *arrow* indicates step 1 of Subheading 3.1).

3.1. Querying the Database by Gene Name

1. On the home page, click the "Search Data" box (Fig. 1): this will bring you to the "Expression database" page.
2. On the "Expression database" page, type the name of your gene of interest into the "Gene" box—as you type, an auto-completion box will appear to list all gene in the database that begin with the letters you have typed so far (this can save typing). When you have finished typing the gene name, click on the "Go" button to the right of the box (Fig. 2).
3. This will lead to a type of summary page, called a Gene Strip (Fig. 3: the right-most column may not be fully visible on very small browser windows and, if this is a problem, try viewing the browser in full-screen mode). The Gene Strip presents several options for navigation.
   (a) The columns most immediately useful are the two summary columns, marked "In situ expression profile" and

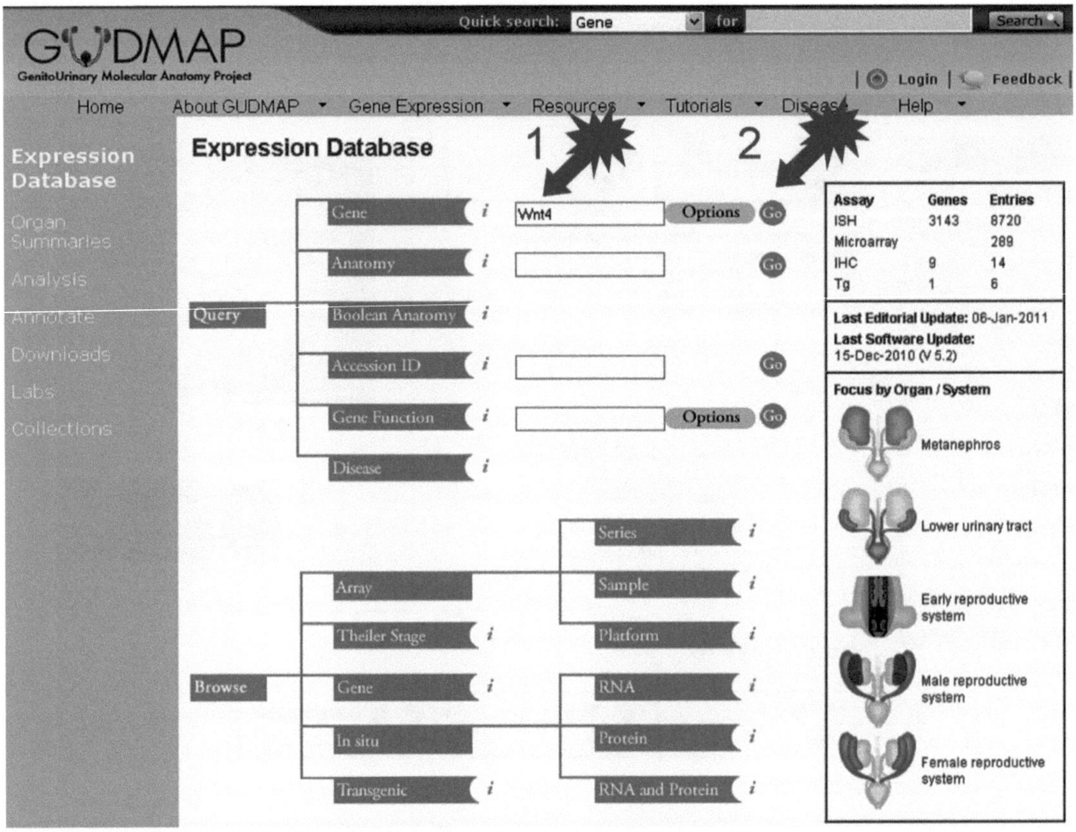

Fig. 2. The expression query page (step 2 of Subheading 3.1).

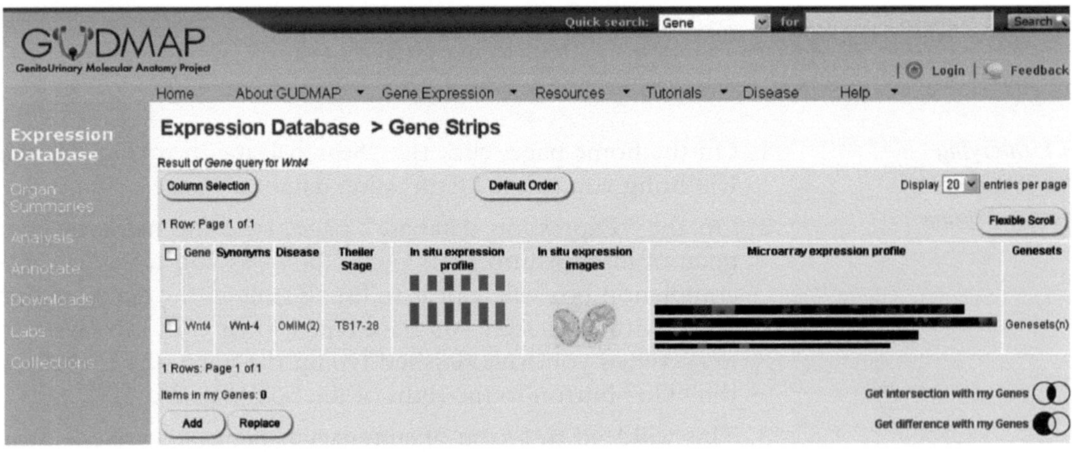

Fig. 3. An example of a Gene Strip summary (step 3 of Subheading 3.1).

"Microarray expression profile". The "In situ expression profile" provides an instant overview of expression in the six main parts of the urogenital system (mesonephros, metanephros, lower urinary tract, early reproductive

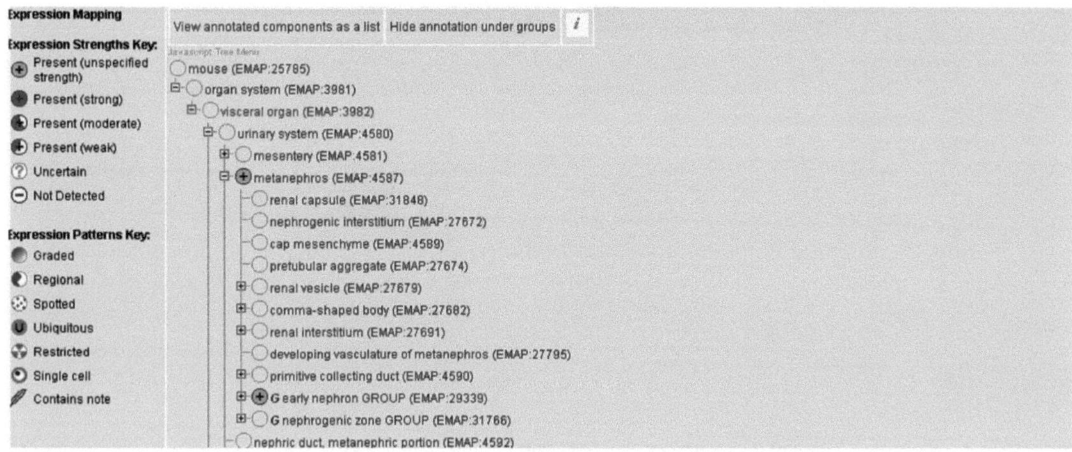

Fig. 4. A display of anatomical annotation of gene expression (see step 3(**b**) of Subheading 3.1).

system, male reproductive system, and female reproductive system; holding the mouse over any of the bars brings up its legend in a small pop-up window). Clicking on any of the small bars brings up a list of entries for that gene, similar to that described in ref. (2) below, but filtered only for that anatomical part. Similarly, clicking on any microarray summary bars brings up microarray information relevant to that anatomical part.

(b) Clicking on the entry in the "Gene" column of the Gene Strip (*Wnt4* in the case of this illustration), will bring up a page with more information on that gene, another view of the Gene Strip, and an index of in situ and microarray entries. Clicking on one of these entries leads to a page with all information about it, including original images and annotations to the ontology; an example of the annotation display is shown in Fig. 4.

(c) Clicking on the Disease column will retrieve information about diseases associated with that gene in the Online Mendelian Inheritance in Man (OMIM) database (http://www.ncbi.nlm.nih.gov/omim).

(d) Clicking on the "Theiler stage" column will bring up a summary table of the number of submissions in the database, and the type (in situ or array), for the gene of interest at each stage in development. Clicking on entries in this table (Fig. 5) leads directly to tables of individual submissions (Fig. 6). The columns on the page illustrated in Fig. 5 allow viewing of all information for a particular entry (the GUDMAP entry details column), another way into the gene information page (the "Gene" column, mentioned in ref. (2) above), another way into the Theiler

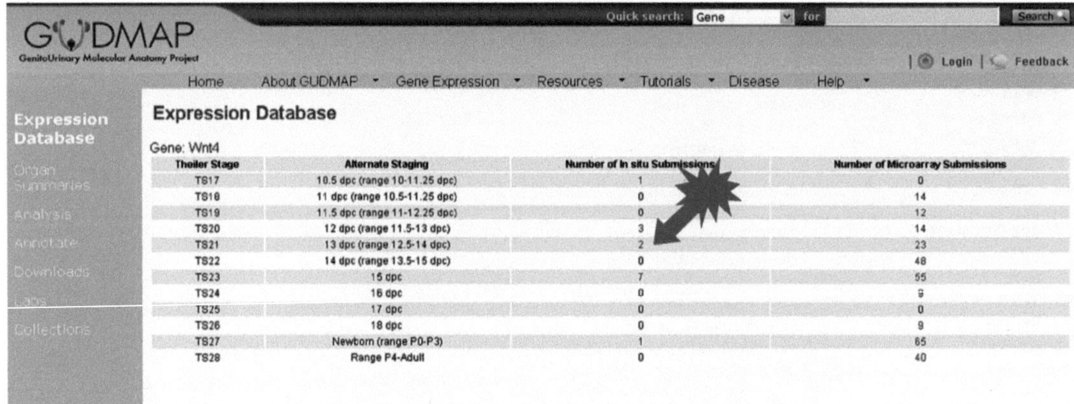

Fig. 5. Entries arranged by stage of development (see step 3(d) of Subheading 3.1).

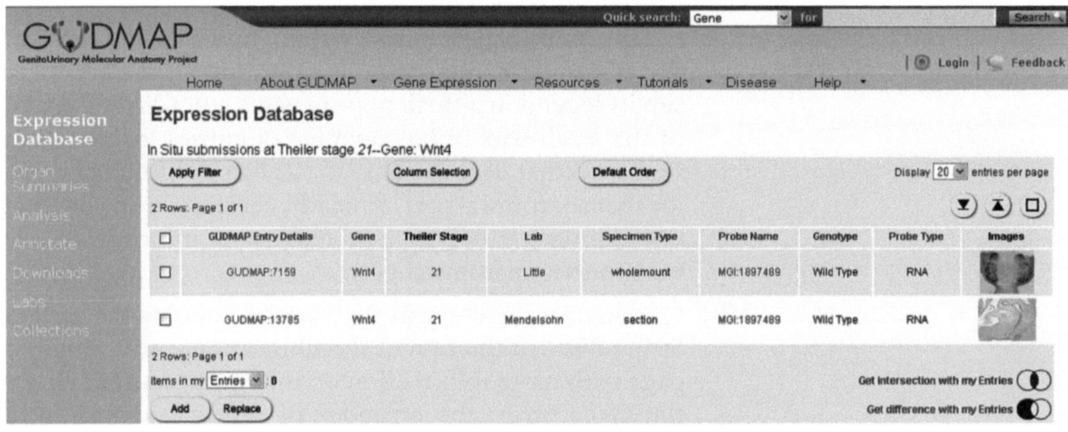

Fig. 6. A table of individual submissions from a query by gene (see step 3(**d**) of Subheading 3.1).

stage information ("Theiler stage" column), a way to see details of the submitting lab, details of the probe, and the in situ images themselves. Clicking on an in situ image will, depending on context, either bring up an image browsing window that allows browsing of an image at high magnification (Fig. 7) or bring up a list of relevant images, each of which can then be clicked to view.

(e) (Back to the Gene Strip page reached in step 3): Clicking on a microarray brings up heatmap illustrations (colour-coded representations of expression intensity) of gene expression in tissues examined (Fig. 8). The actual raw values can be downloaded, if the user desires, and explored using various generic array analysis tools available outside GUDMAP.

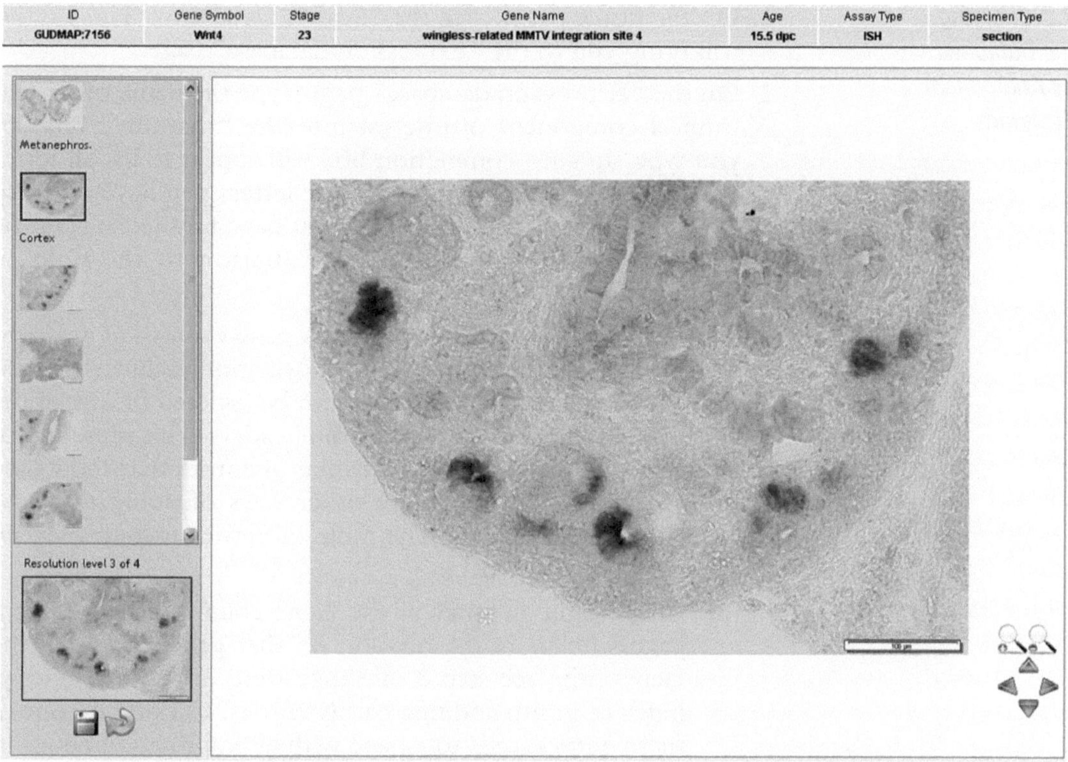

Fig. 7. The GUDMAP image viewer, allowing zooming, panning etc. of original images (step 3(**d**) of Subheading 3.1).

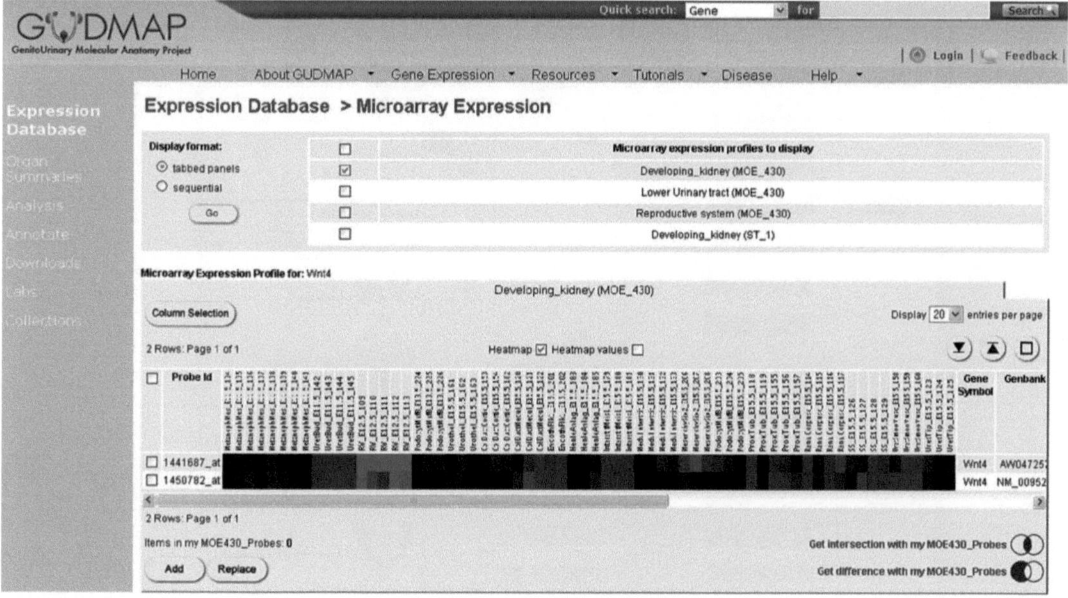

Fig. 8. A heatmap view of microarray gene expression data (step 3(**e**) of Subheading 3.1).

3.2. Querying the Database by Anatomical Structure

1. On the home page, click the "Search Data" box (Fig. 1): this will bring you to the "Expression database" page.
2. On the "Expression database" page, type the name of an anatomical component of interest into the "anatomy" box—as you type, an auto-completion box will appear to list all terms in the ontology that begin with the letters you have typed so far (this can save typing). When you have finished typing the anatomy term, click on the "Go" button to the right of the box (Fig. 9).
3. This brings up list of all entries with gene expression information for that structure (Fig. 10; information includes annotation as "not detected"). The list can be ordered by any of the columns, by clicking on the column headers. This is useful, for example, as a way to prioritise listing of entries that show only positive expression (there are other ways of doing this—see Subheading 3.3 below). The table of entries provides several ways to explore the data.
   (a) Clicking on an entry in the Gene column takes you to a page with more information on that gene, a view of the Gene Strip (see step 3 of Subheading 3.1 above), and an index of in situ and microarray entries. Clicking on one of these entries leads to a page with all information about it, including original images and annotations to the ontology; an example of the annotation display is shown in Fig. 4.

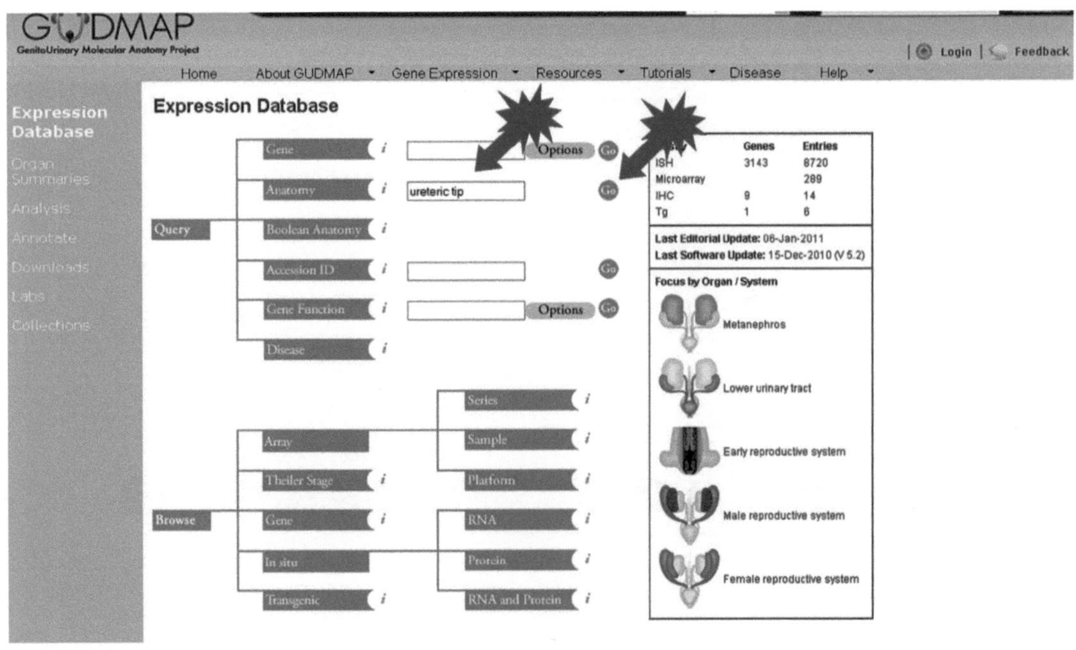

Fig. 9. Launching a query for gene expression in a named anatomical location (step 2 of Subheading 3.2).

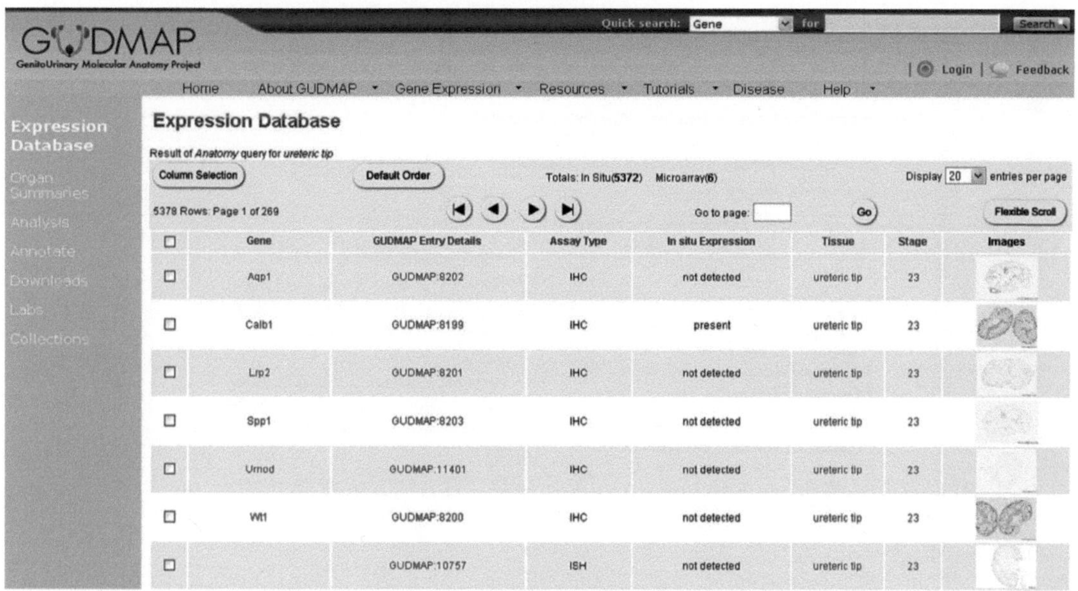

Fig. 10. Result of searching for genes expressed in the ureteric tip (step 3 of Subheading 3.2: only part of the results table is shown here).

(b) Clicking on the "GUDMAP entry details" column shows all information for a particular entry (see Note 3). For in situ data, this includes thumbnail images, which can be clicked to launch a powerful image browser (Fig. 7), annotation to the anatomical ontology (Fig. 4) and experimental details. For microarray data, there are download links to the original data, and extensive experimental details.

(c) Clicking on the "stage" column brings tutorial information about the definition of that stage.

(d) Clicking on the contents of the "images" column returns a complete list of thumbnail images for that entry, plus annotation and experimental information (this column is unfilled in microarray entries).

3.3. Multiple Anatomical Criteria-Based Queries

The database allows more complex searches for genes that are expressed in some places and not others, or at some times and not others. For example, to search for genes expressed in ureteric bud tip, but not ureteric bud trunk,

1. On the home page, click the "Search Data" box (Fig. 1): this will bring you to the "Expression database" page.
2. On the "Expression database" page, click the Boolean Anatomy box. This brings up a Boolean Anatomy Search page (Fig. 11).
3. Enter an anatomical term, either by typing in the box (an autocomplete feature will pop up), and the ontology below will expand in the right place, or by expanding the ontology tree

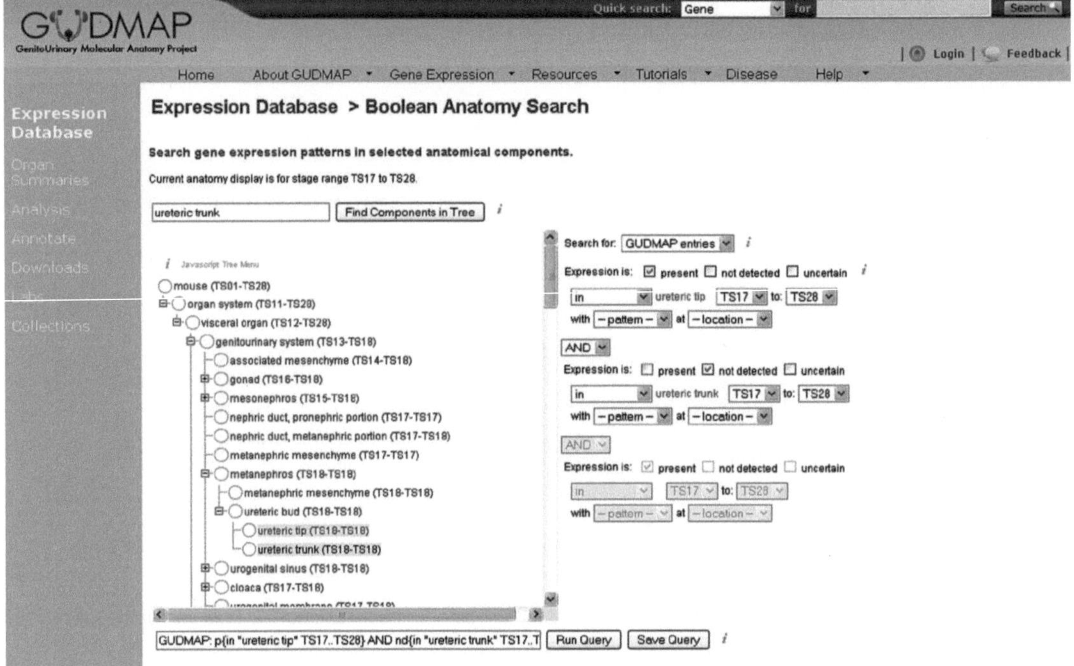

Fig. 11. Setting up a Boolean anatomy search for genes expressed in ureteric bud tip but not the ureteric bud trunk (steps 2 and 3 of Subheading 3.3).

directly, as one would expand a directory tree in GNU/Linux, Mac OSX, or Windows. Click on a tissue of interest (in this case, ureteric tip), and select choices for the tissue being present, absent etc., and any stage range. Next, enter the second tissue of interest as you entered the first one. Again, select whether you need expression present or absent, etc., and any stage range. Finally, select the Boolean function (default = AND). As you enter these choices, a string query appears in the box at the bottom of the page; it is possible to write this string query directly and skip the above stages, but this requires considerable familiarity with the language and with the names of anatomical parts. Figure 11 shows the completed query page.

4. Click "run query", and be prepared to wait a few seconds, longer if the query is really complex. A page will appear that is structured like the output of a simple query, but with only entries that satisfy the Boolean criteria being listed.

3.4. Querying by Gene Function

The database has a gene annotation table that categorises each gene with all of the different Gene Ontology descriptor terms that have been linked to that gene. This allows for lists of genes to be made, saved, and used to form subsequent queries based on the user-selected category of gene function.

1. On the home page, click the "Search Data" box (Fig. 11): this will bring you to the "Expression database" page.

2. On the "Expression database" page, type a biological function, such as one of those defined by the "GO" gene ontology (6), into the Gene function box, and click on "go" next to the box. (For example beginning to type the first few letters of "sequence-specific DNA binding transcription factor activity" will cause a drop-down list of terms that include that specific one and it can then be selected from to auto-complete the query).
3. The result will bring up a list of entries for all genes in the database that are associated, in the GO database, with that function. The format of the list is similar to that described in step 3 of Subheading 3.2 above.
4. From the list of gene that appears, the ones that the user selects from that list to Save to their list of genes then can be clicked on directly, and then the general results page "Gene Strip Summary" is brought up and than this can be browsed to jump to in situ images or microarray gene expression profiles of each of the Affymetrix probesets that are associated with that gene over any of the various Gudmap microarray datasets.

3.5. Querying for Lists of Genes that Have Been Associated with Specific Sample Types Based on Microarray Data Expression Profiles

The database has a number of lists and will be updated over time—of results from published or unpublished mining of the microarray data. These lists are named by sample type or gene expression pattern cluster and consist of microarray probeset identifiers and corresponding genes that have been said to be enriched in their expression in particular samples. These lists and corresponding heatmaps can be viewed on the web site or downloaded as Excel worksheets for further analysis and study.

1. On the home page, click the "Gene Expression" link (Fig. 1): and then choose "Query/Browse Database".
2. On the "Expression database" page, click the "Analysis" link to go to a view of the different sample groups and the specific samples within them. For example, click on the Developmental Kidney folder and then the AffyMOE430 folder that currently has a list of 19 different probeset lists (Fig. 12).
3. For each described gene list, clicking the name of the gene list brings up the corresponding list in the Gudmap heatmap viewer similar to Fig. 8, but in this case, with many more rows corresponding to each of the probes and all of the genes associated with those probes arranged in a hierarchically clustered view. Adjacent probesets and genes are those that exhibit highly similar patterns of expression across the series of sample from which the cluster was derived.
4. From the link labelled "Download" in step 2 of Subheading 3.6 above, the corresponding Excel worksheet that represents that cluster can be downloaded directly for further analysis.

Expression Database > Microarray Analysis

Gene List	Lab	Summary	Number of Probes	Java Treeview	Source File
⊟-□ Studies					
⊟-□ **Developmental Kidney**		Developmental Kidney			
⊟-□ **Affy MOE430**		Developmental Kidney			
⊟-□ **Brunskill et al** (Dev Cell(2008) 15(5):781-91)					
-Top-ranked - all components	Bruce Aronow	223 probesets	223	Treeview	download
-K-means clustered	Bruce Aronow	7,599 probesets	7599	Treeview	download
-Metanephric Mesenchyme	Bruce Aronow		378		download
-Ureteric Bud	Bruce Aronow		667		download
-Ureteric Tip Region	Bruce Aronow		540		download
-Cap Mesenchyme	Bruce Aronow		374		download
-Renal Vesicle	Bruce Aronow		526		download
-S-shaped Body	Bruce Aronow		642		download
-Renal Corpuscle	Bruce Aronow		521		download
-Proximal Tubules	Bruce Aronow		640		download
-Anlage Loop of Henle	Bruce Aronow		576		download
-Cortical Collecting Duct	Bruce Aronow		416		download
-Medullary Collecting Duct	Bruce Aronow		411		download
-Cortical & Nephrogenic Interstitium	Bruce Aronow		473		download
-Medullary Interstitium	Bruce Aronow		441		download
-Urothelium	Bruce Aronow		651		download
-Ureteral Smooth Muscle	Bruce Aronow		343		download
-102_SS	Bruce Aronow	S-shaped body	102	Treeview	download
-110_RV	Bruce Aronow	Renal Vesicles	110	Treeview	download
⊞-□ Affy ST_1.0		Developmental Kidney			
⊞-□ Lower Urinary Tract		Lower Urinary Tract			
⊞-□ Reproductive System		Reproductive System			
⊞-□ Gonadal Tissues		Gonadal Tissues			
⊞-□ Marker Genes		Marker Genes			
⊞-□ Disease Genes		Disease Genes			

Fig. 12. Browsing lists of microarray probesets that represent clusters of gene mined from the overall microarray data that are enriched in different sample compartments (step 2 of Subheading 3.5).

3.6. Combinatorial Searches Across Different Categories of Gene-Associated Information

The database is equipped with a facility for saving the results of a specific query, and then using that list to compare with the results of a new search. For example, to find a list of genes expressed in mesonephric mesenchyme, but not metanephric mesenchyme:

1. Run a search for genes annotated from in situ hybridization analyses as being expressed in mesonephric mesenchyme (for example, by using the method in Subheading 3.3 to search for only entries showing expression present in mesonephric mesenchyme). Adjust the number of entries to display per page to 100 (box top left of page), and then select all genes (ticking the box in the column header above the individual tick boxes means "select all").
2. Scroll to the bottom of the page and click ADD to "my entries".
3. Go back and run a search for all genes involved in "cell fate commitment" using the method described in Subheading 3.4. Adjust the number of entries to display per page to 100

(box top left of page), and then select all genes (ticking the box in the column header above the individual tick boxes means "select all").

4. Scroll down. Click "Get intersection with my entries" (bottom right of page). In this example, at the time of writing, one gene is returned (tgfb1i1).

3.7. Using Ready-Run Analyses of Microarrays

As well as providing access to raw microarray data, the GUDMAP database makes some ready-run analyses available, particularly for the sake of people who want to gain valuable information from arrays without undertaking a lot of training in bioinformatics. The analyses themselves are performed by experienced bioinformaticians (identified for each individual entry). To illustrate the use of stored analyses, this section uses them to identify genes, expression of which is particularly enriched in the ureteric bud.

1. From the home page, click on the "Search Data" box (or, equivalently, click the "Gene Expression" tab and click on "Query/Browse database").
2. Type "ureteric bud" in the Anatomy box and click "Go".
3. Click on "Analysis".
4. Expand the "Developmental Kidney" directory (because we are interested in ureteric bud, which is in the kidney). Expand the Affy MOE430 directory that appears, and then expand a directory of analyses that appears within: in this case, we choose the Brunskill example.
5. Click on "Ureteric Bud".
6. After a moment, the computer will return a "gene list" for the ureteric bud—that is, a list of the genes, expression of which is most enriched in the ureteric bud compared to their expression in other tissues. The ones that show most enrichment are at the top (Fig. 13). The methods used to make these gene lists are explained in help files within GUDMAP ("view microarray analysis help").
7. The menu reached at step 5 also allows the users to download an excel spreadsheet of the data to run their own analyses. Figure 14 shows a section of such a spreadsheet, the ureteric bud data highlighted automatically (and the data ordered by the ureteric bud gene list), and Wnt6 data highlighted in a box by the user of the spreadsheet.

3.8. Submitting Data to the GUDMAP Database

For its first few years, the GUDMAP database accepted data only from a limited number of laboratories that were funded as part of the GUDMAP consortium. Now we are in a position to accept data from other contributors, and are indeed very keen do to so. The Editorial Office of the GUDMAP project supports several methods

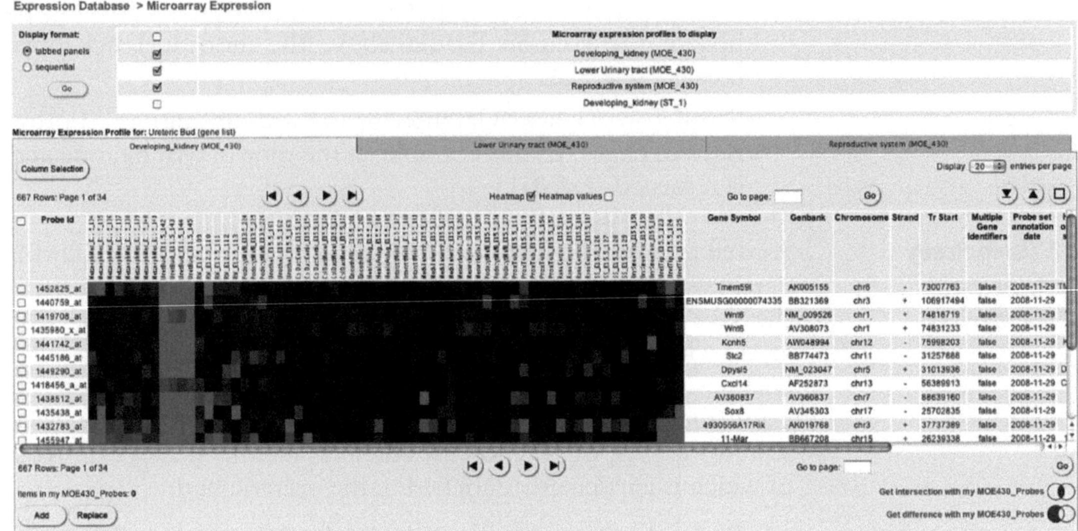

Fig. 13. A "gene list" for transcripts revealed by microarray analysis to be highly enriched in ureteric bud (step 6 of Subheading 3.7).

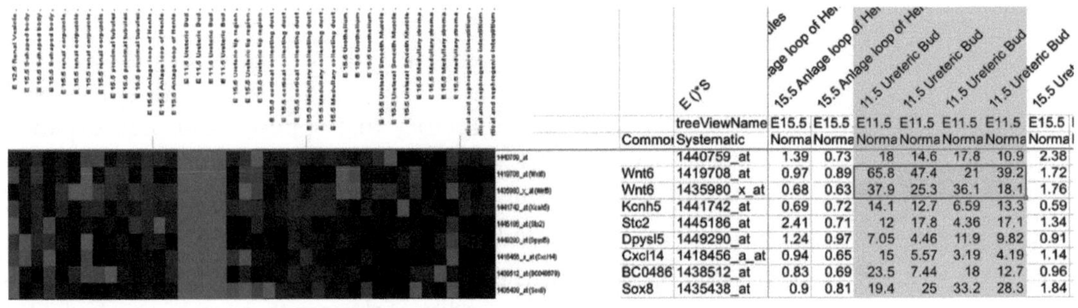

	E()*S	...age loop of He...	15.5 Anlage loop of He...	15.5 Anlage loop of He...	11.5 Ureteric Bud	11.5 Ureteric Bud	11.5 Ureteric Bud	11.5 Ureteric Bud	15.5 Ure...
	treeViewName	E15.5	E15.5	E11.5	E11.5	E11.5	E11.5	E15.5
Commoi	Systematic	Norma	Norma	Norma	Norma	Norma	Norma	Norma
	1440759_at	1.39	0.73	18	14.6	17.8	10.9	2.38
Wnt6	1419708_at	0.97	0.89	65.8	47.4	21	39.2	1.72
Wnt6	1435980_x_at	0.68	0.63	37.9	25.3	36.1	18.1	1.76
Kcnh5	1441742_at	0.69	0.72	14.1	12.7	6.59	13.3	0.59
Stc2	1445186_at	2.41	0.71	12	17.8	4.36	17.1	1.34
Dpysl5	1449290_at	1.24	0.97	7.05	4.46	11.9	9.82	0.91
Cxcl14	1418456_a_at	0.94	0.65	15	5.57	3.19	4.19	1.14
BC0486	1438512_at	0.83	0.69	23.5	7.44	18	12.7	0.96
Sox8	1435438_at	0.9	0.81	19.4	25	33.2	28.3	1.84

Fig. 14. A section of a downloaded spreadsheet (step 7 of Subheading 3.7).

for submission of new data, and can provide tools for online annotation and considerable direct help and training. Submitters of new data are strongly encouraged to make contact with the editorial office, using the email address gudmap-editors@gudmap.org, to discuss their plans, as early in the project as possible.

4. Notes

1. The GUDMAP database has been tested on GNU/Linux (OpenSUSE and Ubuntu) running Firefox 3.6, Mac OSX running Firefox 3.6, Safari 5, Chrome 6, and Camino 2.0.4, Windows XP running Firefox 3.5.3 and Internet Explorer 6, and Windows Vista running Firefox 3.6.1, Chrome 6, Safari 5.0.2, and Internet Explorer 8.

2. If making a bookmark for GUDMAP, please use the URL form http://www.gudmap.org rather than the IP form (e.g. 192.107.168.132); the URL form is more stable across hardware updates and migrations.
3. Note that there can be more than one GUDMAP entry for a particular gene (this just means that more than one experiment has reported information for that gene).

Acknowledgements

The GUDMAP database is funded by the National Institute of Digestion, Diabetes, and Kidney Disease (NIDDK), NIH, and the National Institute of Child Health and Human Development.

References

1. Little MH, Brennan J, Georgas K et al (2007) A high-resolution anatomical ontology of the developing murine genitourinary tract. Gene Expr Patterns 7(6):680–699
2. Baldock RA, Bard JB, Burger A et al (2003) EMAP and EMAGE: a framework for understanding spatially organized data. Neuroinformatics 1:309–325
3. Brazma A, Hingamp P, Quackenbush J et al (2001) Minimum information about a microarray experiment (MIAME)-toward standards for microarray data. Nat Genet 29:365–371
4. Edgar R, Domrachev M, Lash AE (2002) Gene Expression Omnibus: NCBI gene expression and hybridization array data repository. Nucleic Acids Res 30:207–210
5. Deutsch EW, Ball CA, Berman JJ et al (2008) Minimum information specification for in situ hybridization and immunohistochemistry experiments (MISFISHIE). Nat Biotechnol 26: 305–312
6. Ashburner M, Ball CA, Blake JA et al (2000) Gene ontology: tool for the unification of biology. The Gene Ontology Consortium. Nat Genet 25:25–29
7. Mugford JW, Yu J, Kobayashi A, McMahon AP (2009) High-resolution gene expression analysis of the developing mouse kidney defines novel cellular compartments within the nephron progenitor population. Dev Biol 333: 312–323
8. Georgas K, Rumballe B, Wilkinson L et al (2008) Use of dual section mRNA in situ hybridisation/immunohistochemistry to clarify gene expression patterns during the early stages of nephron development in the embryo and in the mature nephron of the adult mouse kidney. Histochem Cell Biol 130:927–942
9. Brunskill EW, Aronow BJ, Georgas K et al (2008) Atlas of gene expression in the developing kidney at microanatomic resolution. Dev Cell 15:781–791
10. Georgas K, Rumballe B, Valerius MT et al (2009) Analysis of early nephron patterning reveals a role for distal RV proliferation in fusion to the ureteric tip via a cap mesenchyme-derived connecting segment. Dev Biol 332:273–286
11. Georgas KM, Chiu HS, Lesieur E, Rumballe BA, Little MH (2011) Expression of metanephric nephron-patterning genes in differentiating mesonephric tubules. Dev Dyn 240: 1600–1612
12. Thiagarajan RD, Georgas KM, Rumballe BA et al (2011) Identification of anchor genes during kidney development defines ontological relationships, molecular subcompartments and regulatory pathways. PLoS One 6:e17286
13. Chiu HS, Szucsik JC, Georgas KM et al (2010) Comparative gene expression analysis of genital tubercle development reveals a putative appendicular Wnt7 network for the epidermal differentiation. Dev Biol 344:1071–1087
14. Rolland AD, Lehmann KP, Johnson KJ, Gaido KW, Koopman P (2011) Uncovering gene regulatory networks during mouse fetal germ cell development. Biol Reprod 84:790–800

Chapter 18

Isolation of High Quality RNA from Embryonic Kidney and Cells

Shifaan Thowfeequ and Odyssé Michos

Abstract

All the mRNAs within a cell and their relative levels are indicative of gene expression within that cell, which is essential for its structure and function in its differentiated state. Therefore, methods for the identification of the specific mRNAs and the quantitation of their levels are invaluable tools for understanding gene expression. Due to high endogenous RNase activity within virtually all living cells, the isolation of good quality RNA with minimal degradation is not a trivial task. This protocol outlines a tried and tested methodology for isolating high quality RNA from embryonic kidneys for various applications including microarray analysis and quantitative reverse transcription PCR (qRT-PCR).

Key words: RNA isolation, TRI reagent, RNeasy kits, RNA quantification, Kidney

1. Introduction

During transcription, messenger RNA (mRNA) is synthesized complementary to the DNA sequence of specific genes. Therefore, the transcriptome, encompassing all the protein coding mRNAs within a cell or tissue, gives a global picture of gene expression within that particular cell or a population of cells in a given tissue type. In subsequent steps, ribosomal RNA (rRNA) and a whole array of transfer RNAs (tRNA) have integral roles in the translation process, thereby synthesizing the polypeptide chains for a whole array of proteins based on the sequences encoded in the different mRNAs. More recently, microRNAs (miRNA) have been implicated to have regulatory roles in gene expression through gene silencing by translational repression; while small nuclear RNAs (snRNA) contribute to the spliceosome that help process the pre-mRNA (1, 2).

Odyssé Michos (ed.), *Kidney Development: Methods and Protocols*, Methods in Molecular Biology, vol. 886, DOI 10.1007/978-1-61779-851-1_18, © Springer Science+Business Media, LLC 2012

Table 1
Typical amount of RNA that can be extracted from a single pair of kidneys at different stages of development

Embryonic stage	Total RNA/ng
E12.5	~300–500
E13.5	~500–700
E14.5	~1,400–1,900
E16.5	~4,500–6,200

For developmental biologists studying organogenesis, gene expression quantitation is vital for the analysis of gene expression patterns during developmental processes such as epithelial branching, cell migration, selective apoptosis, and mesenchymal to epithelial transition events. Currently, well-tested, more reliable, and high-throughput methods for analyzing the transcriptome are in existence, compared to those for the proteome. Therefore, isolation of good quality RNA as a starting material is essential for applications that utilize such transcript or transcriptome based analyses to study gene expression patterns.

This protocol outlines the methodology for extracting total RNA from embryonic kidney samples or cells at a quality that can be used for most molecular biology applications including, but not limited to, quantitative reverse transcription PCR (qRT-PCR), microarray analysis, and RNA-Seq (or whole transcriptome shotgun sequencing) (3, 4) (Table 1). The high sensitivity of these assays demands the ability to isolate ultrapure RNA from small sample sizes.

Endogenous ribonucleases (RNase) present in almost all living cells are eventually responsible for the degradation of RNA (5). Therefore, the key to good RNA isolation is efficient and rapid isolation to inhibit or minimize the effect of RNases. Historically, RNA isolation protocols employed a combination of cationic surfactants, RNase inhibitors, and chaotropic agents that attempt to maintain RNA integrity while dissociating and disrupting cells and cell components (6). This protocol is based on a guanidinium-thiocyanante–phenol–chloroform extraction with notable modifications. The use of TRI® Reagent (Sigma) allows the samples to be stored long term prior to commencing RNA isolation and minimizes the individual chemicals used in the isolation process. The substitution of chloroform by the less toxic 2-bromo-3-chloropropane results in more efficient phase separation and reduces DNA contamination. Finally, the use of the RNeasy kit (Qiagen) allows direct on-column elution, eliminates the need to precipitate and reconstitute the RNA pellet, and selectively excludes tRNA and smaller rRNAs, thereby obtaining a more pure sample of protein-coding mRNAs.

2. Materials

All the solutions should be made in purified deionized water (attained at a resistivity of 18 MΩ cm at 25°C) or using RNase-free analytical grade water, unless stated otherwise. Care must be taken to make all the work surfaces, dissection tools, tubes, homogenizers, pipettes, needles, and other instruments RNase-free. All the reagents can be prepared and stored at room temperature unless otherwise indicated below.

2.1. Obtaining Samples for RNA Isolation

1. Dulbecco's phosphate-buffered saline (PBS) (containing calcium chloride and magnesium chloride).
2. RNase OUT™.
3. TRI® Reagent.
4. Disposable RNase-free tissue homogenizing pellet pestles and Kontes® microtube pellet pestle motor (Fisher-Scientific).
5. Wiretrol®II micropipette with 50-μl capillaries.

2.2. RNA Isolation

1. 25-Gauge needle and 1-ml syringe.
2. 2-ml Phase lock gel (PLG) heavy tubes.
3. 2-Bromo-3-chloropropane.
4. RNase-free water.
5. RNase-free microcentrifuge tubes.
6. RNeasy Mini Kit (Qiagen).
7. β-Mercaptoethanol.
8. 70% (v/v) Ethanol in RNase-free water.

2.3. RNA Quantification

1. Microvolume spectrophotometer such as the Thermo Scientific NanoDrop™ or similar.
2. Agilent 2100 Bioanalyzer (optional).

3. Methods

3.1. Obtaining Samples for RNA Isolation

1. Spray all the dissection instruments with RNase OUT™ and then leave for 5–10 s to allow RNase decontamination to work. Then, thoroughly rinse with purified deionized water to get rid of excess RNase OUT™ (see Note 1).

2. Embryonic kidneys and specific cell populations from embryonic kidneys can be isolated. The dissections should be performed in cold Dulbecco's PBS and the embryos and isolated kidneys/cells should be kept on ice at all times.

3. Rinse the isolated kidneys in ice-cold PBS. Using a Wiretrol micropipette, ensuring minimal residual PBS carryover, transfer the isolated kidneys directly to an RNase-free 1.5-ml microcentrifuge tube containing 500 μl of TRI® Reagent (see Notes 2 and 3). In the case of isolated cells, pellet the cells by centrifuging at 200 × *g*, for 5 min at 4°C and resuspend the pellet in 500 μl of TRI® Reagent (see Note 4).

4. Homogenize the cells for 2 min approximately, using an RNase-free tissue homogenizer attached to a pellet pestle motor or equivalent (see Note 5).

5. The homogenized tissue samples can be frozen and stored at −80°C for up to a year before proceeding with RNA isolation.

3.2. RNA Isolation

1. Remove all the samples from −80°C and gradually thaw on ice.

2. Pass the samples five times through a 25-gauge needle attached to a 1 ml syringe, making sure not to introduce any air bubbles. Top up with TRI® Reagent to obtain a total volume of 1 ml (see Note 6).

3. Stand at room temperature for 5 min to ensure the complete dissociation of nucleoprotein complexes from the nucleic acids.

4. Add 100 μl of 1-bromo-3-chloropropane (BCP) into each tube for every 1 ml of TRI® Reagent used (see Note 7).

5. Vortex thoroughly for 2 min to ensure that the BCP properly mixes with the TRI® Reagent. Then shake at room temperature for 10–15 min.

6. Transfer the samples into prespun (see Note 8) PLG Heavy tubes and shake for a further 5 min at room temperature.

7. Stand the samples at room temperature for 5 min and then centrifuge at ≥12,000 × *g* for 15 min at 4°C. After phase separation, the mixture separates into three phases—a dense red organic phase at the bottom, containing protein, an interphase, containing DNA, and above the PLG, a colorless upper aqueous phase, containing the RNA (see Note 9).

8. Collect the colorless upper aqueous phase into a new RNase-free microcentrifuge tube making sure not to touch the PLG with the pipette tip. From this point on, use the Qiagen RNeasy Mini Kit for the subsequent steps as described below.

9. Add 600 μl RLT buffer (containing 1% (v/v) β-mercaptoethanol) to the samples and mix by triturating several times.
10. Add one volume (volume of supernatant from step 8 plus volume of RLT) of 70% ethanol and mix immediately by pipetting.
11. Immediately transfer the entire sample to an RNeasy spin column in a 2 ml collection tube. Centrifuge for 15 s at ≥8,000 × *g* at room temperature. Discard the flow-through (see Notes 10–12).
12. Add 700 μl of Buffer RW1 to the RNeasy spin column, centrifuge for 15 s at ≥8,000 × *g* at room temperature and discard the flow-through.
13. Add 500 μl Buffer RPE to the RNeasy spin column, centrifuge for 15 s at ≥8,000 × *g* at room temperature and discard the flow-through (see Note 13).
14. Add 500 μl Buffer RPE to the RNeasy spin column and centrifuge at ≥8,000 × *g* for 2 min.
15. Remove the spin columns from the tubes and place in a new 2 ml collection tube. Centrifuge at full speed for 1 min to dry the spin column membrane and to eliminate possible carryover of the buffer or ethanol to the RNA elution steps.
16. Transfer the RNeasy spin columns to a new RNase-free 1.5 ml collection tubes and add 15 μl of RNase-free water directly onto the spin column. Incubate the tubes containing the RNeasy spin columns at 37°C for 2 min before centrifuging. Repeat step 16 with another 15 μl of RNase-free water to obtain a total eluate volume of 28 μl (see Notes 14 and 15).
17. The RNA samples can be stored at −20°C for several weeks or −80°C for even longer, until needed for RT-PCR, microarray analysis or RNA-Seq experiments.

3.3. RNA Quantification

RNA concentrations can be measured on a spectrophotometer such as the Nano Drop that requires minimal sample volume for quantification. The final preparation of RNA obtained by this procedure will be free of DNA and proteins, and should have a 260/280-absorbance ratio (*A*260/280) ≥ 1.8 (see Note 16 and Figs. 1 and 2).

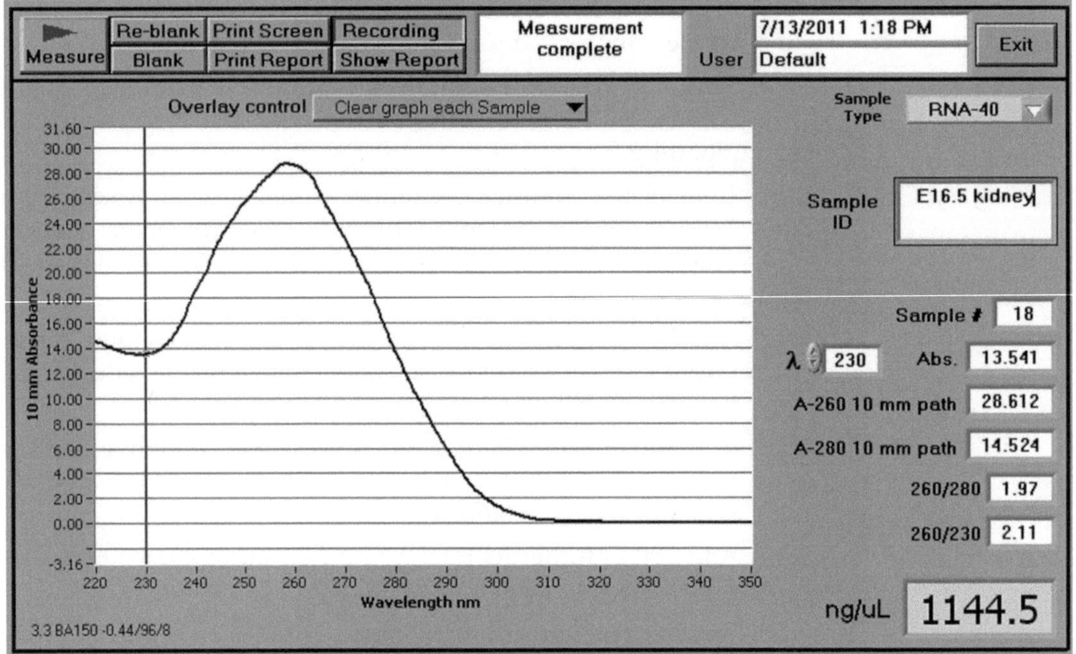

Fig. 1. The Nanodrop showing distinct peak of absorption at 260 nm for RNA. Both *A*260/280 and *A*260/230 are within the acceptable range to be used for microarray analysis. The RNA sample was extracted from a pair of E16.5 kidney.

4. Notes

1. Alternatively if RNase OUT™ is not available, the dissection instruments can be made RNAse-free, by soaking them overnight in 0.5 M NaOH; 0.1% SDS (w/v), with mild shaking and then thoroughly rinsing with purified deionized water.
2. TRI® Reagent is hazardous and its vapors can be dangerous. Hence, all necessary precautions recommended by the manufacturer should be taken at all times, when using this reagent. It is advisable to use a fume hood for Subheadings 3.1 (step 4) and 3.2 (steps 2–8).
3. Although the final volume would be brought up to 1 ml, 500 μl (or less) is initially used in order to prevent splashing during homogenization. This also allows for the pooling of different samples before proceeding with RNA isolation.
4. If isolating RNA from cells obtained by fluorescence-activated cell sorting, the cells can be collected directly from the flow cytometer into tubes containing TRI® Reagent.
5. Alternatively, the samples can be homogenized, by triturating 30 times using a fine pipette tip attached to a P200 Gilson

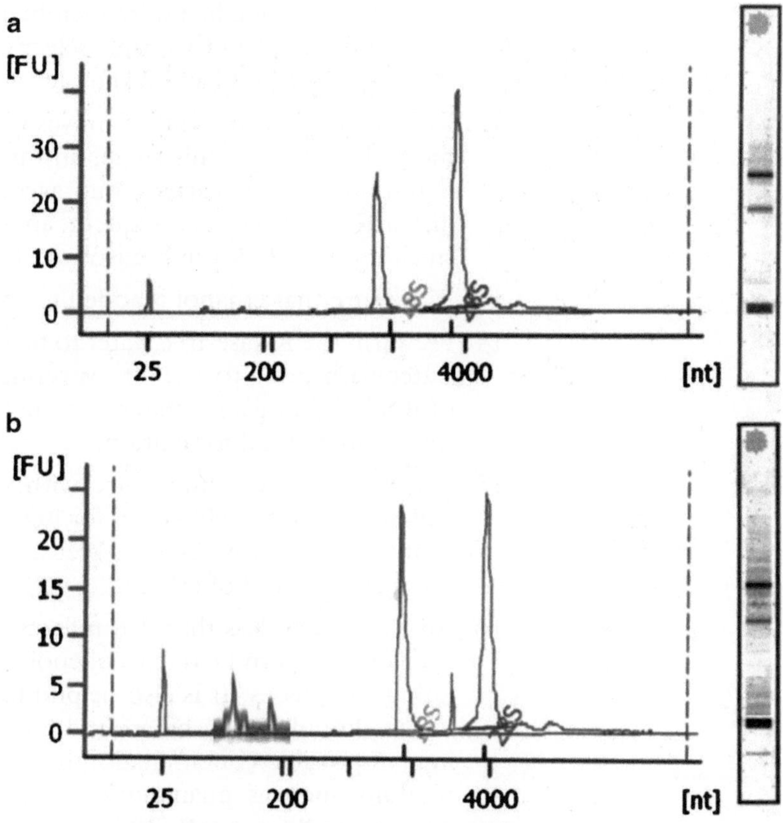

Fig. 2. The Bioanalyzer profile for good quality, intact total RNA (**a**) has distinct peaks for 28S and 18S ribosomal subunits (ideally the peak for 28S being twice the size of that for 18S). The *smaller peak* is the marker. For more degraded RNA, *additional peaks* might be present between or to the left of the ribosomal RNA peaks depending on the extent of degradation (**b**). This can be reflected in the electrophoresis run profile for both the samples (*right of the plots*). All the RNA samples were extracted from E13.5 kidneys.

pipette or by passing in and out of a 1-ml syringe through a 25-gauge needle. Avoid air bubbles while doing so.

6. At this stage, different samples can be combined if necessary, but do not exceed a total volume of 1 ml.
7. Chloroform could be used instead at a concentration of 200 μl for every 1 ml of TRI® Reagent used. However BCP is less toxic than chloroform and is better at reducing DNA contamination of the RNA during phase separation.
8. PLG Heavy tubes need to be prespun prior to use by centrifuging at 200 × *g* for 1 min at room temperature.
9. DNA and protein can be isolated from interphase and the organic phase according to manufacturer's instructions for TRI® Reagent.
10. At this stage, multiple samples can be combined by passing through the same column, before proceeding to step 3.2.12.

11. The columns contain a silica membrane to which RNA, longer than 200 bases bind to, thus selectively excluding tRNA and smaller rRNA (5.8S and 5S) molecules.
12. RNeasy column efficiently removes DNA without DNase treatment. However at this stage, an optional on-column DNase digestion can be carried out according to manufacturer's instructions, if the subsequent applications are sensitive to small traces of DNA in the isolated RNA.
13. Make sure that ethanol is added to Buffer RPE before use.
14. Prewarm the RNase-free water to be used for elution in a 37°C water bath prior to use. If expecting a higher concentration of RNA (≥30 μg), a greater volume (30–50 μl) of RNase-free water can be used for elution.
15. For higher yield, elute twice with two separate volumes of RNase-free water. However, for higher concentration of RNA (but with compromised yield) reuse the eluate from step 16 for the second round of elution.
16. An *A*260/280 less than 1.8 reflects protein contamination in the sample or can be due to phenol contamination when separating the phases. It is also helpful to look at the *A*260/230, which should ideally be around 2.0. A lower *A*260/230, ≤1 implies possible contamination by residual phenol or chaotropic salts such as guanidinium isothiocyanate. Samples with ratios of ≥1.8 for *A*260/280 and ≥2.0 for *A*260/230 generally perform better for microarray than samples with lower ratios. If expecting higher concentrations of RNA, for more accurate measurements the RNA can be diluted tenfold in 10 mM Tris–HCl, pH 7.5, prior to measuring the concentration.

References

1. Bartel DP (2004) MicroRNAs: genomics, biogenesis, mechanism and function. Cell 116: 281–297
2. Bessonov S, Anokhina M, Will CL, Urlaub H, Lührmann R (2008) Isolation of an active step I spliceosome and composition of its RNP core. Nature 452:846–850
3. Brunskill EW, Aronow BJ, Georgas K et al (2008) Atlas of gene expression in the developing kidney at microanatomical resolution. Dev Cell 15:781–791
4. Wang Z, Gerstein M, Snyder M (2009) RNA-Seq: a revolutionary tool for transcriptomics. Nat Rev Genet 10:57–63
5. D'Alessio G, Riordan JF (1997) Preface. In: D'Alessio G, Riordan JF (eds) Ribonucleases, structures and functions. Academic, San Diego, pp 15–19
6. Chomczynski P, Sacchi N (1987) Single-step method of RNA isolation by acid guanidinium thiocyanate-phenol-chloroform extraction. Anal Biochem 162:156–159

Chapter 19

Laser Capture

S. Steven Potter and Eric W. Brunskill

Abstract

This chapter describes detailed methods used for laser capture microdissection (LCM) of discrete subpopulations of cells. Topics covered include preparing tissue blocks, cryostat sectioning, processing slides, performing the LCM, and purification of RNA from LCM samples. Notes describe the fine points of each operation, which can often mean the difference between success and failure.

Key words: Laser capture, Laser capture microdissection, Tissue purification, Small sample analysis, Gene expression profiling

1. Introduction

For many research projects the purity of the starting biological sample being investigated is of the utmost importance. For example, in studies of the molecular events driving kidney development, there is great power in being able to divide the entire kidney into discrete subcomponents. The higher the resolution of the analysis the better one is able to assign molecular processes that emerge to specific compartments and cell types. In particular, a microarray-based analysis of the total developing kidney might identify expression of genes involved in Wnt signaling. But the results would not determine which cell types are sending signals, and which are receiving them. On the other hand, an analysis of gene expression patterns in the multiple individual distinct compartments of the developing kidney would identify precise ligand and receptor expression patterns for each element (1). This clearly yields a much more useful set of data. Indeed, there are many situations in the study of development and disease where there is great advantage to be gained through the analysis of small regions of a sample.

Odyssé Michos (ed.), *Kidney Development: Methods and Protocols*, Methods in Molecular Biology, vol. 886,
DOI 10.1007/978-1-61779-851-1_19, © Springer Science+Business Media, LLC 2012

For example, one the first applications of laser capture technology was in the study of tumors, which can exhibit significant morphological heterogeneity (2).

Laser capture microdissection (LCM) allows the purification of discrete subregions of a sample, in some cases even down to single cell resolution. There are multiple variations of the methodology. In its earliest form, a transparent thermoplastic film is placed over a tissue section and a near infrared (IR) (3) wavelength laser is used to heat the region above the cells of interest. This melts the film onto the cells, creating an adhesion that allows the cells to be purified as the film is removed (4). Other versions use a fine ultraviolet (UV) wavelength laser beam to cut out and isolate the region of interest from a tissue section (5–7). This chapter focuses on a combination system made by Applied Biosystems/Arcturus, which uses both IR and UV lasers for microdissection, although most of the principles discussed would equally apply to any commercial LCM product.

The ArcturusXT and Arcturus Veritas instruments combine IR/UV lasers and can be used with special polyethylene naphthalate (PEN) plastic membrane slides. In one preferred format the PEN membrane covers a glass slide, with the tissue sections then placed on top of the membrane. A UV laser is used to cut around the cells of interest, through both the membrane and the tissue (Fig. 1). The chief advantage of this system is that the region to be purified is not directly attached to the glass slide, thereby facilitating easy removal. An overlying thermoplastic membrane is melted onto the region to be captured using the IR laser, and then when this membrane is lifted from the slide it carries with it both the isolated cells and their underlying PEN membrane. This strategy can achieve very reproducible LCM purification of selected regions.

One important advantage of LCM is the excellent preservation of the in vivo properties of the cells purified. The tissue of interest is rapidly removed and frozen during the embedding process. This contrasts with competing procedures, such as fluorescent activated cell sorting (FACS), which requires cell dissociation procedures that can sometimes result in significant perturbation of gene expression patterns (3).

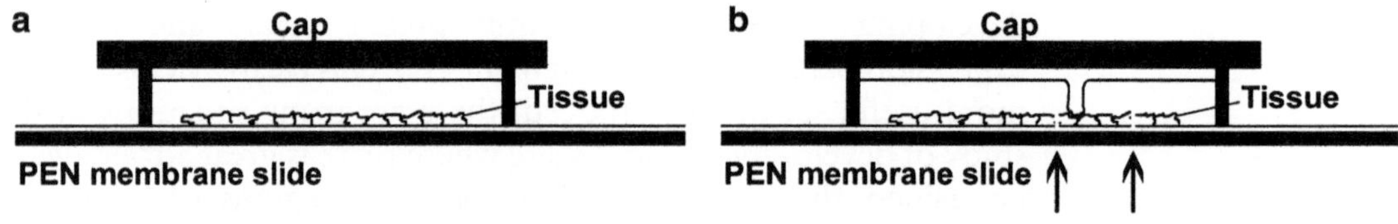

Fig. 1. Laser capture principle. (**a**) Polyethylene naphthalate (PEN) membrane slide is shown with tissue on the membrane. A Cap is shown over the tissue, suspending a thermoplastic membrane above the cells of interest. (**b**) The *arrows* point to positions where the ultraviolet laser has been used to cut through the PEN membrane and the overlying cells at the border of the region of interest. In addition, the overlying membrane has been heated with the IR laser to create a melt spot with the cells to be captured.

2. Materials

2.1. Equipment

1. Laser capture machine, Arcturus XT or Arcturus Veritas (Applied Biosystems), including inverted microscope. Similar machines are available from Zeiss, Leica, and other suppliers.
2. Cryostat. Microm HM520 (Thermo Scientific), or equivalent.
3. –80°C freezer.

2.2. Supplies

1. PEN membrane glass slides (Arcturus, LCM0522).
2. Poly-L-lysine.
3. 2-Methylbutane.
4. Acetone.
5. CapSure HS LCM Caps (Arcturus, LCM0214).
6. OCT (Sakura Finetek Corp., 4583).
7. Liquid nitrogen.
8. Xylene.
9. 100% Ethanol.
10. Qiagen RNeasy Micro RNA purification kit (Qiagen).
11. Fluorescein labeled peanut agglutinin (PNA) (Vector lab).
12. Mayer's hematoxylin.
13. Cryomolds.
14. Eosin Y solution.
15. Scott's Tap Water Substitute Blueing Solution.
16. Qiagen RNeasy Micro Kit (Qiagen).
17. Ovation Pico WTA System (Nugen, 3300-12).
18. WT-Ovation One-Direct Amplification (Nugen, 3500).

3. Methods

3.1. Preparing Tissue Blocks

1. Rapidly dissect out tissue of interest, such as embryonic kidneys, and store briefly in ice-cold PBS (see Note 1).
2. Process through OCT only as many kidneys, or other tissues, as you plan to freeze in one block at a time (see Note 2).
3. Place kidneys in precooled OCT in a 60 mm plate cooled with ice.
4. Quickly mix kidneys in with OCT using a sterile pipette tip, then transfer carefully to a new 60-mm plate with cold OCT,

quickly mix again, and place in a mold with ice-cold OCT covering the bottom. Transfers can be made with a pipetman and a 1-ml pipette with the end enlarged by slicing the tip off with a razor.

5. Cover kidneys with additional OCT and position kidneys, or other tissues of interest, near each other in the mold, in a central position, not too near the top.
6. Immediately freeze in 2-methylbutane in a pyrex beaker resting in liquid nitrogen. The 2-methylbutane should be frozen solid. Hold the tinfoil mold with forceps to keep vertical and gently move in a circular motion against the surface of the 2-methylbutane to improve thermal contact (see Note 3).
7. When the OCT is completely frozen, place the mold in dry ice and then store for long term in either a –80°C or a liquid nitrogen freezer.

3.2. Cryostat Sectioning

Throughout this procedure be very careful not to cut yourself on the sharp blades used in the cryostat. Wear gloves throughout to reduce RNase contamination.

1. Place specimen block in the chamber for 5–10 min to temperature equilibrate. Remove tissue OCT block from the mold. Place chuck that has been at room temperature in chamber and let cool a minute, but not too much. Place OCT on chuck and let cool a minute, but not freeze, and then place tissue OCT block on chuck, and let freeze in position. One can place additional OCT around the base and spread with gloved finger to help hold the block in place.
2. The temperature of the cryostat is critically important. Set to –15°C chamber and –15°C specimen (see Note 4).
3. Begin sectioning. Use the trim setting of 40–60 μm to remove most excess OCT, until tissue is visible. When close to the tissue of interest change to 7–10 μm sections (see Note 5).
4. Collect sections on membrane slides (see Note 6). Collect 5–10 sections per slide. It is important that the sections are placed in the central region of the slide, as the LCM machine cannot work on sections near edges. It is also important, however, to space the sections so that the Cap can be placed on each section without overlapping another one (see Note 7). Try to work fast, as the RNA in one section can be degrading while the other sections are being collected.
5. Freeze the slides quickly with dry ice and store at –80°C.
6. Clean up the cryostat. Remove dirty blade, brushes, OCT, etc.

3.3. Processing Slides

A limitation of LCM is the relatively poor histology of cryostat sections. This is particularly true when no additional staining procedure is used. Nevertheless, in some cases the structure of interest is so well demarcated that no special stains are necessary. One example would be the glomerulus of the kidney. A good general rule is to use as small a number of processing steps as possible. The more steps, the more opportunity for the RNA to diffuse out of the sample and the greater the likelihood of RNA degradation. Another general rule is the colder, the better, as this also reduces RNAse activity. Also, the less exposure to water, the better, since RNAs dissolve in water, causing losses from the tissue section, and ribonucleases require water. Therefore, the more the sample is maintained in a dehydrated state, the better the RNA recovery and the better the resulting RNA integrity.

With these recommendations in mind we present three variations of a protocol for processing slides for LCM. The first is a very straightforward procedure, with a minimum of steps, for use when very obvious structures are to be isolated. The second procedure adds lectin staining which can greatly assist the identification of more subtle structures. The third procedure incorporates hematoxylin and eosin staining, which can provide even more detailed structural definition.

1. Remove the slide from –80°C and immediately place on a room temperature metal surface, such as a slide warmer with the heat turned off. After a few seconds, move the slide to a new position, again at room temperature, to promote gentle warming to room temperature. Let the slide sit 2–3 min.
2. Fix the sample by placing in an ice-cold 1:1 solution of acetone and 75% ethanol for 2 min.
3. To dissolve OCT transfer to room temperature 70% ethanol, with gentle dipping of the slide for 1–2 min.
4. Transfer to fresh 70% ethanol, with gentle dipping, for 15–30 s. If no staining is required then go straight to 95% ethanol, step 7, for lectin staining go to step 5, and for hematoxylin and eosin staining go to step 6.
5. For lectin staining place the slide on an ice-cold metal block and flood the surface sections with lectin staining solution. PNA lectin provides a nice pan epithelial stain that can be very useful for distinguishing structures. Each lectin will need to be optimized for concentration and staining time to achieve the best signal to noise ratio. For PNA a good starting point is 5 μl/ml of 1/10 PBS diluted with autoclaved water. Stain for 6 min. Then rinse in ice-cold 1/10 PBS, 2 × 10 s with gentle dipping, and then 1 × 3 min. Gently dip in 70% ethanol and continue with dehydration series, step 7.

6. For LCM compatible H&E staining (8) take slides from 70% ethanol (step 4) and successively dip in water: 10 s, Mayer's hematoxylin: 15 s, water: 10 s, Scott's Tap Water Substitute: 10 s, 70% ethanol: 10 s (optional), eosin: 3–10 s, and then go to dehydration series, step 7.
7. Gently dip in 95% ethanol: 10 s, and repeat in fresh 95% ethanol: 10 s.
8. Further dehydrate with gentle dipping 2× in 100% ethanol: 45 s each.
9. Xylene with gentle dipping 2 × 1.5 min.
10. Air-dry in vertical position. Then, proceed immediately to LCM.

3.4. LCM Procedure

The LCM should be carried out as quickly as possible to minimize RNA degradation. The rate of RNA degradation is tissue specific and can be tested simply by allowing slides processed for LCM to sit at room temperature for variable time periods and then purifying the RNA from the sections on the slides and determining levels of RNA integrity on an Agilent Bioanalyzer. The processed slides are dehydrated, which significantly reduces RNAse activity. We have found that for embryonic kidneys RNA loss is minimal after 30 min and acceptable for up to 1 h. For other tissues with higher levels of endogenous RNAse, however, RNA degradation can occur much more quickly.

The details below are specific to the Arcturus Veritas machine, but the principles also apply to other platforms.

1. Turn the LCM machine on, activate the Veritas software, insert username and password, and click start a new session.
2. Load slides and caps, fill in relevant information on pop-up windows, and click OK.
3. Roadmap low power magnification images appear that show where the tissue sections on the slides are located. Double-click on a section to provide a higher power image of the region of interest.
4. Use the mouse to place a Cap over the region of interest. Ideally, the tissue should be centrally located and not in contact with the support struts of the Cap (see Note 7).
5. Drag a region without tissue to the center of the field. Double-click the mouse to fire the IR laser. Adjust the aim by left clicking the mouse and using "capture laser is here" function.
6. Adjust the power and duration of the IR laser to achieve an optimal melt spot when the laser is fired. A blurred circle that cannot be focused indicates that the Cap plastic was not melted sufficiently to extend down to the PEN slide. In this case, the

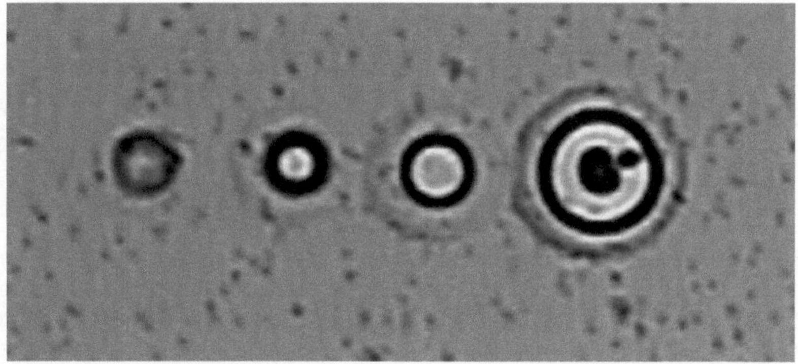

Fig. 2. Ideal infrared (IR) laser melt spots. A series of spots generated with the IR laser are shown. The *blurred spot* on the far *left* indicates insufficient heating to melt the thermoplastic membrane to create a genuine melt spot. The membrane remains suspended above the sample. The next spot is small, but would work well for capturing minute samples of just one or a few cells. The *third spot* is generally ideal for excellent attachment of the thermoplastic membrane to the sample tissue. The *far right spot* is quite large, but could be effective for collecting large samples, where maximal contact is useful.

power and/or duration of the laser pulse needs to be turned higher (Fig. 2). An ideal melt spot is a sharp black line circle with a clear center. This shows that the Cap plastic was heated sufficiently to melt, descend to the PEN slide membrane and form a region where the Cap and slide plastics melted together. It is very important that an appropriate melt spot is formed (see Note 8).

7. Return to the tissue region of interest and from the menu bar activate the UV cutting laser. Adjust the aim using the mouse activated drop down menu function (cutting laser is here).
8. The power of the UV laser needs to be properly adjusted from the window on the left. A "low" power setting of 3–5 is typically appropriate (see Note 9).
9. Click "capture image" to get a photograph of the tissue section before LCM. It is generally advisable to capture images before, after using the UV cutting laser, and after separating the sample of interest from the slide, to thoroughly document the tissue sample that was taken.
10. Use the mouse to draw a line around the tissue of interest.
11. Activate the UV cutting laser, which will then cut along the line drawn with the mouse (Fig. 3).
12. Use the menu bar to return to the IR capture laser. Click the hand. Use manual setting. Automatic setting will trigger a large number of melt spots, creating "plastic sandwich" problems (see Note 10).
13. Double-click the mouse to create a melt spot on the tissue of interest (see Note 10). One variant of the LCM procedure just

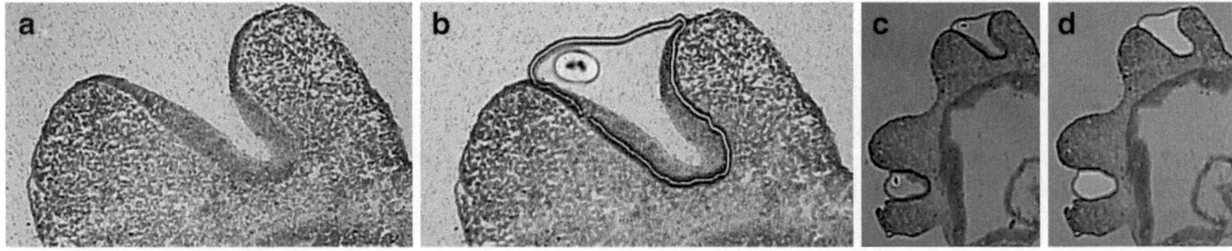

Fig. 3. Laser capture microdissection example. (**a**) A cryostat section showing E10.5 embryonic developing craniofacial region. (**b**) The ultraviolet cutting laser was used to cut around the cells of the olfactory pit. The infrared laser was used to generate a large melt spot, showing melting of the thermoplastic membrane of the Cap to the membrane of the PEN slide. (**c**) A lower magnification image showing both olfactory pits. (**d**) An "after" image showing both olfactory pits cleanly removed from the tissue section, and now residing on the Cap.

uses the IR capture laser to melt plastic onto the cells of interest. No UV cutting laser is used. Then when the Cap is removed the cells that are attached to the melted plastic are lifted from the surface. An advantage of this method is that since no cutting laser is used there is no UV laser damage to cells. This method, therefore, is sometimes useful for the capture of very small samples, with only a few cells, where the UV laser would of necessity be cutting very near all of the cells of interest. Another advantage is that PEN membrane slides, which again are expensive, are not required. A major disadvantage, however, is that the cells must be pulled off of the underlying surface, and from the flanking cells, to which they are attached. It is often challenging to achieve good "lifting" of the cells of interest.

14. Move the field of view by double-clicking on a region of the roadmap image where there is no tissue, and use the mouse activated "place cap in center of field" function to move the Cap to this position. The image should now show the captured tissue attached to the Cap. (If not, then see Note 11.)
15. Take photographs of the Cap with the captured material as well as the tissue with the region of interest removed.

3.5. Processing Caps

1. The laser capture tissue now residing on the Cap can be used for transcription profiling, via RNA-Seq or microarrays, or for DNA analysis or proteomics. For example, RNA can be purified using the Zymo ZR RNA MicroPrep kit, and target amplifications for microarray analysis can be performed using Nugen products designed for extremely small samples, such as Ovation Pico WTA System (for samples with just a few nanograms of total RNA), or WT-Ovation One-Direct Amplification (for samples as small as a single cell).

4. Notes

1. Process samples as quickly as possible. The more time that passes before freezing, the greater the chance of RNA degradation.
2. The OCT is hyperosmotic and tends to absorb the water from the tissue it touches, which can in particular ruin the edges of the tissue of interest. Nevertheless, be sure to carefully rinse the PBS away because it can interfere with the sectioning. Leaving the sample in OCT for too long a period, however, can seriously distort tissue morphology.
3. As you move the mold against the surface a melted region of 2-methylbutane will appear. Keep the mold in this melted region, moving it to improve thermal contact and to prevent freezing of the mold into the 2-methylbutane as it continues to cool and refreeze.
4. If the sample is still too brittle, with flaking and shattering during sectioning, then try warming the specimen and chamber temperatures a degree or two.
5. The membrane slides are quite expensive, so use regular slides until tissue is clearly visible, and then switch to membranes slides.
6. We have found that embryonic kidney sections do not adhere well to the membranes of PEN slides. To prevent loss of sections during later processing steps it is necessary to pretreat the slides by dipping in 1/10 dilution of poly lysine, and then air drying in a vertical position.
7. The Caps hold the thermoplastic membrane immediately above the sample section. The Cap rests on struts arranged in a circle around the region of interest on the PEN membrane slide. If these struts rest on tissue then the tissue can stick to them, and end up contaminating the sample. This material is informally referred to as "Cap crap". The best way to avoid Cap crap is to have sections that do not make unintended contact with the Caps. Small sections that can be contained within the strut-encircled region are ideal. Also, it is important to have flat sections, without wrinkles or folds that might extend vertically far enough to contact the membrane of the Cap. Contaminants can be in part addressed using an ablation laser. This is a high intensity laser that is fired at the unwanted material. In our experience, however, the ablation laser will often explode the contaminating material into many small pieces that then are scattered on the Cap. If possible, it is best to simply avoid the contaminating material in the first place.

8. If the melt spot is too small then there might not be sufficient contact for the Cap to lift the UV cut tissue section and underlying PEN membrane from the slide. On the other hand, if the melt spot is too large then it might cover too wide a region and reduce the resolution of the LCM, and/or create "plastic sandwich" problems, as described in Note 10. In some cases, it seems impossible to actually create a melt spot. Instead, only a blurred circle is formed, suggesting that the plastic has not been able to melt all the way down to the tissue section. This can be the result of the cap not lying flat on the PEN membrane slide. In some cases, the struts are on a thickened region of tissue, perhaps a folded part of tissue section, or a part of tissue section that is elevated after coming loose from the membrane. In this case, try moving the Cap to a new region of the slide, where the tissue section is not protruding.
9. If the UV power setting is too low then the PEN membrane and tissue are not completely cut and the sample cannot be separated, or "lifted", from the slide. On the other hand, if the power setting is too high, then it can cause damage of flanking tissue. If large swaths of tissue are being collected then UV damage of the relatively small edge regions may be acceptable. On the other hand, if a small region of only a few cells is being collected, or a single cell layer, then the UV power setting must be kept to a minimum to reduce damage. This is an empirical trial and error process, finding the minimal setting that allows good sample "lifts".
10. It is often advisable to locate the melt spot near an edge of the tissue region to be captured. If the melt spot region is too extensive then this can result in a "plastic sandwich". The captured tissue is trapped between the PEN slide membrane and the melted Cap membrane. This enclosed tissue is difficult to access, which can result in dramatically reduced yields of RNA.
11. Sometimes the sample fails to lift from the PEN slide with the Cap. This can be caused by incomplete cutting with the UV laser, or ineffective melting with the IR laser. One can repeat the cutting with the UV laser. If additional cuts still do not release the sample then the UV laser power may need to be increased. One can also improve the lifting by increasing the melted contact surface with the IR laser. In some cases, the first lift attempt will only remove the cells from the melt spot region, but not carry with it the underlying membrane. In this case it is advisable to remelt to the spot where the cells have been removed. The plastic-to-plastic melt creates a firmer attachment than plastic to cells.

Acknowledgments

This work was supported by NIH grants RC4DK090891, UO1DK070251, and UO1DE020049. We thank Lauren Kadel and Andrew S. Potter for technical assistance with laser capture.

References

1. Brunskill EW, Aronow BJ, Georgas K et al (2008) Atlas of gene expression in the developing kidney at microanatomic resolution. Dev Cell 15:781–791
2. Curran S, McKay JA, McLeod HL, Murray GI (2000) Laser capture microscopy. Mol Pathol 53:64–68
3. Geho DH, Bandle RW, Clair T, Liotta LA (2005) Physiological mechanisms of tumor-cell invasion and migration. Physiology (Bethesda) 20:194–200
4. Emmert-Buck MR, Bonner RF, Smith PD et al (1996) Laser capture microdissection. Science 274:998–1001
5. Kolble K (2000) The LEICA microdissection system: design and applications. J Mol Med 78:B24–B25
6. Micke P, Ostman A, Lundeberg J, Ponten F (2005) Laser-assisted cell microdissection using the PALM system. Methods Mol Biol 293:151–166
7. Schermelleh L, Thalhammer S, Heckl W et al (1999) Laser microdissection and laser pressure catapulting for the generation of chromosome-specific paint probes. Biotechniques 27:362–367
8. Espina V, Wulfkuhle JD, Calvert VS et al (2006) Laser-capture microdissection. Nat Protoc 1:586–603

Chapter 20

Use of In Situ Hybridization to Examine Gene Expression in the Embryonic, Neonatal, and Adult Urogenital System

Bree A. Rumballe, Han Sheng Chiu, Kylie M. Georgas, and Melissa H. Little

Abstract

Studies into the molecular basis of morphogenesis frequently begin with investigations into gene expression across time and cell type in that organ. One of the most anatomically informative approaches to such studies is the use of in situ hybridization, either of intact or histologically sectioned tissues. Here, we describe the optimization of this approach for use in the temporal and spatial analysis of gene expression in the urogenital system, from embryonic development to the postnatal period. The methods described are applicable for high throughput analysis of large gene sets. As such, ISH has become a powerful technique for gene expression profiling and is valuable for the validation of profiling analyses performed using other approaches such as microarrays.

Key words: In situ hybridization, Metanephros, Kidney, Urogenital system, Genitourinary system, Gene expression, mRNA expression

1. Introduction

In situ hybridization (ISH) is a technique to localize the expression of a gene in a particular tissue and at a particular time point either during development or in the adult. ISH can also be used to assess gene expression strength across different cell types and structures within the same tissue. Gene-specific RNA probes (riboprobes) designed to a complementary sequence within the 3′ UTR of a gene bind to and detect mRNA expression in the tissue being hybridized. Here, we describe the use of riboprobes nonradioactively labeled with digoxigenin hybridized in situ to whole embryonic urogenital tracts and cultured kidney explants using whole mount ISH and paraffin sectioned kidneys from the embryonic, neonatal and adult mouse using section ISH (SISH). Bound riboprobes are detected using an anti-digoxigenin antibody conjugated

Odyssé Michos (ed.), *Kidney Development: Methods and Protocols*, Methods in Molecular Biology, vol. 886,
DOI 10.1007/978-1-61779-851-1_20, © Springer Science+Business Media, LLC 2012

to alkaline phosphatase (AP) and visualized through an in situ color reaction with chromogenic substrates of the enzyme. The technique has many different applications. In developmental biology, ISH can be used to locate the cellular and tissue-specific expression pattern of a gene and can be used to perform gene expression profiling across different developmental stages of the embryonic and postnatal urogenital system, including the kidney. Although it can be utilized for the analysis of single genes, ISH has been extremely successful in large-scale gene expression mapping of the kidney (1–3). ISH can also be used to examine abnormal gene expression in genetically altered knockout and mutant mouse strains. In mutant mice, ISH has been successfully used to identify potential downstream gene targets by identifying those genes whose expression is lost or altered when the mutated gene is functionally defective. In this way, regulatory gene networks can be deciphered. ISH is also applicable to kidney pathology, where it can be used to expression profile the kidney and its substructures in mouse models of kidney disease, either genetic or surgical and in other renal pathologies. ISH can also be used to examine the tissues response to experimental perturbations of kidney function, such as via treatment with drugs or after surgical or environmental renal injury. By using specific marker genes of known structures or processes, ISH can be used to compare normal and perturbed renal function and morphological development. Examples of such markers include genes involved in cellular proliferation and the cell cycle; renal transporters; specific markers of renal developmental or the nephron stages (metanephric mesenchyme, cap mesenchyme, and renal vesicle or S-shaped body); ureteric tree branching (including ureteric bud, ureteric tip and collecting duct markers); nephron patterning and segmentation using specific segment markers (such as those marking the subregions of the proximal, distal and loop of Henle tubules, podocytes, glomerular basement membrane and other glomerular structures); and cell-specific markers (such as endothelial, mesangial, mesenchymal, or smooth muscle cells).

Whole mount ISH (WISH) is valuable as a high throughput expression profiling technique for the examination of many genes, across multiple developmental stages and tissue types. In some instances it may be more informative to examine the whole urogenital system or whole kidney, such as during the investigation of mutant phenotypes. However, the kidney is a very complex tissue with a large number of distinct cell types arising during the tubulogenesis, segmentation, and functionalization that occur to form the nephrons. In addition, by approximately 15.5 dpc (days post-coitum) the size of the kidney is such that penetration issues and tissue structure can reduce the accuracy of gene expression information gained via WISH. This is where SISH is advantageous over WISH. Here, we describe two methods for SISH of PFA-fixed paraffin-embedded kidney tissue. SISH has the ability to examine, at a high resolution, distinct cellular elements and allows for a more accurate description of the site of gene expression. In addition, SISH is more effective for investigating gene expression in the larger, more complex neonatal and adult kidneys.

We also describe optional methods for semiautomated WISH and SISH procedures, which utilize specialized robotic systems. These methods have been developed as part of the GenitoUrinary Development Molecular Anatomy Project (GUDMAP) and have been successfully used in the high throughput examination of gene expression patterns in the urogenital system, especially the kidney (4) and form a large component of the GUDMAP database, which is publicly available via the GUDMAP Web site (www.gudmap.org).

We have used the WISH method described here to perform gene expression profiling across different tissues and stages of the embryonic mouse urogenital system. Such tissues have included in vitro cultured kidney explants, whole embryos (9.5 and 10.5 dpc), the early urogenital system (bisected embryos at 10.5 dpc) and female and male urogenital tracts including the kidneys, gonads, mesonephroi, ureters, bladder, and genital tubercle/ external genitalia (11.5, 12.5, 13.5, 14.5, and 15.5 dpc). Using WISH, we have successfully investigated the development of the genital tubercle in the mouse (5), identified nephron patterning genes that are expressed in differentiating mesonephric tubules of the male and female reproductive system (6) and profiled the sex-specific expression of genes in the male and female gonad (12). In more high resolution analyses, we have successfully used SISH to examine early nephron patterning within the renal vesicle (7), to validate microanatomic resolution microarray profiling of the developing kidney (8), to identify 37 anchor genes for different compartments of the developing kidney and nephron (3) and to examine the changing profile of critical kidney genes at the cessation of nephrogenesis in the neonatal mouse (9). We have used SISH in high resolution profiling studies for GUDMAP to examine gene expression in the embryonic (15.5 and 17.5 dpc), neonatal (P0, 2, 4, and 6), and adult kidney and in the embryonic (13.5 and 15.5 dpc) and postnatal (P0 and adult) reproductive system (testis, epididymis, ovary, uterus, oviduct, mesonephros, and genital tubercle) and lower urinary tract (ureter, bladder, and urethra) (www.gudmap.org).

Here we describe one WISH method which can be performed either manually or using a robot (semiautomated) and is partially based on previous protocols by Wilkinson and Nieto (10) and Challen et al. (11). Two SISH methods are described, one method developed for manual SISH and the second method for semiautomated SISH, and are based on the previously described methods by Wilhelm et al. (12) and Rumballe et al. (13), respectively. The semiautomated SISH protocol can also be performed manually without the use of a robot and using the same materials and procedure.

2. Materials

All ISH methods require DIG-labeled antisense riboprobes and the ISH methods presented here have been optimized for riboprobes of 500–800 bp in length generated via PCR from a DNA template (mouse cDNA or DNA clone) (see Notes 1, 2 and 3). The procedure we use for generating riboprobes is described in detail on the GUDMAP Web site which can be accessed on the Little Group Protocols via the Project Protocols link on the GUDMAP Resources page http://gudmap.org/Resources/index.html. All solutions should be prepared in clean, baked (2 h at 180°C) glassware or sterile plastic ware and using ultrapure water (RO) of 18 MΩ-cm at 25°C to ensure no contamination from RNases.

2.1. Materials for Whole Mount In Situ Hybridization

1. Stock solutions for WISH:
   (a) 20× SSC: 3 M NaCl, 0.3 M Na citrate, pH 5.
   (b) 5% CHAPS.
   (c) 1 M Tris–HCl (solutions at pH 7.4, 7.6, and 8.0).
   (d) 5 M NaCl; 1 M $MgCl_2$; 0.5 M EDTA; and 10% Tween 20.
2. Solutions for WISH prehybridization (see Note 4):
   (a) Phosphate buffered saline (PBS).
   (b) 4% Paraformaldehyde (PFA) in PBS prepared fresh on the day of use.
   (c) PBTX: 1× PBS, 0.1% Triton X-100.
   (d) Methanol/PBTX series: 25, 50, 75, and 100% methanol diluted with PBTX.
   (e) 0.2 M NaOH (optional for robot cleaning).
   (f) PBT: 1% Tween 20 in PBS.
   (g) 6% Hydrogen peroxide in PBT.
   (h) 10 μg/ml Proteinase K (Roche, 3115879) in PBTX prepared fresh before use.
   (i) 0.2% Glutaraldehyde—4% PFA in PBTX.
   (j) TBTX: 0.05 M Tris–HCl pH 7.5, 0.15 M NaCl, and 0.1% Triton X-100.
3. Solutions for WISH hybridization (see Note 4):
   (a) WISH hybridization buffer: 50% formamide, 5× SSC, 2% blocking powder, 0.1% Triton X-100, 0.5% CHAPS, 1 mg/ml torula yeast RNA, 5 mM EDTA, and 50 μg/ml heparin.

4. Solutions for WISH posthybridization (see Note 4):
   (a) TBTX: 0.05 M Tris–HCl pH 7.5, 0.15 M NaCl, and 0.1% Triton X-100.
   (b) Solution 1: 50% formamide, 5× SSC, 0.1% Triton X-100, and 0.5% CHAPS.
   (c) 2× SSC.
   (d) Solution 1: 2× SSC stringency series (100, 75–25, 50–50, and 25–75%).
   (e) 2× SSC: 0.1% CHAPS.
   (f) 0.2× SSC: 0.1% CHAPS.
   (g) WISH preblocking solution: 10% heat-inactivated sheep serum, and 2% BSA in TBTX.
   (h) Preabsorbed anti-Digoxigenin (DIG) antibody bound to AP (Roche, 11093274910): 18 mg of mouse embryo powder is placed in a 10 ml tube with 10% heat-inactivated sheep serum, 2% BSA in TBTX and 15 μl anti-DIG-AP and incubated at 4°C for 3 h or longer with gentle rocking and centrifuged for 10 min, 4°C at 13,000 rpm. Supernatant is collected and diluted to 50 ml with 10% sheep serum and 2% BSA in TBTX. Preabsorbed antibody can be kept at 4°C and recycled up to three times.
   (i) 0.1% BSA in TBTX.
   (j) NTMT: 0.1 M NaCl, 0.1 M Tris–HCl pH 9.5, 0.05 M $MgCl_2$, and 0.1% Tween 20.
   (k) NBT-BCIP (Roche) in NTMT: 3.5 μl of each substrate per 1 ml NTMT.
   (l) PBS.
   (m) 1% Triton X-100 in PBS.
   (n) 4% PFA in PBS.
   (o) 1% Agarose in PBS (optional for photography).
5. WISH equipment:
   (a) Sterile specimen tubes or tissue culture plates (we routinely use 48 multiwell plates).
   (b) Rocking platform.
   (c) Fume hood.
   (d) Incubator at 65°C (see Note 5).
   (e) Dissecting microscope and camera (we use a Nikon SMZ1500 research stereomicroscope and Nikon DXM1200f, Color 12 megapixel digital camera).
   (f) *Optional for semiautomated WISH*: BioLane HTI Robot and nylon mesh baskets (we use the blue system with the small, 20 basket tray).

2.2. Materials for Section In Situ Hybridization

1. Stock solutions for SISH:
   (a) 50× Denhardt's solution: 0.5 g Ficoll (type 400), 0.5 g polyvinylpyrrolidone, 0.5 g bovine serum albumin (fraction V), and water to 50 ml.
   (b) 20× SSC: 3 M NaCl, 0.3 M sodium citrate, pH 5.
   (c) 5 M NaCl; 1 M $MgCl_2$; 1 M Tris–HCl pH 7.6.
   (d) 1 M Tris–HCl pH 9.5.
   (e) 0.5 M EDTA.
   (f) 10% Tween 20.
2. Solutions for SISH prehybridization (see Note 4):
   (a) Xylene AR grade.
   (b) Ethanol–water series (100, 95, 80, 70, 60, 30% ethanol diluted with water).
   (c) PBS.
   (d) 4% PFA in PBS prepared fresh before use.
   (e) 10 μg/ml Proteinase K in PBS prepared fresh before use.
   (f) Acetylation solution: per 100 ml, mix 1.33 ml triethanolamine with water until dissolved, add 0.175 ml 37% HCl and immediately prior to use add 0.375 ml acetic anhydride.
   (g) NaCl solution: 0.85% [w/v] in water.
   (h) 0.85% [w/v] NaCl in 70% ethanol.
   (i) Additional ethanol solutions (95 and 70% diluted with water).
3. Solutions for SISH hybridization (see Note 4):
   (a) *Semiautomated SISH hybridization buffer*: 50% Formamide, 2× SSC pH 5, 1× Denhardt's solution, 10% dextran sulfate, 0.5 mg/ml salmon sperm DNA, 0.2 mg/ml torula yeast RNA, and water.
   (b) *Manual SISH hybridization buffer*: 50% formamide, 5× SSC, 5× Denhardt's solution, 250 μg/ml yeast RNA, and 500 μg/ml herring sperm DNA.
4. Solutions for SISH posthybridization (see Note 4):

   Semiautomated SISH Solutions Posthybridization
   (a) 5× SSC.
   (b) 50% Formamide, 1× SSC.
   (c) *Optional* TNE: 10 mM Tris–HCl pH 7.5, 500 mM NaCl, and 1 mM EDTA.
   (d) *Optional* 2 μg/ml RNase A in TNE.
   (e) 2× SSC.

(f) 0.2× SSC.

(g) MBST: 100 mM maleic acid, 150 mM NaCl, and 0.1% Tween-20, pH 7.5.

(h) Automated SISH blocking buffer: 2% Blocking Reagent (Roche, 11096176001), 20% heat-inactivated sheep serum in MBST.

(i) 1:1,000 anti-Digoxigenin (DIG) antibody bound to AP (Roche 11093274910) diluted in automated SISH blocking buffer.

(j) NTMT: 0.1 M NaCl, 0.1 M Tris–HCl pH 9.5, 50 mM $MgCl_2$, and 0.1% Tween20.

(k) 2 mM Levamisole in NTMT.

(l) BM Purple (Roche, 11442074001).

(m) PBS.

(n) 4% PFA in PBS.

(o) Aqueous mounting medium.

Manual SISH Solutions Posthybridization

(a) 5× SSC, pH 5.

(b) 0.5× SSC, pH 5.

(c) NT: 150 mM NaCl, 50 mM Tris–HCl, pH 7.5.

(d) Manual SISH blocking buffer: 10% heat-inactivated sheep serum in NT.

(e) 1:1,000 anti-Digoxigenin (DIG) antibody bound to AP (Roche, 11093274910) diluted in 1% heat-inactivated sheep serum in NT.

(f) NBT/BCIP (Roche, 11383213001 and 11383221001) in NTM: 3.5 μl of each substrate per 1 ml NTM.

(g) NTM buffer: 100 mM NaCl, 100 mM Tris–HCl pH 9.5, and 50 M $MgCl_2$.

(h) PBS.

(i) 4% PFA in PBS

(j) Aqueous mounting medium.

5. SISH equipment:

(a) Superfrost Plus® glass slides.

(b) Glass coverslips for slide 22 mm × 50 mm.

(c) Glass/metal slide staining racks.

(d) Glass-staining jars (300 ml).

(e) Fume hood.

(f) Humidified aluminum foil-wrapped slide incubation chambers.

(g) Incubators at 37 and 65°C (see Note 5).

(h) Slide microscope and camera (we use the semiautomated slide System from Olympus and Soft Imaging Systems (BX51 microscope, digital CCD camera, motorized scanning stage and workstation, automated slide loader and slide software) and images captured using Olyvia software (Soft Imaging Systems, Olympus).

(i) *Optional for semiautomated SISH*: Tecan Freedom EVO150 platform GenePaint™ System.

3. Methods

Both WISH and SISH methods begin with fixed kidneys and urogenital tissues isolated from adult, neonatal or embryonic mice (from time-mated pregnant females). We routinely use the outbred CD1 strain. All tissues are dissected in ice-cold PBS and immediately fixed in fresh 4% PFA in PBS overnight at 4°C (see Note 4). Fixed tissues are dehydrated with an alcohol series prior to the in situ hybridization procedure. All ISH methods are carried out at room temperature unless otherwise specified. Prehybridization and probe hybridization steps and the immediate posthybridization washes are carried out at a temperature chosen for optimal probe binding, usually between 55 and 68°C (see Note 5). We routinely use 65°C. Posthybridization wash solutions are preheated to 65°C (or the hybridization temperature). All glassware should be baked (2 h at 180°C) or sterile plastic ware used and all equipment contacting the tissue should be cleaned with 70% ethanol and may be treated with an RNase removal reagent, such as RNase AWAY™ (Invitrogen, 10328011), to eliminate RNase contamination. Within each experiment we utilize at least two control riboprobes, usually one strongly and one weakly expressed gene in your chosen tissue, to monitor experimental quality (see Note 1).

3.1. Whole Mount In Situ Hybridization

The WISH method presented here is essentially identical for manual and semiautomated procedures. However, with semiautomated WISH, some washes are performed in a BioLane HTI Robot. The BioLane system uses nylon mesh baskets to contain the tissues. We routinely use the small, 20-basket robot tray, which limits the experiment to 20 probes per robot run including control probes. However, the system can be altered according to your requirement, as three different tray sizes are available. In each WISH run, we routinely use the following tissues per probe for profiling in the GUDMAP project; two in vitro cultured kidney explants (on filter); two whole embryos at 9.5 dpc, three bisected embryos at 10.5 dpc; one female and one male whole, intact urogenital tract (including the kidneys, gonads, mesonephroi, ureters, bladder, and genital tubercle/external genitalia) at 12.5 or 13.5 dpc. The tissues examined per probe will vary according to your requirements. The WISH procedure may require minor modifications for older and/or larger tissues.

Manual WISH: the entire procedure is performed in individual sterile plastic tubes or multiwell tissue culture plates on a rocking platform, either at room temperature or in a 65°C incubator (see Note 5).

Semiautomated WISH: steps 1–4 are performed in a BioLane HTI robot. Prior to WISH, the nylon mesh baskets and robot tubing are cleaned with 0.2 M NaOH, followed by water using the cleaning program.

1. Fixed embryonic tissues are washed twice in PBTX for 10 min each (see Note 4) and dehydrated using a Methanol/PBTX series (25, 50, 75, and 100% methanol in PBTX) for 20 min each, followed by two washes in 100% methanol for 20 min each. Tissues are stored in 100% methanol at -20°C.
2. Prior to WISH, rehydrate tissues using a methanol/PBTX series (100, 75, 50, 25% methanol in PBTX) for 5 min each, followed by washes in PBTX for 10 min and PBT for 5 min.
3. The tissues are then incubated in 6% hydrogen peroxide in PBT for 60 min and washed for 5 min in PBT followed by two 5 min PBTX washes.
4. Digest the tissues with 10 μg/ml Proteinase K in PBTX for 20 min (or as appropriate for the tissue type). Stop digestion by washing twice with PBTX, 5 min each.
5. *Optional for semiautomated WISH*: remove baskets from robot tray and place into the individual wells of a tissue culture plate.
6. Fix tissues in 0.2% glutaraldehyde—4% PFA in PBTX for 20 min, followed by two 10 min washes in PBTX (see Note 4).
7. Prehybridization: Add 0.5 ml WISH hybridization buffer to each tube/well. Incubate at 65°C for 2 h (see Note 5).
8. Prepare 0.2–0.4 μg/ml of each DIG-labeled riboprobe diluted in 0.5 ml WISH hybridization buffer in 1.5-ml plastic tubes (see Notes 1 and 4).
9. Hybridization: aliquot diluted probes into individual tubes/wells containing your tissue and incubate overnight at 65°C (see Notes 4 and 5).

   Semiautomated WISH: steps 10–12, *posthybridization washes, anti-DIG-AP binding, and postantibody washes, are performed in a BioLane HTI robot.*
10. Posthybridization washes are performed at 65°C and include a Solution 1—2× SSC stringency series (100, 75–25, 50–50, and 25–75%) for 5 min each followed by two washes in

2× SSC—0.1% CHAPS for 10 min each, two washes in 0.2× SSC—0.1% CHAPS for 5 min each and two washes in TBTX for 10 min each (see Note 4).

11. Tissues are prepared for anti-DIG-AP antibody binding by incubating in WISH preblocking solution for 2 h at room temperature. Replace preblock with preabsorbed antibody and incubate at 4°C overnight.
12. Postantibody washes include five washes in 0.1% BSA in TBTX for 30 min each, followed by two TBTX washes for 10 min each and three NTMT washes for 10 min each.
13. *Optional for semiautomated WISH*: remove baskets from robot tray and place into individual wells of a tissue culture plate.
14. Incubate tissue in color substrates NBT/BCIP in NTM, in the dark, at room temperature (see Note 6). Monitor color development every 30 min (see Note 7). Allow color development to continue until signal detected is sufficient for imaging (1–30 h).
15. Once color development is complete, wash the tissue in distilled water to stop the color reaction. Follow this with an overnight wash in 1% Triton X-100 in PBS at 4°C. Additional washes in 1% Triton X-100 in PBS can be performed at 4°C for several days to remove excessive color (see Note 8). Wash three times in PBS for 5 min to remove Triton X-100.
16. Fix tissues with 4% PFA in PBS for 30 min (see Note 4). Remove fixative by washing three times with PBS for 5 min each. Samples are stored in PBS at 4°C in individual 2 ml tubes.
17. Photograph tissue suspended in PBS in a tissue culture dish with a base of 1% agarose in PBS (which produces a blue background) using a dissecting microscope and camera (see Note 9). Examples are shown in Fig. 1.

3.2. Section In Situ Hybridization

Two methods are given for SISH, one for manual and one for semiautomated SISH. With semiautomated SISH, the majority of steps are performed in a Tecan Freedom EVO150 platform (GenePaint™ System). Some steps are the same for both methods and for other steps both the procedure and solutions differ. Italicized text indicates when the step is specific to either the manual or automated method. In addition, the semiautomated SISH method can also be performed manually without the use of a robot, using the same materials and steps.

1. Fixed kidneys are washed in PBS (see Note 4), dehydrated using an ethanol series to a final solution of 70% ethanol and processed into paraffin blocks as soon as possible. Embed 1–2 adult kidneys and 5–8 embryonic kidneys per block. During embedding, kidneys are oriented such that adult kidneys are sectioned

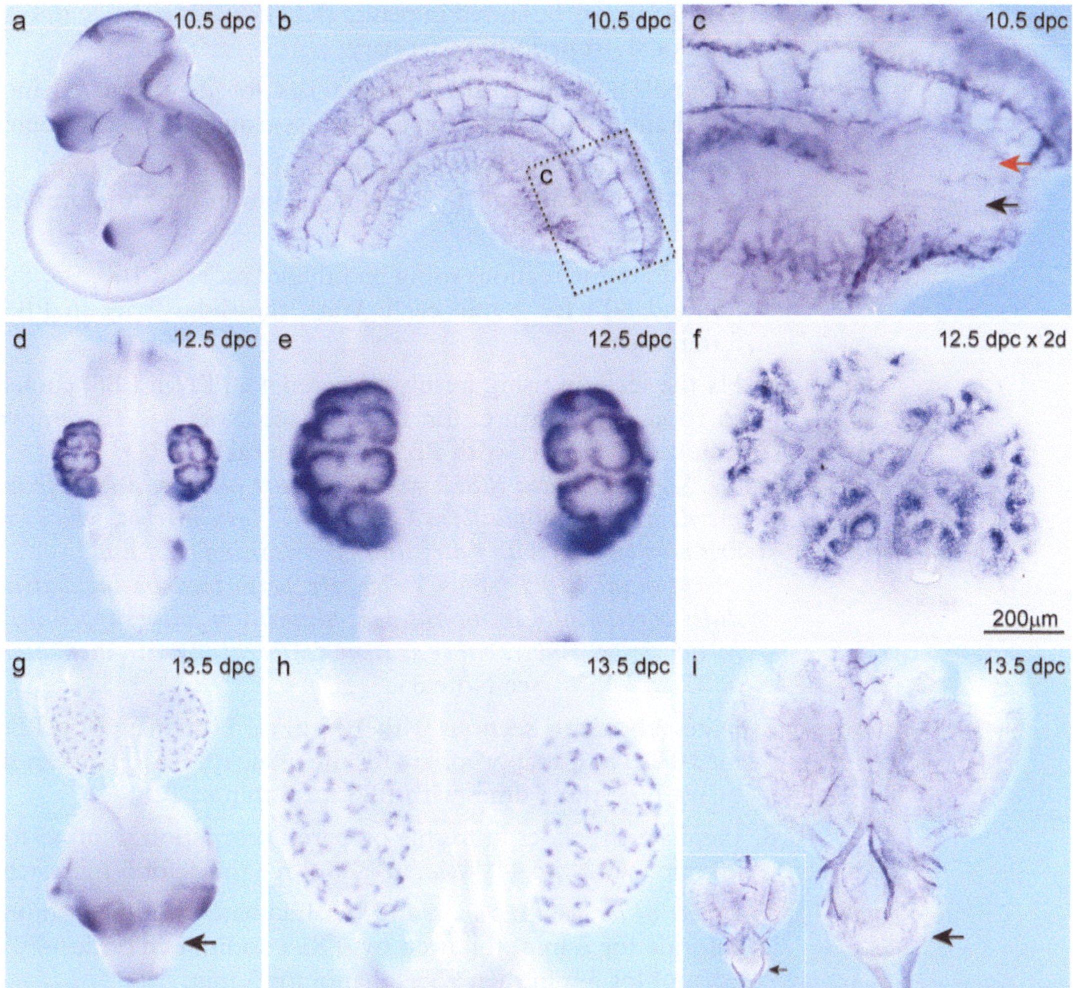

Fig. 1. Whole urogenital tissues hybridized with mouse riboprobes using the semiautomated WISH method visualized with NBT/BCIP. (**a**) *Tcfap2b* expression in a 10.5 dpc whole embryo. (**b**, **c**) *Cd34* expression in the developing vasculature of a bisected 10.5 dpc embryo. The hind limb is present and the caudal tail end of the embryo is on the *right*. The mesonephros, metanephric mesenchyme (*red arrow*), and nephric duct (*black arrow*) are visible and enlarged in (**c**). (**d**, **e**) *Crym* expression in the cap mesenchyme of the kidney at 12.5 dpc. Images of the whole urogenital tract (**d**) and kidneys (**e**) are shown. The tract also includes gonads, mesonephroi, ureters, and bladder. (**f**) *Wnt4* expression in a 12.5 dpc kidney cultured in vitro for 2 days (using the method described in ref. 11. (**g**, **h**) *Hs3st3b1* expression in early nephrons of the kidney at 13.5 dpc. The whole urogenital tract is shown in (**g**) and includes gonads, mesonephroi, ureters, bladder (not seen) and genital tubercle (*black arrow*) and the kidneys, which are enlarged in (**h**). (**i**) *Cd34* vasculature expression in the 13.5 dpc urogenital tract without the external genitalia allowing the bladder to be visualized (*black arrow*). The *inset image* shows the reverse side of the urogenital tract and the gonads (testes in this male specimen).

transversely and embryonic kidneys sagittally. These orientations provide optimal resolution of all regions of the kidney. Kidneys are stored in paraffin blocks at room temperature.

2. Prior to SISH, paraffin embedded tissue is sectioned at 7 µm onto Superfrost Plus® slides and air-dried completely before use.

The slides may be stored in plastic slide boxes at room temperature for short periods if necessary.

3. Assemble individual glass-staining jars for dewaxing, ethanol rehydration, and fixation, in a fume hood and label accordingly.
4. Dewax sections by immersing slides in xylene for 10 min (see Note 4). Repeat with fresh xylene solution for an additional 10 min.
5. Dehydrate the sections using an ethanol series of 100, 95, 80, 60, and 30% for 1 min each. Wash the slides twice in PBS, 5 min each.
6. Fix the sections using freshly prepared 4% PFA in PBS, cooled to room temperature, for 10 min (see Note 4). To remove fixative, wash twice with PBS for 5 min each.

   Semiautomated SISH: steps 7–25 *are performed in a Tecan Freedom EVO150 platform GenePaint™ System robot, which has first been cleaned with water using the cleaning program.*

   Manual SISH: steps 7–25 *are performed by incubating slides horizontally in humidified, aluminum foil-wrapped slide incubation chambers either at room temperature or in incubators at 37 and 65°C* (see Note 5).
7. Digest the tissue sections with 10 μg/ml Proteinase K in PBS for 10–20 min as appropriate for the tissue type. Stop digestion by washing three times with PBS for 5 min each.
8. Incubate the slides in freshly prepared acetylation solution for 10 min (see Note 4). Wash in PBS three times for 5 min each.
9. *Optional for semiautomated SISH*: Incubate in 0.85% sodium chloride for 3 min, followed by 0.85% sodium chloride—70% ethanol for 5 min then 95% ethanol for 5 min.
10. Prehybridization: incubate the slides with preheated SISH hybridization buffer (semiautomated or manual) for 1–3 h at 65°C (see Note 4).
11. Prepare 0.5–1 μg/ml of DIG-labeled riboprobe diluted in SISH hybridization buffer (semiautomated or manual) in a 1.5–2-ml plastic tube (see Notes 1 and 4). *Optional: Heat to 85°C for 5 min and store on ice until prehybridization of slides is complete.* Minimum probe volumes required per slide: *200 μl for manual SISH and 500 μl for semiautomated SISH.*
12. Hybridization: aliquot diluted probes onto the slides and hybridize at 65°C, overnight (minimum of 10 h) (see Notes 4 and 5). *For manual SISH carefully wipe the outside edges of the slides using lint-free tissues, taking care not to touch the tissue sections, and cover sections with either glass coverslips or parafilm squares during hybridization.*

    Posthybridization washes, anti-DIG-AP binding, and postantibody washes are different for manual and automated SISH methods. For the manual SISH method, go directly to step 19.

Steps 13–18 *are for the semiautomated SISH method only*:

13. After hybridization, wash the slides in 5× SSC (pH 5) at 65°C for 5 min, and then with 50% formamide, 1× SSC (pH 5) solution at 65°C for 20 min (see Notes 4 and 5).
14. *Optional step if concerned about RNases*: incubate with TNE for 10 min at 37°C, then with 2 μg/ml RNase A in TNE for 15 min at 37°C and wash in TNE for 10 min at 37°C.
15. Wash the slides with 2× SSC (pH 5) for 20 min at 65°C, with 0.2× SSC (pH 5) for 20 min at 65°C and 0.2× SSC (pH 5) for 20 min at room temperature. Wash the slides with 1× MBST for 5 min.
16. Prepare sections for anti-DIG-AP antibody binding by incubating the slides in automated SISH blocking buffer for 60 min. Replace blocking buffer with 1:1,000 anti-DIG-AP diluted in automated SISH blocking buffer and incubate for 2 h.
17. To remove unbound antibody, wash the slides in MBST three times for 5 min each.
18. Reduce background with 10-min incubation in 2 mM levamisole in NTMT. Disassemble slide chambers in NTMT solution. Go to step 23 for AP color reaction.

Steps 19–22 *are for the manual SISH method only:*

19. After hybridization, wash the slides with 5× SSC (pH 5) at 65°C for 5 min, then with 0.5× SSC (pH 5) at 65°C for 60 min, followed by 0.5× SSC (pH 5) at room temperature for 10 min.
20. Wash the slides twice in NT buffer for 10 min each.
21. Incubate the slides in manual SISH blocking buffer (10% heat-inactivated sheep serum in NT) for 60 min to prepare for anti-DIG-AP antibody binding. Replace with 1:1,000 anti-DIG-AP in 1% heat-inactivated sheep serum in NT overnight at 4°C.
22. Remove unbound antibody with three washes in NT for 10 min each, followed by a 10-min NTM wash. Go to step 23 for AP color reaction.

    Steps 23–25 *are the AP color reaction steps for both manual and semiautomated SISH methods and are performed by incubating slides horizontally in humidified, aluminum foil-wrapped slide incubation chambers.*

23. Carefully wipe away excess wash solution from the outside edges of the slides using lint-free tissues, taking care not to touch the tissue sections. Incubate tissue with color substrate in the dark at room temperature. *For the semiautomated SISH method we use BM Purple. For the manual SISH method we use NBT/BCIP in NTM.* Monitor color development every 60 min (see Note 7). Allow color development to continue until signal detected is sufficient for imaging (4–100 h). Long incubations

require the addition of new color substrate solution to ensure that the tissue does not dry out. Once color development is complete, wash the tissue in PBS (see Note 8).

24. Fix tissues with 4% PFA in PBS for 20 min and remove fix by washing twice with PBS for 10 min each (see Note 4).
25. Mount with aqueous mounting medium using glass coverslips and photograph using a slide microscope and camera (see Note 9). Examples are shown in Fig. 2. Store mounted slides in storage boxes.

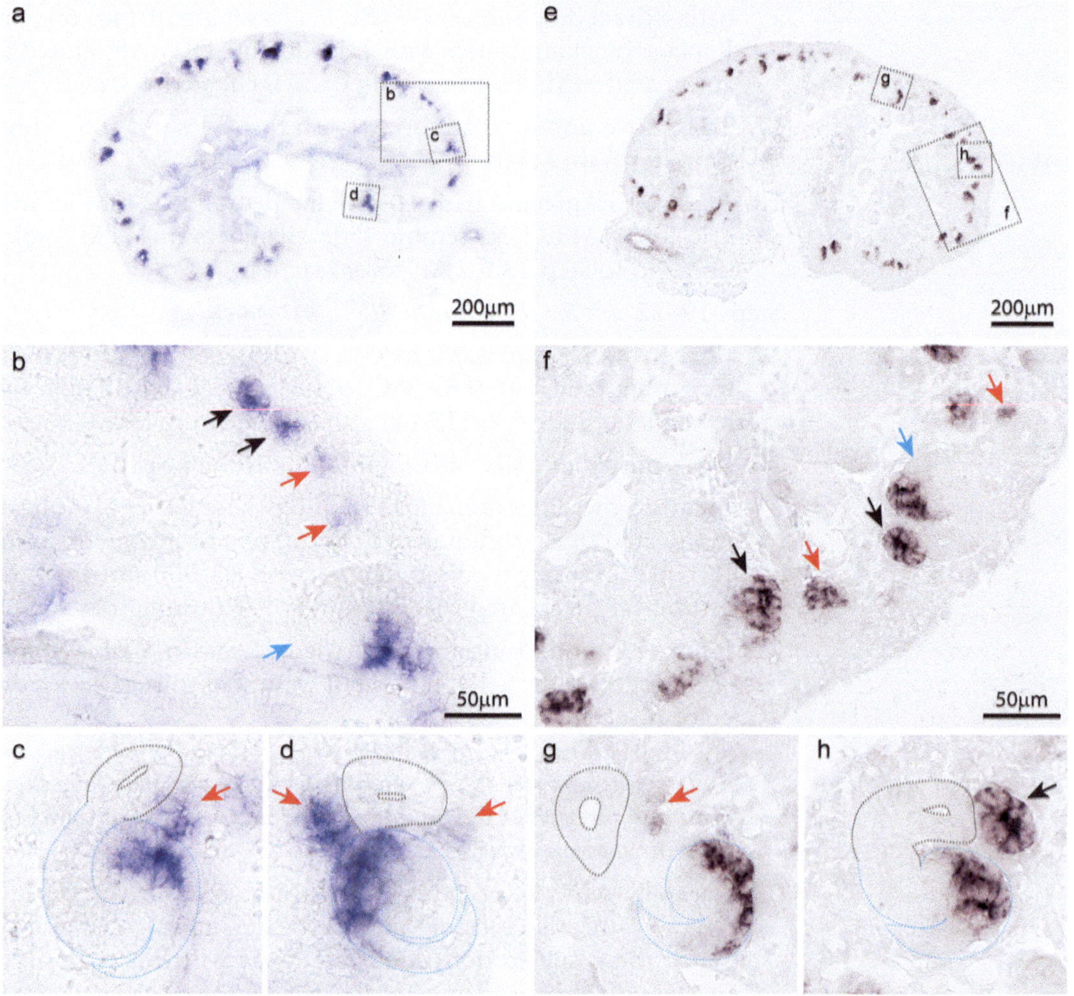

Fig. 2. Mouse embryonic kidney sections (15.5 dpc) hybridized with a *Wnt4* riboprobe using the semiautomated SISH method visualized with BM purple (**a–d**) and the manual SISH method visualized with NBT/BCIP (**e–h**). *Arrows* indicate *Wnt4* expression in pretubular aggregates (*red arrows*), renal vesicles (*black arrows*), and S-shaped bodies (*blue arrows*). In the high magnification images (**c**, **d** and **g**, **h**), ureteric tips are outlined in *black* and S-shaped bodies in *blue*.

4. Notes

1. In order to assess the sensitivity and quality of each ISH experiment, it is imperative to include two or more riboprobes as positive controls, with differing expression strengths (strongly and one weakly expressing genes). For kidney (15.5, 17.5 dpc, and neonatal), we routinely use *Wnt4* (strong), *Wnt7b* (moderate), and *Shh* (weak) riboprobe controls. The control genes will vary depending on your tissue type and stage.
2. When designing riboprobes, longer riboprobes produce a stronger ISH signal; however, they are usually more difficult to amplify using PCR. For validation of microarray expression analyses, riboprobes are designed to amplify a region corresponding to the microarray probeset. For more details refer to the GUDMAP Web site (http://gudmap.org/Resources/index.html).
3. In some instances, ISH may be less sensitive at detecting gene expression compared to microarray procedures. This must be taken into account when using ISH as an approach for the validation of microarray data.
4. The preparation and use of solutions containing xylene, formamide, triethanolamine, acetic anhydride, levamisole, and PFA should be performed in a fume hood.
5. The temperature chosen for probe hybridization may need to be modified according to your probe requirements. Optimal hybridization will usually occur between 55 and 68°C. Ensure that the prehybridization and heated posthybridization washes are carried out at the modified temperature.
6. Alternative color substrates can be used for each method (NBT/BCIP or BM purple); however, postantibody solutions and washes may need to be altered. The color development is faster with NBT/BCIP. When BM purple is used for SISH, aqueous mounting media must be used to prevent precipitation of the color substrate. When NBT/BCIP is used with the manual SISH method, it produces a more purple color than the blue color seen when used with the WISH method. In whole mounted tissue, NBT/BCIP is used as the preferred substrate because it produces a more specific signal than BM purple.
7. Monitor color development regularly (every 30 min for WISH, 60 min for SISH). Color development will vary depending on the probe and tissue type and requires much longer incubation times for SISH compared to WISH. If necessary, tissues may be incubated over several days either at room temperature or 4°C, depending on the rate of color development. If there is no background staining with a particular probe, the color

reaction should be incubated as long as possible to ensure that all hybridization sites are identified. This is especially critical for genes, which show strong expression in one region and weak expression in a different region of the same tissue/organ.

8. For very dark staining tissues that have been left in color substrate too long or which show high background staining, washes in 1% Triton X-100 in PBS can be performed at 4°C to remove excessive color. Follow with at least three washes in PBS for 5 min each to remove residual Triton X-100. In whole mounted tissues, these detergent washes also improve the intensity of blue color when using NBT/BCIP.

9. To assist with the analysis of gene expression patterns in the embryonic and adult kidney when using SISH, we have previously developed a method for dual SISH/immunohistochemistry (13, 14). This protocol utilizes the known expression patterns of seven antibody markers, which together identify the six stages of early nephron development, the tubular nephron segments, and the components of the renal corpuscle in both the embryonic and adult kidney.

Acknowledgments

This work was supported by NIH NIDDK grant to M.H.L. (DK070136). M.H.L. is a Principal Research Fellow of the National Health and Medical Research Council of Australia.

References

1. Takemoto M, He L, Norlin J et al (2006) Large-scale identification of genes implicated in kidney glomerulus development and function. EMBO J 25(5):1160–1174
2. Raciti D, Reggiani L, Geffers L et al (2008) Organization of the pronephric kidney revealed by large-scale gene expression mapping. Genome Biol 9(5):R84
3. Thiagarajan RD, Georgas KM, Rumballe BA et al (2011) Identification of anchor genes during kidney development defines ontological relationships, molecular subcompartments and regulatory pathways. PLoS One 6(2):e17286
4. Little MH, Brennan J, Georgas K et al (2007) A high-resolution anatomical ontology of the developing murine genitourinary tract. Gene Expr Patterns 7(6):680–699
5. Chiu HS, Szucsik JC, Georgas KM et al (2010) Comparative gene expression analysis of genital tubercle development reveals a putative appendicular Wnt7 network for the epidermal differentiation. Dev Biol 344(2):1071–1087
6. Georgas KM, Chiu HS, Lesieur E, Rumballe BA, Little MH (2011) Expression of metanephric nephron-patterning genes in differentiating mesonephric tubules. Dev Dyn 240(6):1600–1612
7. Georgas K, Rumballe B, Valerius MT et al (2009) Analysis of early nephron patterning reveals a role for distal RV proliferation in fusion to the ureteric tip via a cap mesenchyme-derived connecting segment. Dev Biol 332(2):273–286
8. Brunskill EW, Aronow BJ, Georgas K et al (2008) Atlas of gene expression in the developing kidney at microanatomic resolution. Dev Cell 5:781–791
9. Rumballe BA, Georgas KM, Combes A et al (2011) Nephron formation adopts a novel spatial topology at cessation of nephrogenesis. Dev Biol 360(1):110–122

10. Wilkinson DG, Nieto MA (1993) Detection of messenger RNA by in situ hybridization to tissue sections and whole mounts. Methods Enzymol 225:361–373
11. Challen G, Gardiner B, Caruana G et al (2005) Temporal and spatial transcriptional programs in murine kidney development. Physiol Genomics 23(2):159–171
12. Wilhelm D, Hiramatsu R, Mizusaki H et al (2007) SOX9 regulates prostaglandin D synthase gene transcription in vivo to ensure testis development. J Biol Chem 282:10553–10560
13. Rumballe B, Georgas K, Little MH (2008) High-throughput paraffin section in situ hybridization and dual immunohistochemistry on mouse tissues. CSH Protoc 5030:1. doi:10.1101/pdb.prot5030
14. Georgas K, Rumballe B, Wilkinson L et al (2008) Use of dual section mRNA in situ hybridisation/immunohistochemistry to clarify gene expression patterns during the early stages of nephron development in the embryo and in the mature nephron of the adult mouse kidney. Histochem Cell Biol 130(5):927–942

Chapter 21

Detection of β-Galactosidase Activity: X-gal Staining

Sally F. Burn

Abstract

X-gal staining is a rapid and convenient histochemical technique used to detect reporter gene expression. A prerequisite is the creation or acquisition of transgenic reporter mouse lines, in which the bacterial LacZ gene has been knocked into the gene of interest or placed under the control of regulatory elements corresponding to the gene of interest. Expression is marked by a dark blue stain and can be detected at the single cell level, providing a robust visual readout of gene expression in the developing kidney. Here, we describe the methodology, applications, and limitations of this technique.

Key words: Gene expression, Reporter, Transgenic, β-Galactosidase, X-gal, LacZ, Embryo, Staining

1. Introduction

1.1. Chemistry of X-gal Staining Reaction

X-gal staining (also often referred to as LacZ staining) is a relatively simple and rapid method to perform. It is also a very informative technique, particularly in the fields of molecular biology, genetics, and developmental biology. X-gal staining is central to cell lineage-tracing studies and can also be used as readout of gene expression.

The technique utilizes the bacterial (*Escherichia coli*) LacZ gene, which encodes the β-galactosidase enzyme (commonly referred to as β-gal). β-Galactosidase catalyzes the hydrolysis of β-galactosides into monosaccharides. One such β-galactoside is X-gal (5-bromo-4-chloro-3-indolyl-beta-D-galactopyranoside), an organic compound. β-Galactosidase cleaves X-gal into galactose and 5-bromo-4-chloro-3-hydroxyindole; this second compound is then oxidized into 5,5′-dibromo-4,4′-dichloro-indigo. As its name suggests, this final product is blue in color. X-gal staining therefore provides a visual assay of LacZ activity. Thus, we also can use this blue stain as a marker of our gene of interest, by placing the LacZ gene under the control of this gene.

Odyssé Michos (ed.), *Kidney Development: Methods and Protocols*, Methods in Molecular Biology, vol. 886,
DOI 10.1007/978-1-61779-851-1_21, © Springer Science+Business Media, LLC 2012

1.2. LacZ Reporter Mice

Transgenic LacZ reporter mice are generated in three main ways: (1) LacZ is targeted into the endogenous gene or locus of interest (LacZ knock in); (2) a plasmid containing LacZ under the regulatory control of genetic enhancer elements of interest is randomly integrated into the genome; (3) LacZ is introduced into the genome in one of the previous two ways but is only expressed following Cre-mediated recombination. In the first two methods, LacZ is expressed wherever the gene or regulatory elements being studied are active. In the final method, LacZ is expressed at these sites only when Cre recombinase removes sequences inhibitory to expression; furthermore, assuming the gene driving LacZ is ubiquitously expressed (as in the case of the Rosa26 locus), the LacZ gene is also expressed in all the descendants of the cell in which its expression was induced. The use of Cre permits tissue-specific and/or temporal control of LacZ expression. Tissue-specificity is conferred by placing Cre under the control of specific genetic elements. Temporal control is achieved by using an inducible Cre, for example CreERT2, a form of Cre fused to a modified estrogen receptor. Following exposure to Tamoxifen (a synthetic estrogen), the CreERT2 fusion protein is released from cytoplasmic sequestration and can translocate to the nucleus where it mediates recombination to remove a "stop sequence" and allow expression of LacZ (1). Cre-expressing lines are often used in conjunction with a ubiquitously expressed Cre-inducible LacZ, such as that in the R26R mouse (2). Thus, the spatial and temporal specificity of expression is controlled by the Cre line in this situation.

1.3. Uses for X-gal Staining

The first transgenic LacZ mice were reported over 20 years ago (3, 4). Since then, many lines have been generated and used to answer important questions about mammalian embryonic development. Two major uses for X-gal staining are (1) to characterize expression of a gene and (2) to trace the lineage of cells during development. Gene expression may be examined either by knocking LacZ into the gene of interest, and thus getting a readout of the full endogenous expression pattern, or by placing LacZ under the control of regulatory elements associated with the gene of interest. The latter method facilitates the dissection of the regulatory landscape around a gene, and is useful when trying to identify specific regulatory regions required for specific components of the full expression pattern. If expression of a LacZ reporter is specific to a certain cell type or structure within the kidney, it can be used as a marker of that tissue in subsequent studies.

Cell lineage tracing is a key technique in developmental biology. By employing a suitable LacZ reporter, often in conjunction with a Cre transgene, a group of progenitor cells and all its clonal descendants can be marked. Understanding the origins and developmental history of a specific cell type is a major area of interest in developmental biology.

X-gal staining has been employed in many studies of kidney development. A common use for the technique is to examine expression in the developing kidney of the gene of interest. A good example of this can be found in a recent paper by Lu et al. (5), in which they examined expression of the Etv4 and Etv5 transcription factors using transgenic LacZ knock-in mice. Furthermore, the regulation of Etv4 and Etv5 by GDNF was revealed by culturing kidneys heterozygous for Etv4lacz or Etv5lacz with GDNF-soaked beads and examining X-gal stain levels. In addition to expression of individual genes, the activity of whole signaling pathways can be visualized using LacZ-based reporters that respond to a specific signal or transcription factor. For example, the BAT-gal (β-catenin activated transgene driving β-galactosidase) reporter provides a readout of activity of the canonical Wnt signaling pathway, which can be detected in whole, sectioned, or cultured kidneys (6, 7). Examples of X-gal staining in the kidney are provided in Fig. 1.

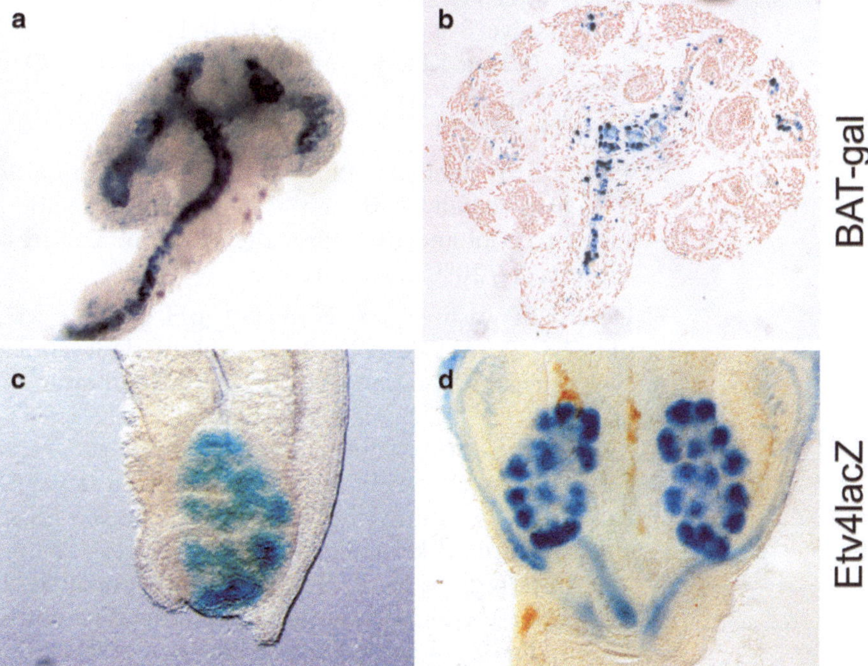

Fig. 1. Examples of X-gal staining in embryonic kidneys. (**a**, **b**) Staining for *BAT-gal* expression reveals activity of the canonical Wnt signaling pathway in the UB (**a**: whole E12.0 kidney; **b**: sectioned E13.5 kidney). (**c**, **d**) X-gal detection of Etv4lacz activity confirms expression of *Etv4* in the UB tips and, to a lesser extent, the MM (**c**: E12.5 kidney cultured for 2 h; **d**: E12.5 urogenital ridge cultured for 24 h). Different preparation and analysis techniques may be employed to obtain the optimal expression pattern. For example, staining can be performed on whole (**a**) or cultured kidneys (**c**, **d**); stained whole kidneys may also then be sectioned (**b**).

2. Materials

2.1. LacZ Reporter Mice

The three main types of transgenic LacZ reporter mice were outlined in the introduction. Many transgenic LacZ reporter mouse lines already exist. The online database of mice available from the JAX or MMRRC mouse repositories can be searched for such mice: http://jaxmice.jax.org/findmice/index.html or http://www.mmrrc.org/. For a broader search of virtually all published mouse strains, consult Mouse Genome Informatics: http://www.informatics.jax.org/. Furthermore, many of the targeted ES cells generated by the several gene targeting and gene trap consortia can be obtained and used to generate transgenic LacZ mice: http://www.knockoutmouse.org/. If a suitable transgenic reporter does not already exist then a strategy can be devised to generate one. However, this is a complex and lengthy technique, and lies outside the scope of this chapter.

2.2. Solutions and Materials for Preparation of Tissue

1. Phosphate buffered saline (PBS): 137 mM NaCl, 2.7 mM KCl, 10.14 mM Na_2HPO_4, 1.76 mM KH_2PO_4, in double-distilled water (ddH_2O).

   Dissolve 8 g NaCl, 0.2 g KCl, 1.44 g Na_2HPO_4 (anhydrous), 0.24 g $KH_2PO_4 \cdot H_2PO_4$ in 800 ml ddH_2O; adjust pH to 7.4 with HCl (see Note 1), then bring to a final volume of 1 L with ddH_2O.
2. 4% Paraformaldehyde (PFA) in PBS: 2 g PFA in 50 ml PBS.

   Dissolve fully with the assistance of heat and agitation. Allow to cool and then filter the solution. Use fresh or store aliquots at –20°C for future use.
3. Detergent wash: 0.1 M Na_2HPO_4 pH 7.3, 0.1 M NaH_2PO_4 pH 7.3, 2 mM $MgCl_2$, 0.1% sodium deoxycholate, 0.02% Nonidet P-40, 0.05% bovine serum albumin (BSA), in ddH_2O.

   Prepare 500–1,000 ml depending on requirements. Detergent wash can be kept for months at 4°C. As a guide, wells on a 24-multiwell culture plate need 0.5 ml solution to cover a cultured kidney or individual E11.5–E13.5 kidney or urogenital region (UGR); 1 ml solution for pooled E11.5–E13.5 kidneys or UGRs; 1 ml solution for individual embryos up to E13.5; 1.5–2 ml solution for older or pooled embryos. Use 3–5 ml of each solution if washing/staining is carried out in a 10-ml scintillation vial.
4. Dissection tools: including, but not limited to, forceps, scissors, and tungsten dissection needles. A Wiretrol is useful for the transfer of isolated kidneys younger than E12.5. Plastic pipettes can be used for older stages. Dissections are performed

in cold PBS in a Petri dish with the aid of a standard light microscope.

5. Containers for samples: samples which need to be kept separate (e.g., if they are of different genotypes) should be placed in individual wells of a 24-multiwell culture plate. If it is not important to keep samples separate then it is more economical to wash and stain pooled samples in one container, for example a plastic capped 10-ml glass bottle or scintillation vial. If genotyping is required, then PCR tubes will be needed for the yolk sac or embryonic tail tissue.
6. Shaker.

2.3. X-gal Staining Reagents

1. Stain solution: 7.2 mM NaCl, 5 mM $K_3Fe(CN)_6$, 5 mM $K_4Fe(CN)_6$, in detergent wash. Prepare 100–250 ml depending on requirements. Store in the dark at 4°C (see Note 2); stain solution can be stored in this way for several months.
2. X-gal: commercially available.

   Prepare and store as per manufacturer's instructions. We reconstitute our X-gal to 50 mg/ml in dimethylformamide and store in aliquots in the dark at −20°C.
3. Just prior to use, add X-gal to stain solution for a final concentration of 0.3 mg/ml. Keep away from light at all times.

2.4. Staining and Analysis Equipment

1. Foil or other material to keep staining reactions concealed from light.
2. 37°C incubator.
3. 4% PFA in PBS.
4. Light stereomicroscope and camera for imaging of fixed staining pattern.

2.5. Sectioning Equipment

1. 25, 50, 75, 85, and 95% ethanol in ddH_2O.
2. 100% Ethanol.
3. Histoclear.
4. 65°C oven.
5. Paraffin wax (molten).
6. Prewarmed tools and molds for mounting.
7. Microtome.
8. Superfrost slides.
9. Slide dryer.
10. Nuclear Fast Red.
11. Mounting medium (Eukitt, DPX, or similar).

3. Methods

3.1. Preparation of Embryos

1. Set up timed mattings of appropriate transgenic LacZ reporter mice (see Note 3). Day E0.5 is counted as the morning on which a vaginal plug is detected. Collect the embryos at the required stage.
2. It is wise to include a positive control tissue if this is the first time that X-gal staining is being performed on a particular mouse line, in order to differentiate between experimental error and a genuine absence of stain. Ideally, fresh control tissue should be obtained from a well-characterized LacZ-expressing line on the same day as the experimental dissections are performed. If this is not possible, then fixed control tissue stored at 4°C may also be used (see Note 4).
3. Dissect embryos in cold PBS using a light microscope. Collect yolk sac or embryonic tail samples in PCR tubes if genotyping is required (see Note 5). If embryos need to be analyzed individually, for example if they are of different genotypes, place them in cold PBS in individual wells of a 24-multiwell culture plate. Wild-type samples may be pooled in a suitable container to reduce the volume of solutions used.

3.2. Dissection of Kidney Tissues

1. The type of dissection required depends on both the embryonic stage and whether the staining pattern will be examined whole mount or in sections. Staining of E9.5–E10.5 nephric ducts should be examined within the context of whole embryos or posterior halves of embryos. Further detail can then be obtained by sectioning the embryo once it has been stained, fixed, and embedded (see Subheading 3.5). Similarly, later stage kidneys can be stained within the embryo and subsequently dissected out or examined in sections. However, penetration of the detergent and stain solutions into the kidney of a whole or half embryo may be incomplete at stages later than E12.5. Staining of whole embryos to examine kidney expression is not recommended for E14.5 or older embryos.
2. If embryos are to be stained whole, decapitate embryos E11.5 or older, to increase stain penetration. Then, proceed to Subheading 3.3.
3. If kidneys are to be isolated for staining, dissect kidneys out. Wild-type kidneys can be pooled for staining; kidneys from embryos of differing genotypes should be placed in individual wells of a 24-multiwell plate. Keep embryos and kidneys in PBS on ice until all are ready for detergent washing. Then, proceed to Subheading 3.3.

4. It is also possible to examine staining in E11.5–E12.5 kidneys after they have been cultured. This technique enhances visibility of staining in distinct structures, such as ureteric bud branches and renal vesicles. Staining of cultured kidneys may also be a useful follow-up to kidney culture experiments. At the end of the culture period, move the filters (on which the kidneys lie) from medium to room temperature PBS. Then, proceed to Subheading 3.3.

3.3. Fixing and Washing

1. Fix tissues in room temperature 4% PFA at room temperature, on a shaker, for the times shown in Table 1 (see Note 6). After fixing cultured kidneys (see Note 7), use a scalpel blade and forceps to cut out a square of filter containing the cultured kidney and remove this piece of filter to a 24-multiwell culture plate for further processing.
2. Wash tissues three times in detergent wash, 20 min each wash, at room temperature on a shaker. Use a plastic transfer pipette to remove and add liquid.
3. During the final detergent wash, add X-gal to the stain solution as described in Subheading 3.3. Only make up the amount of X-gal staining solution that is required that day and keep it in the dark at room temperature until use.
4. Remove final detergent wash, and then add room temperature X-gal staining solution. Ensure tissues are completely covered.

Table 1
Prestaining fixation times

	Time		
Stage	Whole embryo	Isolated kidney/ urogenital region (min)	Cultured kidney (min)
E9.5	45 min	–	–
E10.5	1 h	–	–
E11.5	1 h and 30 min	10	10
E12.5	1 h and 45 min	10	10
E13.5	2 h	15	–
E14.5	2 h and 30 min	20	–
E15.5	–	25	–
E16.5	–	30	–
E17.5	–	35	–
E18.5	–	40	–

5. Cover the 24-multiwell plate or scintillation vial with foil and place at 37°C overnight (see Note 8).

3.4. Fixing and Analysis of Stain

1. The following morning examine the samples for blue stain using a light microscope (see Note 9). If the staining pattern is satisfactory proceed to the next step. Further incubation at 37°C may increase a weak stain. If no stain is detectable then fresh stain can be added and the reaction restarted at 37°C for the rest of the day.
2. Wash out the stain solution with PBS: wash the samples in PBS for 20 min, three times, at room temperature on a shaker. Make sure that the samples are still kept in the dark throughout these washes, as X-gal may still be present.
3. Fix the stain by replacing the final PBS wash with 4% PFA. Leave the samples in fix overnight at 4°C, on a shaker, in the dark (see Note 10). The next day, wash the samples three times with PBS.
4. Image stain patterns using a standard light microscope attached to a camera. Store stained samples in PBS at 4°C in dark.

3.5. Sectioning of Stained Samples

Stained, fixed samples can be further analyzed by sectioning. A full description of wax embedding techniques is outside the scope of this chapter. However, as a general rule, the length of time which stained samples spend in alcohol, clearing agents, and wax should be minimized, while still being long enough to allow full dehydration, clearing, and wax penetration. Lengthy washes may result in loss of X-gal stain. The use of Histoclear, instead of xylene, as the clearing agent is also advisable to retain stain. Finally, slides should be dried at 42°C rather than at higher temperatures. Nuclear Fast Red provides a good counterstain to visualize morphology on sections of X-gal stained tissues. A suitable protocol for embedding stained, fixed E11.5–E13.5 kidneys is as follows:

1. 3 × 10 min washes in PBS at room temperature.
2. Wash for 5–10 min in 25% ethanol (in ddH_2O).
3. Wash for 5–10 min in 50% ethanol (in ddH_2O).
4. Wash for 5–10 min in 75% ethanol (in ddH_2O).
5. Wash for 5–10 min in 85% ethanol (in ddH_2O).
6. Wash for 5–10 min in 95% ethanol (in ddH_2O).
7. 3 × 10 min each in 100% ethanol.
8. 3 × 15 min each in Histoclear (see Note 11).
9. The first two washes are performed at room temperature, the third at 60°C.
10. 5 min wash in 1:1 Histoclear–paraffin wax mix, again at 60°C.
11. 3 × 15–20 min each in melted paraffin wax at 60°C.
12. Embed in fresh molten wax.

4. Notes

1. pH 7.4 is the optimal pH for bacterial β-galactosidase. Lower pH may result in increased background as endogenous β-galactosidase operates at pH 4.0 in certain mammalian tissues (including the adult kidney).
2. Wrap bottles or tubes in foil to protect stain reactions from light.
3. The ideal mating strategy is to obtain a 3–6-month-old stud male, heterozygous for the LacZ reporter or transgene of interest, and mate him with 5–8-week-old wild-type females. Approximately half the embryos in resulting litters will carry LacZ. Homozygous stud males may also be used if it has been established that homozygosity is not detrimental to viability or fertility; this will result in litters in which all embryos carry LacZ. Similarly, the number of embryos carrying LacZ can be increased by mating two heterozygous parents. However, this is only advisable in situations where embryonic expression of the LacZ reporter/transgene has been well characterized and found to be comparable between heterozygous and homozygous embryos. Remember that LacZ knock-ins may ablate gene function and so homozygosity is likely to produce a phenotype. If LacZ expression is to be induced by Cre-mediated recombination then the mating strategy must be adapted to incorporate a suitable Cre recombinase-expressing mouse.
4. Positive control tissue can be obtained in advance and stored for X-gal staining. This is not as desirable as obtaining fresh control tissue but is sometimes necessary. Dissect and fix the tissue as described in Subheadings 3.1–3.3. After fixation, wash the tissue for 20 min, three times each in PBS at room temperature; then store at 4°C in PBS. Replenish stocks of control tissue every 1–2 month. When needed, wash the stored tissue three times in detergent wash and proceed with staining as normal. Note that the intensity of staining will decrease with time spent in storage.
5. Genotyping is necessary when X-gal staining patterns need to be interpreted with respect to genotype. It is also possible to genotype embryos for the LacZ gene. Genotyping for LacZ can be valuable for troubleshooting if no stain is detected, to rule out the possibility of embryos not actually carrying the LacZ gene.
6. It is important to adhere to the fixation times provided. Overfixation reduces β-galactosidase activity.
7. To fix cultured kidneys, remove the PBS from beneath the filter and replace with room temperature 4% PFA for 2 min.

Then, gently add more room temperature 4% PFA on top of the filter for the remainder of the fixation time. Do not shake. Note that the kidneys may float free from the filter if they are cultured for less than 3 h. This is not detrimental to the tissue.

8. It is important that the staining reaction is performed in the dark, as X-gal is light sensitive. Incubation must be at 37°C as this is the temperature at which the β-galactosidase enzyme operates. Stain may begin to appear after a couple of hours but for optimal staining of the full expression pattern samples should be incubated overnight.
9. X-gal stain usually appears as bright blue. However, it is also normal to have a slight green tinge, or even to appear nearly black in regions of extremely high expression.
10. Samples may also be fixed at room temperature if faster fixation is required. Isolated kidneys or UGRs should be fixed for at least 1–2 h, and embryos for at least 2 h.
11. The duration of the Histoclear and subsequent wax incubations must be adjusted to be suitable to the stage being examined. The protocol outlined here is for E11.5–E13.5 isolated kidneys. Kidneys from older embryos will require longer incubations. Wash times should be optimized for the stage of interest.

    As a guide, E17.5 stained fixed kidneys require 15 min washes in each alcohol solution, 20 min Histoclear washes, and 1-h incubations in wax.

References

1. Indra AK, Warot X, Brocard J et al (1999) Temporally-controlled site-specific mutagenesis in the basal layer of the epidermis: comparison of the recombinase activity of the tamoxifen-inducible Cre-ER(T) and Cre-ER(T2) recombinases. Nucleic Acids Res 27(22):4324–4327
2. Soriano P (1999) Generalized lacZ expression with the ROSA26 Cre reporter strain. Nat Genet 21(1):70–71
3. Kothary R, Clapoff S, Brown A et al (1988) A transgene containing lacZ inserted into the dystonia locus is expressed in neural tube. Nature 335(6189):435–437
4. Kothary R, Clapoff S, Darling S et al (1989) Inducible expression of an hsp68-lacZ hybrid gene in transgenic mice. Development 105(4):707–714
5. Lu BC, Cebrian C, Chi X et al (2009) Etv4 and Etv5 are required downstream of GDNF and Ret for kidney branching morphogenesis. Nat Genet 41(12):1295–1302
6. Maretto S, Cordenonsi M, Dupont S et al (2003) Mapping Wnt/beta-catenin signaling during mouse development and in colorectal tumors. Proc Natl Acad Sci USA 100(6): 3299–3304
7. Burn SF, Webb A, Berry RL et al (2011) Calcium/NFAT signalling promotes early nephrogenesis. Dev Biol 352(2):288–298

Chapter 22

Fluorescent Immunolabeling of Embryonic Kidney Samples

Cristina Cebrián

Abstract

This chapter provides a basic protocol to perform fluorescent immunolabeling on embryonic kidney samples. The procedure can be summarized in five steps: permeabilization, primary antibody incubation, washes, secondary antibody incubation, and final washes. This protocol can be used on samples of different origins, from thin sections to whole mounts, just by adjusting incubation times, temperatures, and buffer composition. Despite its simplicity, we have successfully and consistently used this protocol to detect the "usual suspects" in kidney development: CalbindinD-28k, E-cadherin, Pax2, podocalyxin, α-SMA, and Phospho-Histone H3 among others. This protocol also provides a starting point when trying to optimize labeling with a new antibody.

Key words: Embryo, Kidney, Immunolabeling, Antibody, Permeabilization, TSP, Fluorescence, Microscopy

1. Introduction

The development of the vertebrate kidney initiates when the ureteric bud (UB), an outgrowth of the Wolffian duct, invades the neighboring metanephric mesenchyme (MM) inducing it to aggregate, epithelialize, and differentiate into nephrons. Simultaneously, the MM induces the branching of the UB, generating the entire renal collecting tree (1). Therefore, the vertebrate kidney originates—in most part—from three rather undifferentiated cell populations (UB, MM, and stroma) that give rise to more than a dozen cell types in the mature kidney (2). Indeed, the anatomical and cellular complexity of the kidney reflects the myriad of functions of the organ. From a highly specialized filtering structure such as the glomerulus to the complex transport pattern of the epithelial tubules and the fine-tuned regulatory function of the macula densa, these cells have a characteristic gene expression profile and can be

Odyssé Michos (ed.), *Kidney Development: Methods and Protocols*, Methods in Molecular Biology, vol. 886,
DOI 10.1007/978-1-61779-851-1_22, © Springer Science+Business Media, LLC 2012

identified by well-established protein markers. Similarly, specific antigens are present in the progenitor populations throughout renal development. Therefore, given the sequential nature of nephron induction, differentiated glomeruli and renal tubules coexist with undifferentiated progenitors providing an amazing distribution of protein markers.

The UB and the connecting tubule can be labeled with anti-CalbindinD-28k antibodies (3). Pan-cytokeratin and TROMA-1 antigens are also UB specific (4, 5), and anti e-cadherin antibodies are used to label the UB before epithelialization of the nascent nephrons occurs (6). The nephrogenic mesenchyme can be labeled with anti-Pax2, Six2, and Cited1 antibodies, although their expression is somehow restricted to specific domains of the MM and does not completely overlap (7–9). As the progenitor cells undergo differentiation, new structures form and new antigens appear as a consequence of a change in their gene expression pattern (10). WT1 and podocalyxin proteins are detectable in differentiating and mature podocytes as part of the glomeruli (11, 12), Aquaporin-1 antibodies label proximal tubules (13) and uromodulin is present in the thick ascending limb of the loop of Henle (14). A complete list of markers detected during development and in mature nephrons has been analyzed by in situ hybridization and immunohistochemistry by Georgas et al. (15).

Fluorescent immunolabeling was first described by Coons and Kaplan (16) and has become a powerful technique for antigen localization. It is routinely used in the study of renal development and a growing list of antigen-specific antibodies is now available to researchers. This chapter provides a basic protocol for fluorescent immunolabeling on embryonic kidney samples; researchers are encouraged to use it as a starting point and modify it as needed to achieve the desired result. Further optimization is not described in this chapter, but it may involve antigen retrieval (17–19) and/or Tyramide signal amplification methods (20).

2. Materials

2.1. Tissue Samples (See Note 1)

1. 5–10 μm thin frozen or paraffin sections (see Note 2).
2. 50- to 200-μm thick vibratome sections.
3. Whole embryonic urogenital tracts or isolated kidneys (see Note 3).

2.2. Equipment

1. Fluorescence microscope.

2.3. Consumables

1. 1× Phosphate buffered saline (PBS).
2. 4% Paraformaldehyde, freshly made in 1× PBS.

3. 0.1% (v/v) Triton X-100, 0.05% (w/v) Saponin in 1× PBS (TSP).
4. Normal serum (NS) (see Note 4).
5. Primary antibodies (see Note 5).
6. Secondary antibodies: fluorophore-conjugated, affinity purified F(ab′)2 fragment IgG.
7. Aqueous mounting medium (see Note 6).
8. Coverslips.
9. Clear nail polish.
10. Xylene.
11. Ethanol series: 100, 75, 50, and 25% ethanol. Dilute ethanol in 1× PBS.
12. For thin paraffin or frozen section labeling:
    (a) Hydrophobic barrier pen.
    (b) Glass staining jars and holders.
    (c) Humidified chamber (see Note 7).
13. For vibratome sections or whole tissue labeling:
    (a) 12, 24, or 48-multiwell plates.
    (b) 0.4 μm pore size polyester membrane (only for fresh whole tissue, optional).
    (c) Fine brush (only for vibratome sections).
    (d) Microscope slides.
    (e) Platform rotator.

3. Methods

3.1. Prepare the Samples

1. Paraffin sections:
    (a) De-paraffinize and rehydrate the sections following a standard protocol (2×5 min xylene, 2×5 min 100% ethanol, 5 min 75% ethanol, 5 min 95% ethanol, 5 min 50% ethanol, 5 min 30% ethanol, and 2×5 min PBS).
    (b) Dry the area on the slide around the tissue and mark a hydrophobic ring around the sample with a hydrophobic barrier pen. Let the ring dry for a few seconds.
    (c) Wash in 1× PBS for 5 min.
2. Frozen sections:
    (a) Select the slides to be labeled and let them defrost at room temperature for 5 min.

   (b) Mark a hydrophobic ring around the sample with a hydrophobic barrier pen. Let the ring dry for a few seconds.
   (c) Wash in 1× PBS for 5 min, repeat for a total of two washes.

3. Vibratome sections:
   (a) Collect 50–200 μm samples in 1× PBS on 48 or 24-multiwell plates. Keep one section per well if samples are to be analyzed serially.
4. Whole mount tissue:
   (a) Dissect the kidneys or entire urogenital tracts in ice-cold 1× PBS.
   (b) (Optional) Culture the tissue on polyester membranes for a few hours to overnight (see Note 8).
   (c) Rinse in ice-cold 1× PBS.
   (d) Fix with freshly made 4% PFA, with gentle shaking at 4°C (see Note 9).
   (e) Wash with 1× PBS for 10 min, repeat for a total of three washes.

3.2. Immunolabeling

For vibratome sections, free floating whole mounts and on-filter tissues, perform washes and antibody incubations on multiwell plates (see Note 10). For frozen or paraffin sections, perform all washes on glass jars. Permeabilization and antibody incubations on slides should be done in a humidified chamber. See Table 1 for specific conditions.

Appropriate controls should be included, especially when trying new antibodies (see Note 11).

1. Permeabilize and preblock the tissue with TSP containing 10% NS (TSP-NS). This step is optional for thin (5–7 μm) sections but it is highly recommended for thicker sections and whole mounts.
2. Dilute primary antibodies in TSP-NS. Follow manufacturer's directions for dilution range. Discard the permeabilization buffer and replace with primary antibody dilution. Follow Table 1 for times and temperatures. If necessary, the antibody dilution can be collected after incubation and reused. Add sodium azide 0.02% w/v to avoid contamination.
3. Rinse the samples briefly with wash buffer and perform the indicated washes (Table 1).
4. Dilute secondary antibodies in TSP-NS and incubate at the right temperature for the appropriate time (Table 1).
5. Rinse the samples briefly with wash buffer and perform the indicated washes (Table 1).
6. Use a fluorescence microscope to look at the labeling before mounting, being careful not to dry the samples. If background

Table 1
For each type of sample two options are given, with either short or long incubations

		Permeabilization	Primary antibody	Washes	Secondary antibody	Washes
Frozen or paraffin thin sections	*Buffer*	*TSP-NS*	*TSP-NS*	*1× PBS*	*TSP-NS*	*1× PBS*
	Short	10–30 min at RT	1–3 h at RT	3×5 min RT	1–3 h at RT	3×10 min RT
	Long	o/n at 4°C	o/n at 4°C	3×15 min RT	o/n at 4°C	3×20 min RT
Vibratome sections or whole mounts	*Buffer*	*TSP-NS*	*TSP-NS*	*TSP*	*TSP-NS*	*TSP*
	Short	1–5 h at RT	3–5 h at RT	3×10 min RT	3–5 h at RT	3×15 min RT
	Long	o/n at 4°C	o/n at 4°C	o/n at 4°C	o/n at 4°C	o/n at 4°C

As a rule, thicker sections/tissue will need longer incubation time. When labeling is weak, increase antibody incubations' length and/or temperature (up to 37°C). If high background is the issue, reduce temperature of antibody incubations and/or increase length and/or temperature of the washes is high, the samples should be washed further. When needed, samples can be washed beyond the time indicated on Table 1 for up to an overnight at 4°C.

3.3. Mounting of the Samples

1. Paraffin and frozen sections:
   (a) Working one slide at a time, shake off most of the wash buffer, being careful not to dry the sample.
   (b) Add 2–3 drops of mounting medium per slide, on top of the tissue sections.
   (c) Position a coverslip on top of the slide, lower one side first and slowly continue lowering the coverslip until it sits on top of the slide covering the samples. Make sure no air bubbles are trapped between the coverslip and the sample.
   (d) Dry any excess mounting medium and seal the coverslip with clear nail polish.
2. Free floating vibratome sections or in-filter tissue:
   (a) Wash once with 1× PBS.
   (b) Using a fine brush (for vibratome sections) or fine forceps (for filters), transfer the samples to a microscope slide. Several sections can be mounted together in the same slide (see Note 12). For in-filter tissue, trim the filter to fit on the slide and make sure that the explants are facing up.
   (c) Do not allow the samples to dry excessively. If necessary, add a few drops of 1× PBS with the brush to drying sections.
   (d) After positioning the desired number of samples in one slide, add a few drops of mounting medium on top of the tissue and cover with a coverslip.
   (e) Dry any excess mounting medium and seal the coverslip with clear nail polish.

3.4. Storage of the Samples

1. Wait until the nail polish is completely dry before imaging the samples.
2. Make sure that the samples are well sealed and reapply nail polish if necessary.
3. Store the samples at 4°C in the dark. In most cases, labeling will be stable for months, although prompt imaging is recommended.

4. Notes

1. The fixative of choice must be 4% PFA, freshly made in 1× PBS. Fixation time should be adjusted according to tissue size and not extend beyond 24 h at 4°C. Formalin fixation results in antigen masking, so it is not recommended.

2. Best results are obtained with frozen sections. Therefore, whenever possible, choose frozen over paraffin sections for fluorescent immunolabeling.
3. This protocol can be used on renal tissue from any embryonic stage: as early as E10.5, at the inception of kidney organogenesis, and as late as newborn. Early stages, from E10.5 until E13.5, may be more informative when analyzed as whole urogenital tracts. Vibratome, paraffin or frozen sections are usually the best option for later stages.
4. Use NS obtained from the same species in which the secondary antibody is made. That is, if the secondary is a donkey anti-goat antibody, the serum used throughout the immunolabeling should be normal donkey serum.
5. One of the main advantages of fluorescent immunolabeling is the use of multiple antibodies simultaneously, as long as each antibody is obtained from a different species (although the use of fluorophore-conjugated primary antibodies overcomes this limitation). Make the choices on primary and secondary antibodies in advance so there would not be any cross-reactivity, and check the settings of your fluorescence microscope to avoid fluorescence overlap.
6. Avoid mounting media containing phenylenediamine. Some fluorophores weaken or fade when stored in phenylenediamine-containing media http://www.jacksonimmuno.com/technical/techq3.asp.
7. To make a humidified chamber, tape or glue 1 ml plastic pipettes into a 9″×9″ (or any suitable size) plastic dish with a lid. Paper tissue saturated with distilled water is arranged between the pipettes that hold the microscope slides up. Cover the outside of the dish and the lid with aluminum foil to protect the slides from direct light.
8. The manipulation of small, free-floating embryonic tissue is often cumbersome. Alternatively, by allowing the freshly dissected tissue to attach to a polyester membrane for a few hours, multiple tissue samples can be cultured together and be processed for immunolabeling simultaneously. To prevent the tissue from detaching from the membrane during fixation, add 4% PFA only to the bottom of the membrane and incubate at 4°C for 5 min. After 5 min, add enough 4% PFA to completely cover the samples. If a plastic ring holds the membrane, it may be necessary to cut the membrane off the ring before antibody incubation to minimize the volume of diluted antibody.
9. Fixation time depends on the size of the sample; E10–E12 urogenital tracts can be fixed in as little as 3 h or as long as overnight. Larger tissues should always be fixed overnight. In any case, do not extend fixation time beyond 24 h.

10. Larger wells allow for easier manipulation of the tissue and larger washing volumes; however, they also require larger volumes of antibody dilutions. In general, 24 and 12-multiwell plates provide enough volume for efficient washing of most free-floating samples without requiring too much antibody.
11. When trying a new primary antibody, a tissue of known reactivity towards the antibody should be included as positive control. A negative control should be also included to test for the specificity of the primary antibody; substitute NS (from the same species where the primary antibody was raised) for the antibody.
12. Samples can be visualized directly in the multiwell plates if an inverted fluorescence microscope is available. However, imaging and storage improves when the samples are mounted on microscope slides. Mounting vibratome sections can be tricky and requires some practice. It is relatively easy to manipulate the sections with a fine brush if they are still embedded in agarose. A notch on the agarose block provides orientation and several consecutive sections can be mounted in one slide. Moisture is the key; make sure that the brush is soaked and the slide has a drop of buffer while transferring and orienting the section. Once the section is in the desired location and orientation, use some tissue to dry the area around the agarose. That will lock the sample in position to some extent.

References

1. Saxén L (1987) Organogenesis of the kidney. Cambridge University Press, Cambridge [Cambridgeshire], NY
2. Brenner BM, Rector FC (2008) Brenner & Rector's the kidney, 8th edn. Saunders Elsevier, Philadelphia
3. Davies J (1994) Control of calbindin-D28K expression in developing mouse kidney. Dev Dyn 199:45–51
4. Vega QC, Worby CA, Lechner MS, Dixon JE, Dressler GR (1996) Glial cell line-derived neurotrophic factor activates the receptor tyrosine kinase RET and promotes kidney morphogenesis. Proc Natl Acad Sci USA 93:10657–10661
5. Lehtonen E, Virtanen I, Saxen L (1985) Reorganization of intermediate filament cytoskeleton in induced metanephric mesenchyme cells is independent of tubule morphogenesis. Dev Biol 108:481–490
6. Cho EA, Patterson LT, Brookhiser WT, Mah S, Kintner C et al (1998) Differential expression and function of cadherin-6 during renal epithelium development. Development 125:803–812
7. Dressler GR, Douglass EC (1992) Pax-2 is a DNA-binding protein expressed in embryonic kidney and Wilms tumor. Proc Natl Acad Sci USA 89:1179–1183
8. Ohto H, Takizawa T, Saito T et al (1998) Tissue and developmental distribution of Six family gene products. Int J Dev Biol 42:141–148
9. Plisov S, Tsang M, Shi G et al (2005) Cited1 is a bifunctional transcriptional cofactor that regulates early nephronic patterning. J Am Soc Nephrol 16:1632–1644
10. Brunskill EW, Aronow BJ, Georgas K et al (2008) Atlas of gene expression in the developing kidney at microanatomic resolution. Dev Cell 15:781–791
11. Rackley RR, Flenniken AM, Kuriyan NP et al (1993) Expression of the Wilms' tumor suppressor gene WT1 during mouse embryogenesis. Cell Growth Differ 4:1023–1031
12. Schnabel E, Dekan G, Miettinen A, Farquhar MG (1989) Biogenesis of podocalyxin – the major glomerular sialoglycoprotein – in the newborn rat kidney. Eur J Cell Biol 48: 313–326
13. Sabolic I, Valenti G, Verbavatz JM et al (1992) Localization of the CHIP28 water channel in rat kidney. Am J Physiol 263:C1225–C1233

14. Bachmann S, Koeppen-Hagemann I, Kriz W (1985) Ultrastructural localization of Tamm-Horsfall glycoprotein (THP) in rat kidney as revealed by protein A-gold immunocytochemistry. Histochemistry 83:531–538
15. Georgas K, Rumballe B, Wilkinson L et al (2008) Use of dual section mRNA in situ hybridisation/immunohistochemistry to clarify gene expression patterns during the early stages of nephron development in the embryo and in the mature nephron of the adult mouse kidney. Histochem Cell Biol 130:927–942
16. Coons AH, Kaplan MH (1950) Localization of antigen in tissue cells; improvements in a method for the detection of antigen by means of fluorescent antibody. J Exp Med 91:1–13
17. Syrbu SI, Cohen MB (2011) An enhanced antigen-retrieval protocol for immunohistochemical staining of formalin-fixed, paraffin-embedded tissues. Methods Mol Biol 717:101–110
18. Pavlakis E, Chalepakis G (2008) pH-dependent antigen unmasking in paraformaldehyde-fixed tissue cryosections. Appl Immunohistochem Mol Morphol 16:503–506
19. Long DJ 2nd, Buggs C (2008) Microwave oven-based technique for immunofluorescent staining of paraffin-embedded tissues. J Mol Histol 39:1–4
20. Merz H, Malisius R, Mannweiler S et al (1995) ImmunoMax. A maximized immunohistochemical method for the retrieval and enhancement of hidden antigens. Lab Invest 73:149–156

Chapter 23

Immunohistochemical Staining of dpERK Staining During Early Kidney Development

Xuan Chi and Odyssé Michos

Abstract

Signaling through the ERK/MAPK pathway within the Wolffian duct and ureteric bud epithelium is critical for kidney induction and branching morphogenesis. ERK signaling is activated by receptor tyrosine kinase such as RET and FGFR2. This protocol describes a method to detect the diphosphorylated form of ERK (dpERK) on paraffin embedded tissue of early mouse embryo.

Key words: dpERK, Immunostaining, Paraffin section, Wolffian duct, Kidney

1. Introduction

The extracellular signal-regulated kinase (ERK) family of MAP kinase is activated by hypertrophic stimuli and activated ERK induces a variety of downstream responses including gene transcription, translation and cytoskeletal rearrangement, promoting cell proliferation and survival. Diphosporylated form of ERK1 and ERK2 (dpERK) is an established indicator of receptor tyrosine kinase (RTK) signaling (1, 2) and has been used to map active RTK domains within Drosophila, Xenopus, zebrafish, and early mouse embryos (3–8), using antibodies specific to dpERK. ERK signaling remains active during organogenesis, but in a more restricted fashion. An example is dpERK expression during early kidney development, anti-dpERK specifically stains the domain in the Wolffian duct that will form the ureteric bud tip (9). Here, we describe immunohistochemical staining for dpERK on frozen mouse sections, in order to delineate the spatial and temporal pattern of active ERK signaling during later mouse development, which can map the active ERK signaling domain at the cellular resolution and semiquantitatively.

Odyssé Michos (ed.), *Kidney Development: Methods and Protocols*, Methods in Molecular Biology, vol. 886, DOI 10.1007/978-1-61779-851-1_23, © Springer Science+Business Media, LLC 2012

2. Materials

2.1. Cryosection

1. Sucrose: 30% in PBS.
2. Tissue-Tek OCT compound.
3. Superfrost Plus microscope slides.
4. Cryostat and accessories.

2.2. Immunohistochemistry

1. 4% PFA, make it up fresh on the day of use.
2. 10× PBS without calcium, magnesium, diluted to 1× before use.
3. PapPen.
4. PBT: 0.1% Triton X-100 in 1× PBS.
5. Methanol (MeOH) series: 25, 50, 75% in PBT and 100%.
6. Ethanol (EtOH) series: 70, 95% in dH_2O and 100%.
7. 30% Hydrogen peroxide.
8. Blocking solution: 3% normal goat serum in PBT.
9. Primary antibodies: monoclonal anti-diphosphorylated ERK-1&2 antibody (Sigma, M8159, mouse IgG1).
10. Secondary antibodies: goat anti-mouse IgG1 (SouthernBiotech, 1070-08).
11. VECTASTAIN® Elite ABC reagents (with peroxidase as the enzyme) (Vector Laboratories).
12. DAB peroxidase substrate kit (Vector Laboratories).
13. Permanent mounting media.
14. A transmitted light (brightfield) microscope, equipped with ×10 and ×40 lenses.

3. Methods

3.1. Cryosection

1. Dissect the embryos out in ice-cold PBS. Count the number of pairs of somites your embryo has and use this to stage the age of embryos precisely. Transfer the embryos to cold 4% PFA to preserve endogenous dpERK signals.
2. For mouse embryos at E10 or earlier, fix them in 4% PFA for 3 h at 4°C. For embryo older than E10.5, fix them in 4% PFA overnight at 4°C.
3. Briefly wash with PBT and store in 100% MeOH (can be stored long term).

4. When ready to section, reverse the MeOH gradient back to PBT:

   Each wash is 10 min at room temperature with shaking.

   (a) 75% MeOH—PBT.

   (b) 50% MeOH—PBT.

   (c) 25% MeOH—PBT.

   (d) PBT.

5. 30% Sucrose in PBT overnight at 4°C. The embryos will first float and gradually sink to the bottom of the container.
6. Embed the embryos in OCT Tissue-Tek compound.
7. Freeze in a dry ice—isopentane bath (–70°C).

3.2. Cryosectioning

Cut cryosections at 10 μm, dry on slide warmer (50°C) for 1 h. Depending on the target cells/organs, you can choose to cut transverse (cross), sagittal or frontal sections. While sectioning, follow the structure of the target organ closely under a microscope by its unique morphology or by an adjacent landmark structure. For example, to section the Wolffian ducts and ureteric buds within an E10.5 (37 somites) embryo, the embryo is cut at anterior edge of the hind limb bud and cross-sectioned. On the section, a round Wolffian duct structure can be observed under a bright field microscope that gives rise to a bulging ureteric bud at the posterior end. One can also estimate the position of the Wolffian duct along the longitudinal axis by the shape of the hind limb bud on the section.

The slides can be stored at –80°C with desiccant.

3.3. Immunohistochemical Staining

1. On the first day of staining: take the slides out of freezer and let them dry on a slide warmer for 20 min (See Note 1).
2. Outline with PapPen.
3. Wash the sections in dH_2O twice for 5 min each at RT (See Note 2).
4. Block each section with 500 μl blocking solution for 1 h at RT.
5. Remove blocking solution and add 200 μl primary antibody, diluted 1:100 in blocking solution, to each section, cover slides with coverslips, and incubate overnight at 4°C.
6. Remove antibody solution and wash the sections in PBT three times for 5 min each at RT.
7. Add 500 μl biotinylated secondary antibody (See Note 3) diluted 1:200 in PBT, to each section. Incubate for 2 h at 37°C.
8. Prepare ABC reagent according to the manufacturer's instructions and incubate solution for 30 min at RT before use.
9. Remove secondary antibody solution and wash the sections three times with PBT for 5 min each at RT.

10. Add 500 μl ABC reagent to each section and incubate for 1 h at RT.
11. Remove ABC reagent and wash sections three times in PBT for 5 min each.
12. Add 500 μl DAB substrate solution to each section and monitor staining closely.
13. As soon as the sections develop (which normally takes 2–10 min), immerse the slides in dH_2O.
14. Counterstain with hematoxylin solution (15–30 s) if desired and rinse thoroughly with tap water.
15. Dehydrate the sections through alcohol gradient: incubate sections in 95% EtOH twice for 15 s each. Repeat in 100% EtOH twice for 15 s each.
16. Soak in Histoclear and incubate the sections twice for 5 min each.
17. Mount with permanent mounting media and coverslip.
18. Take photograph of the stained slides with a transmitted light (brightfield) microscope.

4. Notes

1. The primary antibody does not work on paraffin-embedded sections.
2. Antigen retrieval procedures do seem to enhance the signals, particularly when ABC method is not used to amplify the signals. The citrate buffer antigen retrieval procedures have been tested for this protocol and are recommended to use before the blocking solution (in between steps 3 and 4).
3. The primary antibody does work with an immunofluorescence protocol, using fluorophore-labeled secondary antibodies or biotin-conjugated secondary antibodies, followed by fluorophore-conjugated streptavidin.

   Reagents

   (a) Sodium citrate buffer (10 mM sodium citrate, pH 6.0): Add 2.94 g tri-sodium citrate dihydrate salt ($C_6H_5Na_3O_7 \cdot 2H_2O$) to 1 L of dH_2O and mix to dissolve. Adjust pH to 6.0 with 1 N HCl.

   Methods

   (a) Place slides on a rack in 600 ml of sodium citrate buffer in a glass 2-L beaker. Mark a line at the top of the liquid on the beaker.

(b) Microwave until boiling, then boil for 15 min (add dH_2O every 5 min to the marked line).

(c) Cool slides for 30 min in the beaker.

(d) Wash slides in dH_2O twice for 5 min each, followed by a wash in PBS for 5 min.

References

1. Corson LB, Yamanaka Y, Lai KM et al (2003) Spatial and temporal patterns of ERK signaling during mouse embryogenesis. Development 130(19):4527–4537
2. Lunn JS, Fishwick KJ, Halley PA, Storey KG (2007) A spatial and temporal map of FGF/Erk1/2 activity and response repertoires in the early chick embryo. Dev Biol 302(2):536–552
3. Gabay L, Seger R, Shilo BZ (1997) MAP kinase in situ activation atlas during Drosophila embryogenesis. Development 124(18): 3535–3541
4. Christen B, Slack JM (1999) Spatial response to fibroblast growth factor signalling in Xenopus embryos. Development 126(1):119–125
5. Reich A, Sapir A, Shilo B (1999) Sprouty is a general inhibitor of receptor tyrosine kinase signaling. Development 126(18):4139–4147
6. Curran KL, Grainger RM (2000) Expression of activated MAP kinase in *Xenopus laevis* embryos: evaluating the roles of FGF and other signaling pathways in early induction and patterning. Dev Biol 228(1):41–56
7. Sawada A, Shinya M, Jiang YJ et al (2001) Fgf/MAPK signalling is a crucial positional cue in somite boundary formation. Development 128(23):4873–4880
8. Shinya M, Koshida S, Sawada A et al (2001) Fgf signalling through MAPK cascade is required for development of the subpallial telencephalon in zebrafish embryos. Development 128(21): 4153–4164
9. Chi X, Michos O, Shakya R et al (2009) Ret-dependent cell rearrangements in the Wolffian duct epithelium initiate ureteric bud morphogenesis. Dev Cell 17(2):199–209

Chapter 24

Sensing BMP Pathway Activity by Immune Detection of Phosphorylated R-Smad Proteins in Mouse Embryonic Kidney

Javier Lopez-Rios

Abstract

At the onset of mammalian kidney development, the ureteric bud invades the surrounding metanephric mesenchyme, and genetic studies in the mouse have shown that BMP pathway activity has to be antagonized in the vicinity of the epithelium, a task performed by the secreted BMP antagonist Grem1. Here, we describe a short protocol that allows for detection of the pattern of BMP canonical signal transduction by using antibodies that specifically recognize the phosphorylated forms of R-Smad proteins (Smad1, Smad5, and Smad8), which provides a way to monitor overall pathway activity in the mammalian embryonic kidney.

Key words: BMP pathway activity, pSmad, R-Smad, Grem1

1. Introduction

BMP signaling represents one of the major morphogenetic pathways operating during vertebrate embryogenesis. During kidney development, BMPs are required at different stages throughout the formation of the organ, as shown by gene targeting in the mouse (1–7). Moreover, additional genetic experimentation has shown that Grem1, a secreted antagonist of BMP ligands, is required during ureteric bud outgrowth to reduce BMP pathway activity, which allows the epithelium to invade the surrounding metanephric mesenchyme (8–10). In the absence of *Grem1*, ureteric bud growth is stalled leading to kidney agenesis while genetically reducing BMP dosage in Grem1 deficient mutants by inactivating one allele of *Bmp4* (9) or both *Bmp7* alleles (10) is enough to rescue ureteric bud growth and branching. These experiments illustrate that BMP pathway activity has to be tightly modulated during these early events of kidney development.

Odyssé Michos (ed.), *Kidney Development: Methods and Protocols*, Methods in Molecular Biology, vol. 886,
DOI 10.1007/978-1-61779-851-1_24, © Springer Science+Business Media, LLC 2012

Overall BMP pathway activity can be monitored at the cellular level by immunohistochemistry using antibodies that specifically detect the phosphoactivated forms of Smad1, Smad5, and Smad8, the three receptor-regulated Smad (R-Smad) proteins that mediate primary BMP signal transduction (reviewed in refs. 11, 12). BMP homo or heterodimers bind to two type I and two type II membrane receptors, which have serine/threonine kinase activity. When such a complex is assembled, the type II receptor phosphorylates the type I receptor subunits, which upon activation bind and phosphorylate R-Smads on two Ser residues located in their C-terminal region (SxS motif). Phosphorylated R-Smads can then form complexes with Smad4, a co-Smad shared with the rest of the TGFβ transduction machinery, and translocate to the nucleus to regulate the transcriptional targets of the BMP pathway.

Using antibodies that detect the nuclear accumulation of phosphorylated R-Smads allows the detection of cells that are exposed and actively responding to BMP ligands within their environment (Fig. 1) (9, 13, 14). As BMP target genes are generally tissue and context specific, it is sometimes difficult to select a bona fide transcriptional reporter of pathway activity. Therefore, the method described here serves as a measure of primary activation of canonical BMP signal transduction upstream of the transcriptional response.

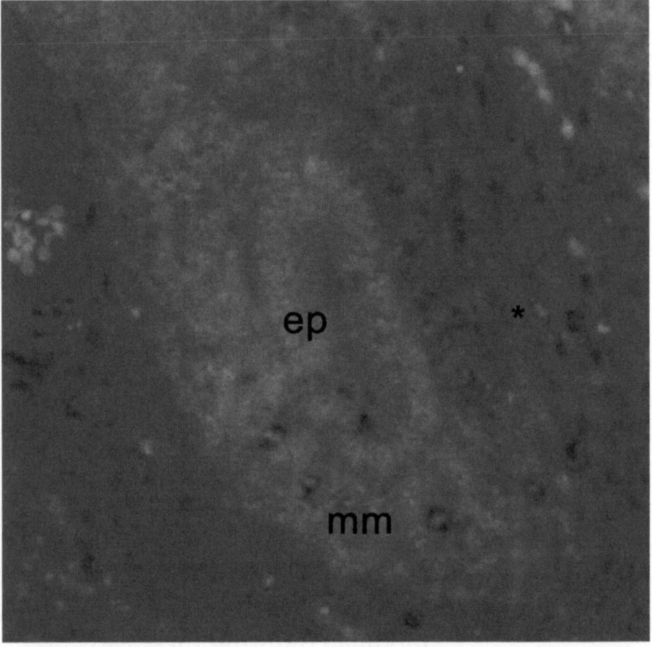

Fig. 1. Immunodetection of phospho-Smad1/5/8 proteins on sections of mouse embryonic kidney at E11.5 (around 50 somites). Nuclear positivity (*dark precipitate*) is seen in the ventral mesenchyme (*asterisk*) while both the epithelium of the ureteric bud (ep) and condensing metanephic mesenchyme (mm) are largely devoid of phospho-Smad 1/5/8-positive cells.

2. Materials

1. Eight to ten micrometer paraffin sections of fixed (4% paraformaldehyde) mouse embryos of the desired age. For ampulla and initial branching stages use E11–E11.75 (40–55 somites (15); sagittal orientation). Collect on Superfrost Plus slides (positively charged), not too close to the edges of the slide.
2. Xylene.
3. 70, 95 and 100% Ethanol, histological grade.
4. PBS (Ca^{2+} and Mg^{2+} free).
5. PBT (PBS, 0.1% Tween 20).
6. Citrate buffer (for antigen retrieval): 10 mM sodium citrate pH 6.0.
7. Plastic box for slides/Coplin jar with lid, autoclave resistant.
8. Portable steam autoclave, with pressure and temperature gauge, working temperature 121°C.
9. Three percent H_2O_2 (dilute 1/10 in deionized water from a 30% stock solution).
10. Humidified incubation chamber for slides.
11. Blocking solution: 5% normal goat serum in PBT.
12. Phospho-Smad1 (Ser463/465)/Smad5 (Ser463/465)/Smad8 (Ser426/428) antibody (Cell Signalling Technology, 9511; IHC validated batch; see Note 1).
13. Biotinylated goat anti-rabbit IgG (Vector Laboratories).
14. Vectastain Elite ABC Kit, Standard (Vector Laboratories).
15. DAB Peroxidase Substrate (Vector Laboratories).
16. Hoechst-33258 staining solution (1:1,600 dilution in PBS from a 8 mg/ml stock solution prepared in PBS).
17. Mounting medium (e.g., Mowiol) and coverslips.

All solutions are made in deionized water.

3. Methods

The following is an immunohistochemistry protocol with antigen retrieval in citrate buffer that works well for the suggested antibodies, requiring an amplification step for optimal results (see Note 2). The critical parameters are the precise timing of the heat-induced epitope retrieval and the quality of the batch of antibody used. Do not allow the slides to dry at any time during the procedure.

To help prevent drying of the sections, it is always a good idea to check with a bubble level that the working area is horizontal. Unless otherwise indicated, all steps are performed at room temperature.

3.1. Deparaffinization and Rehydratation

By total immersion of the sections in the following solutions in serial order:

1. Three times in Xylene for 5 min.
2. Two times in 100% ethanol for 10 min.
3. Two times in 95% ethanol for 10 min.
4. Once in 70% ethanol for 2 min.
5. Twice in water for 5 min.

3.2. Epitope Retrieval

Place the slides in a heat-resistant plastic box/Coplin jar, fill it with unmasking solution up to the top and cover with lid but leave it loose, which prevents excessive evaporation of liquid. Place it in the steam autoclave containing enough water in the bottom (refer to operating instructions). Start the autoclave and when the temperature reaches 121°C (working pressure 15 psi), time 3 min, after which turn off the autoclave. Gently open the steam valve (with great caution to avoid burning yourself or others) to let the steam escape. Alternatively, place the unopened autoclave under running cold water until the pressure is released. When you can safely open the autoclave, take out the box containing the slides and let cool at room temperature for 30 min (see Note 3).

3.3. Inactivation of Endogenous Peroxidase Activity

1. Incubate in 3% H_2O_2 for 15 min.
2. Wash three times for 5 min in water.
3. Wash in PBS for 5 min.

3.4. Blocking

Place the slides in suitable moist incubation chambers and drain off the excess liquid. Immediately add 200–300 μl of blocking solution and incubate for 1 h.

3.5. Primary Antibody Incubation

Drain off the blocking buffer and immediately add 150–200 μl of α-phospho-Smad1/5/8 antibody (1:100–1:200 dilution in blocking buffer, depending on the batch; see Note 1). Incubate overnight at 4°C in a moist chamber.

3.6. Biotinylated Secondary Antibody Incubation

1. Wash three times for 5 min each with PBT.
2. Add 150–200 μl of anti-rabbit biotinylated IgG (1:500 dilution in blocking buffer). Incubate for 30 min.

3.7. ABC Reaction

Prepare the ABC reagent as described by the manufacturer.

1. Add two drops of solution A to 5 ml of PBT and vortex gently.

2. Add two drops of solution B and vortex again.
3. Incubate at least 30 min to allow for the formation of the avidin–peroxidase complexes.

This incubation should be started at the same time as the previous step (3.6).

3.8. ABC Incubation

1. Drain off the solution containing the secondary antibody.
2. Wash three times for 5 min each with PBT.
3. Add 150–200 μl of ABC solution and incubate for 30 min.
4. Wash the sections three times for 5 min in PBT.

3.9. DAB Staining

Add 200–300 μl of DAB solution and monitor signal appearance under a stereomicroscope. Ideally, epitope retrieval and antibody concentrations should be adjusted such that total reaction time is between 5 and 10 min. If staining is too fast, it becomes difficult to stop the reaction in all slides simultaneously. When the desired intensity of the signal is achieved, stop the reaction by draining off the DAB solution and immersing the slide in tap water.

3.10. Counterstaining

1. Incubate the slides for 10 min with Hoechst 33258 staining solution in a Coplin jar in the dark.
2. Wash four times for 3 min each with PBS.
3. Two washes in water for 3 min each.
4. Mount the slides in Mowiol.

3.11. Imaging

Take pictures on a fluorescence microscope equipped with suitable UV excitation and barrier filters to detect Hoechst 33258 signal. The best results are obtained when pictures are taken such that the fluorescent nuclei are detected weakly over a field mainly illuminated by white light. The dark precipitate generated by the DAB quenches the fluorescence emitted by all nuclei, making more obvious the pattern of staining (Fig. 1). Alternatively, bright field and fluorescent pictures can be overlapped using image-processing software.

4. Notes

1. As is always the case in immunohistochemistry, the most critical parameter is the quality of the primary antibody used, and the best commercial antibody available is the one indicated. However, not all batches of this antibody sold by the company are suitable for immune detection of phosphorylated R-Smad1/5/8 in tissue sections, and some may need alternative

epitope retrieval buffers (e.g., 10 mM Tris–HCl pH 9.0, 1 mM EDTA). Other companies also commercialize phospho-specific antibodies recognizing one or more of the R-Smads in the BMP pathway.

2. An alternative for increased sensitivity is the use of HRP-Tyramide amplification systems (TSA Kit, Invitrogen). The use of fluorescence-labeled Tyramide requires determining the appropriate length of epitope retrieval and dilutions of antibodies and substrates, as the gain in sensitivity may also lead to an increase in background. Refer to the manufacturer's instructions.

3. Performing this procedure with a steam autoclave provides a more homogeneous antigen unmasking that the use of conventional microwaves. Make sure that the slides are not too close and are evenly distributed in the box, which is critical for homogeneous retrieval and reproducibility. Make sure that you know how to use the apparatus and refer to its operating manual. Also note that the time of autoclaving has to be empirically determined for each antibody and machine; 3 min is a good starting point. If the staining is too faint try increasing the boiling time, while if too much background develops it can be sign of excessive antigen retrieval.

References

1. Dudley AT, Lyons KM, Robertson EJ (1995) A requirement for bone morphogenetic protein-7 during development of the mammalian kidney and eye. Genes Dev 9(22):2795–2807
2. Luo G, Hofmann C, Bronckers AL et al (1995) BMP-7 is an inducer of nephrogenesis, and is also required for eye development and skeletal patterning. Genes Dev 9(22):2808–2820
3. Oxburgh L, Chu GC, Michael SK, Robertson EJ (2004) TGFbeta superfamily signals are required for morphogenesis of the kidney mesenchyme progenitor population. Development 131(18):4593–4605
4. Oxburgh L, Dudley AT, Godin RE et al (2005) BMP4 substitutes for loss of BMP7 during kidney development. Dev Biol 286(2):637–646
5. Miyazaki Y, Oshima K, Fogo A, Hogan BL, Ichikawa I (2000) Bone morphogenetic protein 4 regulates the budding site and elongation of the mouse ureter. J Clin Invest 105(7): 863–873
6. Miyazaki Y, Oshima K, Fogo A, Ichikawa I (2003) Evidence that bone morphogenetic protein 4 has multiple biological functions during kidney and urinary tract development. Kidney Int 63:835–844
7. Oxburgh L, Brown AC, Fetting J, Hill B (2011) BMP signaling in the nephron progenitor niche. Pediatr Nephrol 26(9):1491–1497
8. Michos O, Panman L, Vintersten K et al (2004) Gremlin-mediated BMP antagonism induces the epithelial–mesenchymal feedback signaling controlling metanephric kidney and limb organogenesis. Development 131(14): 3401–3410
9. Michos O, Gonçalves A, Lopez-Rios J et al (2007) Reduction of BMP4 activity by gremlin 1 enables ureteric bud outgrowth and GDNF/ WNT11 feedback signalling during kidney branching morphogenesis. Development 134(13):2397–2405
10. Gonçalves A, Zeller R (2011) Genetic analysis reveals an unexpected role of BMP7 in initiation of ureteric bud outgrowth in mouse embryos. PLoS One 6(4):e19370
11. Massague J, Seoane J, Wotton D (2005) Smad transcription factors. Genes Dev 19(23): 2783–2810

12. Moustakas A, Heldin CH (2009) The regulation of TGFbeta signal transduction. Development 136(22):3699–3714
13. Witte F, Chan D, Economides AN, Mundos S, Stricker S (2010) Receptor tyrosine kinase-like orphan receptor 2 (ROR2) and Indian hedgehog regulate digit outgrowth mediated by the phalanx-forming region. Proc Natl Acad Sci USA 107(32):14211–14216
14. Tian X, Halfhill AN, Diaz FJ (2010) Localization of phosphorylated SMAD proteins in granulosa cells, oocytes and oviduct of female mice. Gene Expr Patterns 10(2–3):105–112
15. Chan AOK, Dong M, Wang L, Chan WY (2004) Somite as a morphological reference for staging and axial levels of developing structures in mouse embryos. Neuroembryol Aging 3(2): 102–110

Chapter 25

Analysis of In Vivo Transcription Factor Recruitment by Chromatin Immunoprecipitation of Mouse Embryonic Kidney

Claire Heliot and Silvia Cereghini

Abstract

Chromatin immunoprecipitation (ChIP) is a powerful technique for examining transcription factor recruitment to chromatin, or histone modifications, at the level of specific genomic sequences. As such, it provides an invaluable tool for elucidating gene regulation at the molecular level. Combined with high-throughput methods such as second generation sequencing (ChIP-Seq), this technique is now commonly used for studying DNA–protein interactions at a genome-wide scale. The ChIP technique is based on covalent cross-linking of DNA and proteins with formaldehyde, followed by chromatin fragmentation, either enzymatic or by sonication, and immunoprecipitation of protein–DNA complexes using antibodies specific for the protein of interest. The immunoprecipitated DNA is then purified and the DNA sequences associated with the immunoprecipitated protein are identified by PCR (ChIP-PCR) or, alternatively, by direct sequencing (ChIP-Seq). Initially, the vast majority of ChIP experiments were performed on cultured cell lines. More recently, this technique has been adapted to a variety of tissues in different model organisms. We describe here a ChIP protocol on freshly isolated mouse embryonic kidneys for in vivo analysis of transcription factor recruitment on chromatin. This protocol has been easily adapted to other mouse embryonic tissues and has also been successfully scaled up to perform ChIP-Seq.

Key words: Transcription factor, Chromatin immunoprecipitation, ChIP protocol, Mouse, Metanephric kidneys

1. Introduction

Embryonic development and cell-lineage specification occur through the establishment of complex spatio-temporal patterns of gene expression, which are regulated by signaling and transcriptional networks converging on *cis*-regulatory elements. The expression of a gene in a given cell type depends on the interaction of transcription factors with its regulatory sequences and on the acquisition of an appropriate chromatin architecture. In recent years,

Odyssé Michos (ed.), *Kidney Development: Methods and Protocols*, Methods in Molecular Biology, vol. 886, DOI 10.1007/978-1-61779-851-1_25, © Springer Science+Business Media, LLC 2012

analyses integrating transcriptional profiling of loss-of-function mutants with the global identification of sequences to which transcription factors are recruited in vivo have allowed a better understanding of regulatory networks involved in several developmental processes. Moreover, several studies have clearly indicated that the pattern of transcription factor interaction with their target genes evolves during development and therefore cannot be predicted only by in silico motif analysis or by Chromatin Immunoprecipitation (ChIP) experiments using cell lines (1, 2).

ChIP is a useful procedure to identify DNA fragments on which proteins are recruited. This technology is based on covalent cross-linking of proteins and DNA by formaldehyde. After fragmentation of cross-linked chromatin by sonication, DNA fragments containing the protein of interest are immunoprecipitated using a specific antibody. DNA elution and purification allows the identification of the DNA sequences associated with the immunoprecipitated protein. This analysis can be done either by candidate gene approach using PCR amplification to analyze a putative target DNA sequence (ChIP-PCR) or by large-scale approach performing immunoprecipitated DNA sequencing to identify target DNA sequences at a genome scale (ChIP-Seq) (Fig. 1) (3).

Initially, the vast majority of ChIP experiments were performed on cultured cell lines (4, 5). More recently, this technique has been adapted to a variety of tissues in different model organisms (6–8). Here, we describe an in vivo ChIP protocol adapted for the analysis of the HNF1β transcription factor recruitment in early embryonic kidney. After inconclusive tests, with several protocols, we used Zaret's lab chromatin preparation protocol (6). This protocol is optimized to compensate the small size of the embryonic kidney and the relative difficulty to obtain embryos in the mouse model, with the possibility to collect metanephroi from several litters during several days. Moreover, the sonication buffer used allows efficient sonication without compromising IP efficiency. We adapted it for embryonic kidneys by adding homogenization and filtration steps allowing a better cross-linking and increasing the pureness of nuclei (9). The immunoprecipitation protocol is based on the UPSTATE chromatin immunoprecipitation kit, with several modifications. We used Protein A or G Agarose beads blocked exclusively with bovine serum albumin (BSA) (without salmon sperm DNA), since this avoids adding exogenous DNA without increasing the background. This adaptation allows performing ChIP-Seq experiments without using more expensive magnetic beads. We also optimized the wash steps. An overview of our protocol is presented in Fig. 2.

The success of a ChIP experiment critically depends on the chromatin preparation procedure and on the availability of a highly specific antibody against the antigen of interest. During all the steps of chromatin preparation, it is critical to prevent protein

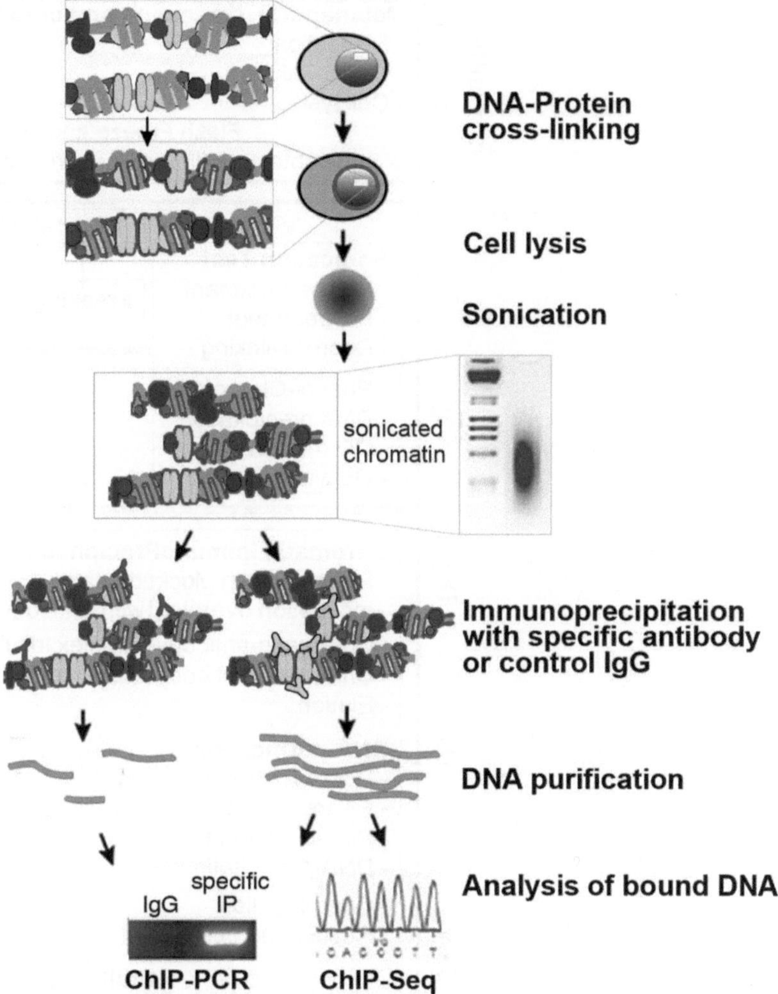

Fig. 1. Chromatin immunoprecipitation (ChIP) in vivo principle. Cells or tissues are treated with formaldehyde to cross-link proteins and DNA. After cell lysis, chromatin is fragmented by sonication. Chromatin is equally separated and incubated with specific antibody or control IgG. Chromatin/protein/antibody complexes are precipitated using agarose-Protein A/G beads. After wash steps, DNA is eluted and purified for further analysis by PCR or sequence. Adapted from Collas and Dahl (3).

degradation and any DNA contamination. Moreover, the chromatin should be adequately fixed and overfixation should be avoided, since this may affect antibody epitope recognition and result in the cross-linking of distant chromatin regions, thus reducing both IP performance and sonication efficiency. The antibody specificity also needs to be tested before ChIP by both immunoprecipitation and Western blot. In addition to these parameters, ChIP experiments performed on heterogeneous cell population have shown that the percentage of chromatin in which the protein of interest is fixed is also critical. When performing ChIP from an embryonic tissue it is

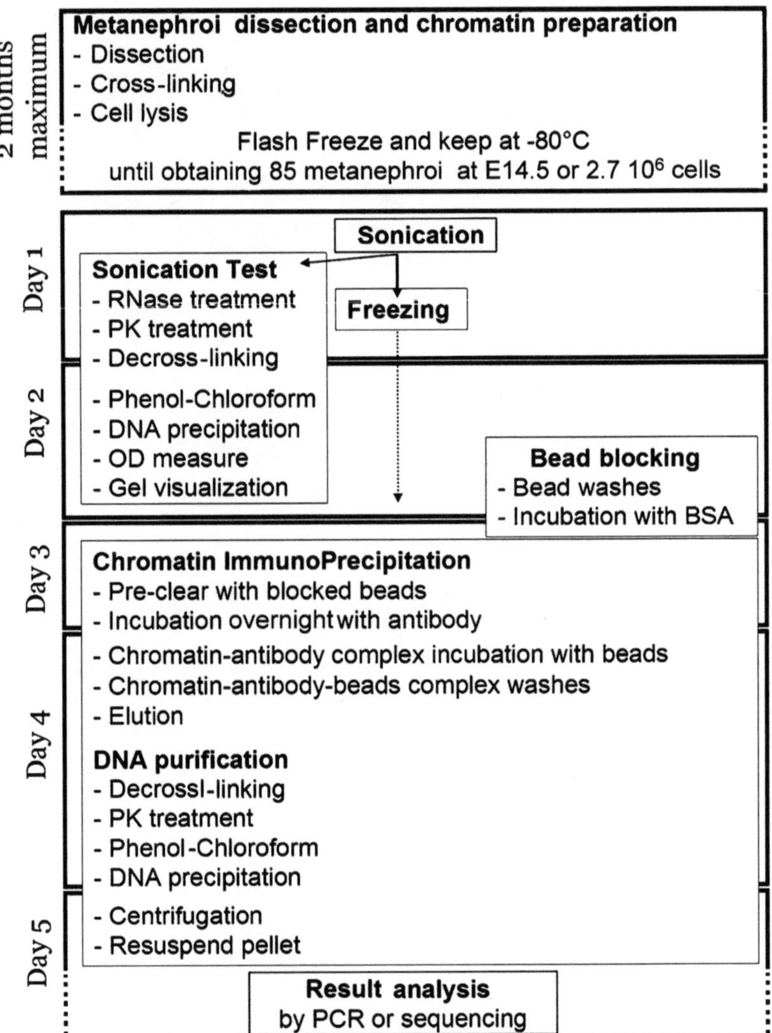

Fig. 2. Protocol overview.

important to select the embryonic stage at which a maximum number of cells express the protein of interest in order to reduce as much as possible the background from nonexpressing cell-types. For the first experiment, we advise to test the chromatin preparation using a previously validated antibody, such as the anti-RNA polymerase II antibody, and a constitutively active target such as the RNA polymerase II site upstream of the beta-actin gene, as described below.

There are several controls to evaluate the specific enrichment in your ChIP experiments. In general, it is used an IgG ChIP control to assay for nonspecific binding to the beads or IgG. In addition, to assess for potential "off-target" bindings of the antibody used, the ideal control would be to compare with a ChIP assay using the same tissue or cell-line, but lacking your transcription factor (i.e., by targeted inactivation or RNAi). When possible it is advisable to include in each experiment a positive control (i.e., a binding site that has been previously identified to be directly bound by your transcription factor) and a negative control (i.e., a genomic sequence that is not bound by the transcription factor).

2. Materials

All material must be DNA free, nuclease free, and free of any plasmid or PCR product. Whenever it is possible, we used commercial solutions, we avoided using laboratory glassware and we used commercial nuclease-free water in all solutions and at all steps. All the equipment was washed and decontaminated before use and we used clean gloves and filter tips during all steps.

2.1. Equipment

1. Centrifuge for microcentrifuge tubes, 15 ml, and 50-ml falcon tubes.
2. Water bath.
3. 1-ml Glass dounce homogenizer with loose and tight pestles (Wheaton).
4. 100-μm filter.
5. Orbital shaker rotator.
6. Cell counting chamber.
7. BioRuptor sonicator (Diagenode).
8. 15 ml high-clarity, and 50-ml polypropylene conical tubes.
9. 1.5- and 2-ml centrifuge microtubes.
10. Siliconized 1.5-ml centrifuge tubes.
11. Syringe and needle (26-gauge).
12. Set of pipetman exclusively used for ChIP experiments.
13. Real-time PCR System (StepOnePlus Life technologies).

2.2. Buffers for Chromatin Preparation

1. 0.5 M benzamidine stock solution: prepare in water, aliquot, and freeze at −20°C.
2. Protease inhibitors 50× stock solution: dilute one protease inhibitor cocktail tablet (Roche, 11697498001) in 1 ml water. Aliquot and freeze at −20°C.

   Protease inhibitors and benzamidine must be added just before use and the number of thawing's must be limited. Phosphatase inhibitors may also be required if the protein of interest is phosphorylated.
3. Dissection buffer: DMEM or HBSS.
4. PBS: prepare by diluting 10× PBS with distilled water.

5. 2% Formaldehyde in PBS, freshly prepared just before use.
6. 1.25 M Glycine in PBS prepared just before use.
7. 5 M Sodium chloride (NaCl).
8. 10% Sodium deoxycholate (DOC).
9. 1 M Tris–HCl, pH 8.
10. 20% SDS.
11. 10% IgePal CA-630 (NP40) in water. Keep at –20°C.
12. 0.5 M EDTA.
13. RIPA buffer: 50 mM Tris–HCl, pH 8, 15 mM NaCl, 0.5% DOC, 0.1% SDS, 0.5% NP40, 5 mM EDTA. Aliquot into 1 ml and keep at –20°C.
14. Nuclear lysis buffer (NLB): 50 mM Tris–HCl, pH 8.5 mM EDTA. Keep at room temperature.

2.3. Buffers for Immunoprecipitation Procedure

1. 1 M Tris–HCl, pH 8.1. Prepare from Trizma base.
2. 10% Triton X-100 in water. Keep at –20°C.
3. 20 mg/ml bovine serum albumin (BSA) prepared in water. Aliquot and keep at –20°C.
4. Protein A Agarose or Protein G Agarose.
5. 5 M lithium chloride (LiCl) prepared in water.
6. ChIP dilution buffer (50 ml): 16.7 mM Tris–HCl, pH 8.1, 167 mM NaCl, 0.01% SDS, 1.2 mM EDTA, and 1.1% Triton X-100. Keep at 4°C.
7. Low-salt immune complex wash buffer (50 ml): 20 mM Tris–HCl, pH 8.1, 150 mM NaCl, 0.1% SDS, 2 mM EDTA, 1% Triton X-100. Keep at 4°C.
8. High-salt immune complex wash buffer (50 ml): 20 mM Tris–HCl, pH 8.1, 500 mM NaCl, 0.1%SDS, 2 mM EDTA, and 1% Triton X-100. Keep at 4°C.
9. LiCl immune complex wash buffer (50 ml): 10 mM Tris–HCl, pH 8.1, 1 mM EDTA, 1% DOC, 1% NP40, and 250 mM LiCl. Keep at 4°C.
10. Tris–EDTA (TE) buffer prepared from 100× stock solution. Keep at 4°C.
11. Sodium bicarbonate ($NaHCO_3$).
12. Antibodies: anti-RNA polymerase II (Millipore, 05-623B). For this antibody, use protein G Agarose beads. Anti-HNF1β H-85 (Santa-Cruz, sc-22840). Normal rabbit IgG (Santa-Cruz, sc-2027) used as control.

2.4. Buffers for DNA Purification and qPCR Amplification Steps

1. DNase-free RNase.
2. 1 M Tris–HCl, pH 6.5. Prepare from Trizma base.
3. 10 mg/ml proteinase K in water.

4. Phenol–chloroform solution.
5. 100% Ethanol.
6. 20 mg/ml Glycogen.
7. 7.5 M Ammonium acetate.
8. Fast SYBR Green PCR Master Mix (Life technologies, 4385612).
9. Primers for mouse β-actin promoter amplification: Forward: 5′-GCAGGCCTAGTAACCGAGACA-3′ and Reverse: 5′-AGTTTTGGCGATGGGTGCT-3′ (10).

Primers for amplification of mouse control region in SMA (Actin aortic smooth muscle): Forward: 5′-tctcacgctcggctgttaaa-3′, Reverse: 5′-agcgcctgtatcaaccctaa-3′. Primers for amplification of HNF1β binding site: Wnt9b s+14132. Forward: 5′-acaggggcccgttaaacatt-3′ and Reverse: 5′-gtcaggctccgagggtttc-3′.

3. Methods

To prevent DNA contamination and protein degradation, all steps are performed under DNA free and nuclease free conditions and samples are maintained on ice or at 4°C during rotation and centrifugation steps, before the elution steps.

3.1. Dissection and Chromatin Preparation

1. Just before dissection, prepare and keep on ice:
   (a) 1 ml dissection buffer with 2 mM benzamidine to keep tissues during dissection.
   (b) 10 ml of 2 mM benzamidine in PBS.
   (c) 2 ml of PBS plus protease inhibitors.
   (d) 1.25 M glycine solution in PBS with benzamidine.
   (e) 125 mM glycine solution prepared by diluting 1.25 M glycine in PBS.
   (f) 1 ml RIPA plus protease inhibitors.
   (g) 100 μl NLB plus protease inhibitors.
   (h) Place dounces, pestles, and two microcentrifuge tubes on ice.
   (i) Place the filter (100 μm) on a 50-ml tube at -20°C.
   (j) Cool down centrifuges (4°C) and switch on water bath (25°C).
2. Prepare 2% formaldehyde solution in PBS plus benzamidine. Keep at RT and protected from light. (Caution: always manipulate solutions containing formaldehyde and perform cross-linking procedure inside an extraction hood.)

3. Dissect kidneys from E14.5 mouse embryos in DMEM or HBSS and collect them into a microcentrifuge tube containing DMEM or HBSS with 2 mM benzamidine. To prevent protein degradation and to preserve native chromatin state, embryos and dissected kidneys must be maintained on ice and dissection needs to be performed as quickly as possible. The entire procedure should not take more than 1 h to collect 2 L (around 50 E14.5 metanephroi). If more than 60 metanephroi are pooled, increase solution volumes for fixation and disruption (RIPA) steps (see Note 1).
4. Remove dissection buffer and wash twice with 1 ml PBS containing 2 mM benzamidine.
5. Remove PBS and add 250 μl of PBS with 2 mM benzamidine. Transfer to a dounce and homogenize embryonic kidneys on ice with a loose pestle until tissue is homogenized.
6. Transfer the dounce into the 25°C water bath under the hood and add 250 μl of 2% formaldehyde solution. Incubate 15 min and homogenize every 2 min using a pestle (see Note 2).
7. To quench formaldehyde, add 55.6 μl of 1.25 M glycine solution (final concentration 0.125 M), homogenize and incubate on ice for 5 min. Transfer to a cold microcentrifuge tube and wash the dounce with 0.125 M glycine solution to recover a maximum of homogenized cross-linked lysate.
8. Centrifuge at 572×*g* at 4°C for 5 min, carefully remove the supernatant, and wash the pellet with 1 ml PBS with protease inhibitors. Repeat this step once.
9. Resuspend the pellet in 300 μl of RIPA buffer and transfer to a dounce. Homogenize by 20–30 strokes with a tight pestle (avoid to remove the pestle from the liquid at each stroke, in order to limit bubble formation). To remove remaining pieces of tissue and connective tissue, transfer the homogenate to a 100-μm filter placed on a 50-ml tube, collect the filtrate by centrifugation, and transfer to a microcentrifuge tube. Wash the former tube, dounce, and filter by repeating homogenization and filtration steps with 300 μl of RIPA and pool the filtrates.
10. Preserve 5 μl to count nuclei and visualize tissue disruption.
11. Centrifuge for 5 min at 572×*g* at 4°C and resuspend the pellet in NLB. Use 2 μl of NLB by harvested metanephros. Incubate on ice for at least 10 min and freeze in liquid nitrogen. Store at –80°C (for maximum 2 months) until obtaining around 85 metanephroi at E14.5 or 2.7×10^6 nuclei.

3.2. Sonication

1. Prepare on ice NLB with protease inhibitors:
   (a) Place the syringe and needle at –20°C.
   (b) Wash the BioRuptor sonicator metallic bar in a 15-ml Falcon tube with water by sonication (3×2 min at 200 W) (see Note 3) and transfer it to a new tube on ice.

2. Thaw on ice the cross-linked kidney chromatin preparations:
   (a) Pool them using the syringe and needle (26-gauge) and transfer them to a cold 15-ml Falcon sonication tube.
   (b) Wash microcentrifuge tubes and syringe with NLB.
   (c) Add the wash to the chromatin lysate to reach a final volume of 495 μl.
   (d) Add 5 μl of 20% SDS (final concentration 0.3%).
   (e) Keep on ice for at least 10 min.
3. Ensure that SDS is not precipitated.

   Place the metallic bar into the chromatin tube and sonicate chromatin lysate to an average size of 200–800 bp. This requires to be empirically optimized (both cycle number and power settings), since different tissues or cells require different sonication conditions (see Note 4).

   In the initial experiment, use 600 μl of lysate and perform a time course to identify the optimal conditions by removing 20 μl at 0, 4, 8, 12, 16, and 20 sonication cycles (each cycle is 10 s "ON" at 200 W and 2 min 30 s "OFF").

   Between two sonication cycles, keep the tube for 30 s in cold water with salt and for at least 2 min on ice in order to limit the increase in temperature due to the sonication. According to the result of the first experiment, choose the appropriate cycle number to obtain DNA fragments between 200 and 800 bp (Fig. 3).
4. After sonication, centrifuge for 15 min at 15,493×*g* at 4°C to remove cell debris and high size chromatin fragments.
   (a) Transfer the supernatant to a new tube and remove 20 μl for the sonication test.
   (b) Flash-freeze in liquid nitrogen and keep the chromatin preparation at −80°C, or directly proceed to IP step 2(c) (see Note 5).
5. Use the 20 μl (sonication test) to analyze average DNA fragments size.
   (a) Add 1 μl RNase and incubate for 30 min at 37°C.
   (b) Add 0.1 mg (5 μl) proteinase K and incubate at 45°C for 3 h.
   (c) De-cross-link by incubation at 65°C for at least 4 h. Proteinase K treatment and de-cross-linking are usually performed in a PCR thermocycler.
6. Perform phenol–chloroform extraction:
   (a) Add 50 μl TE and one volume (75 μl) phenol–chloroform.
   (b) Vortex and centrifuge for 15 min at 15,493×*g* at 4°C.
   (c) Transfer the aqueous phase into a new tube.

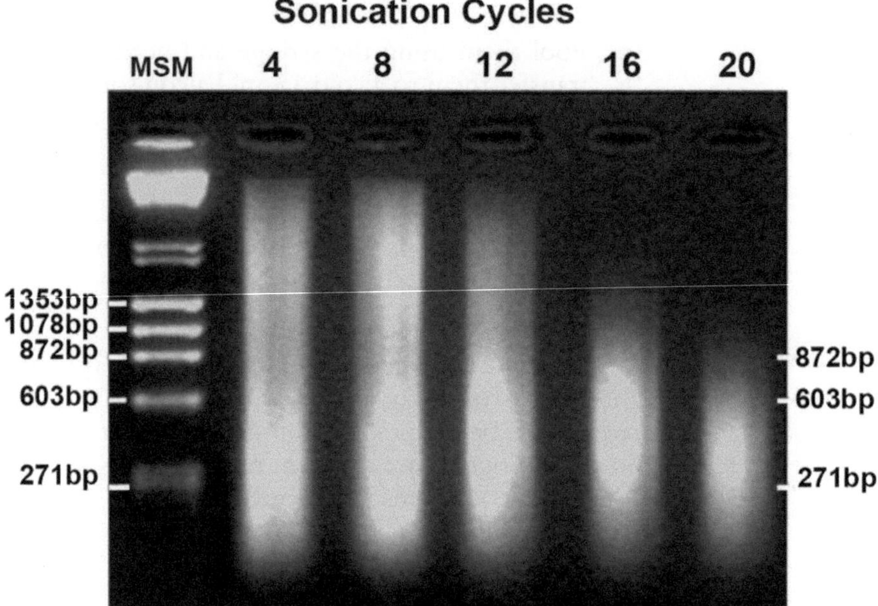

Fig. 3. Analysis of DNA sonication profile. After dissection and chromatin preparation, chromatin from 85 metanephroi at E14.5 is sonicated using BioRuptor in 600 μl of NLB 0.3% SDS. Each sonication cycle is composed by 10 s "ON" at 200 W, 30 s in cold water, and 2 min on ice. Chromatin samples kept at 4, 8, 12, 16, and 20 cycles, are treated with RNase and Proteinase K, de-cross-linked and purified by phenol–chloroform extraction followed by ethanol precipitation. Samples are separated by electrophoresis in a 1% agarose gel. According to this profile, 16 sonication cycles appear adapted for ChIP-PCR experiments. *MSM* molecular size marker in base pairs (bp).

(d) Add 75 μl of TE to the phenol–chloroform phase, vortex, and centrifuge.

(e) Pool the two aqueous phases.

7. Precipitate DNA:

   (a) Add 10 μg (0.5 μl) glycogen, 75 μl (0.5 vol) of 7.5 M ammonium acetate and 562.5 μl (2.5 vol) of ethanol 100%.

   (b) Mix and incubate for 45 min at −80°C.

8. Centrifuge 45 min at 15,493×*g* 4°C.

   (a) Discard the supernatant.

   (b) Wash the pellet with 80% ethanol.

   (c) Centrifuge for 10 min at 15,493×*g* at 4°C and discard the supernatant.

   (d) Resuspend the pellet in 20 μl TE by gentle agitation.

9. Measure the optic density (OD) at 260 nm.

This value will be used to calculate the DNA concentration of chromatin preparation (see Note 6). Load 300 ng in 1% agarose gel (Fig. 3).

If the sonication profile reveals higher fragments size than expected, you can perform one or two additional sonication cycles and centrifugations, as described before, just before performing the preclear step.

3.3. Immunoprecipitation

1. The day before IP, block Protein A/G agarose beads (see Note 7) with BSA as follows: prepare ChIP dilution buffer with 1 mg/ml BSA. Vortex agarose beads and remove 150 μl using a cut tip. Centrifuge for 1 min at 91×*g* at 4°C, discard the supernatant and wash three times the beads with 1 ml ChIP dilution buffer by gently mixing and centrifuging as before. Transfer the beads into a 15-ml Falcon tube and block by incubating overnight at 4°C with 10 ml of ChIP dilution buffer with 1 mg/ml BSA, under rotation. Measure the volume of packed beads. Centrifuge beads for 1 min at 91×*g* at 4°C and resuspend with one volume of ChIP dilution buffer with 1 mg/ml BSA.
2. Thaw the sonicated chromatin on ice and place the equivalent of 100–160 μg DNA (see Note 8) into a 15-ml Falcon tube; complete to 400 μl with NLB if necessary. Add 3.6 ml of ChIP dilution buffer and 70 μl of blocked beads. Preclear chromatin by incubating for 2 h at 4°C under rotation (see Note 9).
3. Centrifuge chromatin for 1 min at 91×*g* 4°C. Take the supernatant (avoid touching the beads) and equally split it into two 2 ml microcentrifuge tubes (~1.940 ml per tube). Transfer the equivalent of 10% of the chromatin (194 μl) in a 1.5-ml microcentrifuge tube as input (keep input in the fridge until DNA purification). Add into one tube the specific antibody (quantity must be empirically defined) and into the second tube a control IgG antibody or no antibody. We use 3–3.5 μg of HNF1β antibody and the same quantity of normal rabbit IgG for 50 μg of chromatin.
4. Incubate overnight at 4°C.
5. Add 40 μl of protein A/G agarose beads (vortex and use a cut tip to add exactly the same bead quantity in each tube) and incubate for 1 h at 4°C under rotation.
6. Centrifuge for 1 min at 91×*g* at 4°C and discard the supernatant (do not touch the beads, keep a minimum of 2 mm liquid above). Wash beads with 1 ml low-salt wash buffer. Incubate under rotation for 5 min at 4°C and centrifuge for 1 min at 91×*g* at 4°C.
7. Discard the supernatant (do not touch the beads) and repeat low-salt wash for 10 min. Centrifuge and perform two additional washes of 5 and 10 min with respectively 1 ml of high-salt wash buffer and then 1 ml of LiCl buffer. Wash once for 10 min with 1 ml TE (see Note 10).

8. To decrease background, change the tube before elution. Resuspend beads with 500 μl TE and transfer to a new siliconized tube. Prevent bead loss by washing the tube and the tip with TE, perform an additional wash (5 min) and then centrifuge for 1 min at 91×*g* at 4°C.

3.4. Elution and DNA Purification

1. Freshly prepared elution buffer: 0.1 M $NaHCO_3$ and 1% SDS.
2. Discard the supernatant and maintain the same volume of residual TE compared to the pellet. Add 200 μl elution buffer, vortex and incubate under rotation for 15 min at RT. Centrifuge for 2 min at 91×*g*.
3. Keep 200 μl of supernatant into a new 1.5-ml siliconized tube. Reelute beads by adding 100 μl elution buffer, vortex and incubate for 15 min at RT under rotation. After centrifugation, pool the eluates.
4. Reverse cross-linking between DNA and proteins in ChIPed and input material by adding respectively 12 μl and 8 μl of 5 M NaCl and incubating at 65°C for at least 4 h.
5. Add 6 μl of 0.5 M EDTA (4 μl for input), 12 μl of 1 M Tris–HCl pH 6.5 (8 μl for input) and 5 μl of 10 mg/ml proteinase K. Incubate for at least 2 h at 45°C.
6. Add 300 μl phenol–chloroform and after a 15-min centrifugation at 15,493×*g* at 4°C, transfer the aqueous phase (above) to a new 2-ml tube and reextract the phenol phase by adding 100 μl TE. Vortex, centrifuge, and pool the aqueous phases.
7. Precipitate DNA by adding 0.5 vol (200 μl) of 7.5 M ammonium acetate, 5 μl of 20 mg/ml glycogen, and 2.5 vol (1.5 ml) of ethanol 100%. Vortex and place overnight at −20°C.
8. Centrifuge 1 h at 15,493×*g* at 4°C, remove the supernatant, and wash the pellet with 80% ethanol. Centrifuge for 10 min at 15,493×*g* at 4°C.
9. Resuspend the pellet in 30 μl TE by agitation for 20 min and transfer in a siliconized tube. Wash the former tube with 25 μl TE. The immunoprecipitated DNA prepared from 50 to 80 μg in a final volume of 55 μl can be used immediately or kept frozen at −20°C.

3.5. Polymerase Chain Reaction

For the detection of specific DNA fragments, commonly used procedures are conventional semiquantitative PCR and quantitative PCR.

In general, PCR analysis of a ChIP experiment on a specific DNA region is based on comparison of signal, or cycle threshold (Ct), of control/IgG versus specific IP (11). This comparison allows calculating the fold enrichment for the amplified DNA region. To ensure that background is equivalent in control and specific IP, we chose to normalize this result by the fold enrichment obtained for a negative control region. As a negative control, we used a genomic region in the aortic smooth muscle actin (SMA) gene, expressed in embryonic kidney. This region does not present HNF1β binding site (12). As a positive control of IP efficiency, we used the β-actin promoter in anti-RNA Pol II ChIP. We describe here a protocol for relative qPCR quantification: all values were compared to a reference DNA (13). For this external reference, we used a pool of input diluted at 1:1,000 because Ct of this dilution is similar to Ct obtained for IgG control IP.

Even if qPCR analysis is more precise, semiquantitative PCR can be used for the first experiments (Fig. 4a) (see Note 11).

1. Design primers encompassing the region of interest to amplify a product of 50–80 bp.
2. The PCR conditions must be empirically established.

   Perform qPCR in 25 μl: 12.5 μl of fast SYBR green master mix (Life technologies), 0.25 μl of each primer at 20 μM, 5 μl DNA, and 7 μl water.
3. qPCR efficiency is determined using standard curves realized using diluted 10% input (1:40; 1:200; 1:1,000; and 1:5,000). PCR efficiency must be similar for a negative control locus and the locus of interest. Ensure using melt curve, that primers do not dimerize and that there is only one amplification product.
4. Determine the initial DNA quantity required for PCR. In our hands, control Ct is similar to Ct obtained using reference DNA (input 10% diluted 1:1,000). This input dilution must be detectable with Ct around 30.
5. Make amplification of control IP, specific IP, input 10% (or 1:1,000 dilution of this input), reference DNA and water. All points are in duplicate except the negative control, which is in triplicate (since it is used for background normalization) (see Note 12).
6. For each DNA sample (control IP, specific IP, input and reference DNA) calculate the difference (dCt) between Ct obtained for the locus of interest and Ct obtained for the negative control locus. To obtain the ddCt, subtract to each dCt, the dCt obtained for the reference DNA. The relative quantity is defined as 2(-ddCt). The relative quantities of different samples can be compared directly or expressed in input percentage. An example of qPCR result analysis is presented in Fig. 4b1.

In general, the enrichment depends on several parameters: chromatin preparation and cross-linking efficiency, the antibody used, the percentage of cells in which the IP protein is recruited to the tested region and the strength of its binding. Variations in these parameters induce very large differences in ChIP results ranging from an enrichment of 100× for histone modification analysis on homogeneous cell cultures to ×3 for transcription factor recruitment in vivo. Classically, an enrichment lower than 2 is considered as background. Amplifying HNF1β binding region Wnt9b s + 14123

PCR with primers framing the *Wnt9b* s+14132 HNF1B binding region :

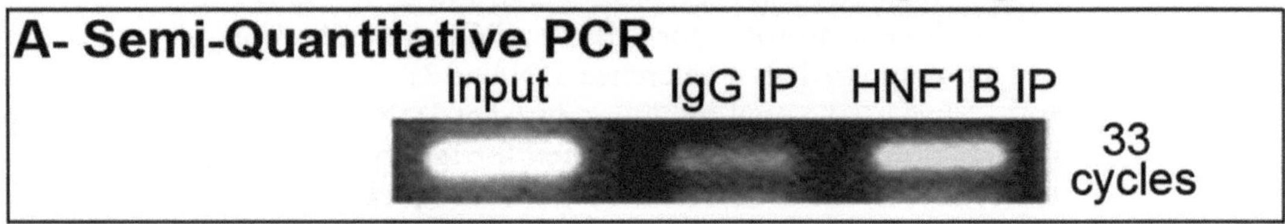

B- Quantitative PCR

1-

	Sma control region		*Wnt9b* s+14132 target region				relative quantity	Fold enrichment	% of input DNA
	Ct	average Ct	Ct	average Ct	dCt	ddCt	2-ddct	Compared to control IP	
control IP	34.8 34.5 34.9	34.7	34.8 34.3	34.5	-0,18	0.31	0.81		0.01%
HNF1B IP	34.3 34.5 34.8	34.5	30.9 30.8	30.9	-3.67	-3.18	9.08	11.24	0.14%
input 0.01%	32.50 32.74 32.35	32.5	32.63 32.79	32.7	0.18	0.67	0.63		0.01%
ref DNA	34.75 33.63 33.38	33.9	33.3 33.6	33.4	-0.49	0.00	1.00		0.02%

2-

3-

Fig. 4. Polymerase chain reaction amplification of the *Wnt9b s*+ 14132 region shows that HNF1B is recruited on this region in vivo. (**a**) Semiquantitative PCR analysis allows visualization of Wnt9b s + 14132 region enrichment. (**b**) Table showing an example of qPCR analysis. Cycle threshold (Ct) obtained for each sample (control IP, HNF1B IP, input and reference DNA) in amplification of the negative control region (Sma) and of the region of interest (Wnt9b s + 14132), are reported. dCt of the reference DNA is highlighted in *gray*. By pooling five independent experiments, we observed a ×15 (+/−2.5) enrichment of this region in immunoprecipitated DNA when compared to the IgG control IP (*left panel*). The same results expressed as input percentage are reported in the *right panel*. 0.01% (+/−0.001) of the *Wnt9b* s + 14132 DNA was nonspecifically precipitated in IgG experiments while In HNF1B CHIP, this region represented 0.14% (+/−0.03) of the input, thus demonstrating the specific IP by the HNF1B antibody. Error bar represents SEM of five independent experiments and is expressed as arbitrary units in the *left panel* and as percentage of input in the *right panel*.

(9), we observed an enrichment superior to 10 in HNF1β immunoprecipitated DNA compared to the control IgG IP (Fig. 4b2). This result could also be expressed as input percentage. We observed that this region represents 0.01 and 0.14% of input in IgG control IP and in HNF1β IP respectively (Fig. 4b3).

PCR analysis allows visualization of protein binding on one genomic locus. In order to analyze the binding sites of a protein on genomic scale, ChIP-Seq must be performed. The present protocol has been successfully scaled up to perform ChIP-Seq (see Note 13).

4. Notes

1. It is possible, but not recommended, to freeze dissected material directly, before performing formaldehyde cross-linking.
2. A long cross-linking time (more than 30 min) may be necessary for proteins that interact indirectly with DNA. However, this decreases sonication efficiency.
3. Depending on the sonicator used, the sonicator bar or probe tip are often contamination sources. After washing and UV treatment, three sonications of 2 min in water allow fragmentation of any potential contaminating DNA.
4. The sonication procedure is relatively difficult to calibrate, since it depends on the sonicator, the solution in which nuclei are resuspended, the tissue or cell type, the pureness of nuclei, and, to a lesser extent, the concentration of nuclei. We prefer to sonicate in 0.3% SDS instead of 1% SDS as usually used (although it decreases the sonication efficiency) because under these conditions, we observe better antibody reaction. In addition, the use of NLB hypotonic buffer allows decreasing SDS concentration without affecting significantly the sonication efficiency.

   BioRuptor manufacturer's instructions recommend to use ice in sonication bath and to make 30 s "OFF" cycles. However, the presence of ice decreases the sonication efficiency and reproducibility. We chose to use ice-cold water in the bath and to keep the BioRuptor in a cold room (4°C). Between two cycles, we keep tubes on cold salt-water and then on ice, for 30 s and 2 min, respectively. Moreover, since the first seconds of sonication are the most efficient in decreasing fragments size, it is advisable to increase the number of cycles instead of the length of each cycle.
5. DNA fragment size influences the ChIP result: sonicated chromatin between 100 and 300 pb is advised for ChIP-Seq but this increases background, very likely due to PCR efficiency or unspecific coating of DNA extremities on beads. We have set up conditions to obtain the majority of DNA fragments between 300 and 800 bp.

6. The initial DNA quantity is essential for the reproducibility of the ChIP results. Most protocols measure OD at 260 nm to roughly calculate DNA concentration in the crude sonicate. Freezing after the sonication step allows a verification of the sonication profile and a more precise quantification of DNA concentration.
7. The type of beads (Protein A or Protein G) depends of the species and the subclass of the antibody of interest. See manufacturer's instructions or, alternatively, pool protein A/protein G agarose beads.
8. Initial chromatin requirement depends on transcription factor abundance. Using an antibody anti-RNA polymerase II, 10–20 μg of DNA per IP is sufficient. For a transcription factor, increasing the initial DNA quantity to 50–80 μg allows for a better reproducibility.
9. If the background observed is too high, the preclear step can be repeated.
10. If high background is observed, increase the number of low salt washes. The doubling of wash steps used here is optimized for anti-HNF1β, but this may be not necessary for anti-pol II antibody.
11. For the first experiments, semiquantitative PCR allows to test more targets sequences with more easily designed primers. Semiquantitative PCR conditions can be optimized (initial immunoprecipitated DNA quantity and number of cycles required) using 1:1,000 diluted input. In general, we use 1/10 eluted DNA for each amplification and 33, 36, and 39 cycles. For more precise analysis, radioactive PCR can also be used to detect PCR products with fewer cycles.
12. In ChIP experiments, the amount of DNA recovered is usually very low, particularly in control IP (0.2 ng by IP). Thus, Ct obtained for background normalization is very high and may lead to poor reproducibility (duplicates with Ct differences superior than 0.5). In order to improve the results of the control Ct, we perform the amplification of the negative region in triplicates.
13. We successfully adapted this protocol for ChIP-Seq analysis. For this experiment, we started with 425 metanephroi at E14.5 and applied the protocol described above. Sonication was performed in five tubes to maintain the chromatin concentration during sonication. Four sonication cycles were added, in order to obtain smaller fragments. After the preclear step, all supernatants were pooled and the IP was done in nine independent tubes. Only one control IP was realized for nine specific IPs. We repeated this protocol to obtain 30 ng of DNA, which were subjected to deep sequencing according to

Illumina manufacture recommendations. Claire Heliot, Stephanie Legras, Irwin Davidson and Silvia Cereghini (Inserm U969 & CNRS-Université Pierre et Marie Curie UMR7622-Paris France).

Acknowledgments

We thank I. Talianidis (Biomedical Sciences Research Center Al. Fleming, Greece.), K. Zaret (University of Pennsylvania School of Medicine, Philadelphia, USA), L. Sachs (UPMC CNRS UMR7221, Paris France), and E. Havis (CNRS UPMC UMR 7622, Paris, France) for their advice during optimization of the ChIP experiment. We thank S. Schneider-Maunoury and C. Haumaitre (UPMC, CNRS UMR 7622 and INSERM U969, Paris, France) for critical reading of the manuscript. This work was supported by Inserm, CNRS, Universite Pierre et Marie Curie and ARC (N° 3911) grants. C. H. is a recipient of a PhD student fellowship from Ministere de la Recherche et de la Technologie and from ARC.

References

1. Cao Y, Yao Z, Sarkar D et al (2010) Genome-wide MyoD binding in skeletal muscle cells: a potential for broad cellular reprogramming. Dev Cell 18:662–674
2. Xu J, Watts JA, Pope SD et al (2009) Transcriptional competence and the active marking of tissue-specific enhancers by defined transcription factors in embryonic and induced pluripotent stem cells. Genes Dev 23: 2824–2838
3. Collas P, Dahl JA (2008) Chop it, ChIP it, check it: the current status of chromatin immunoprecipitation. Front Biosci 13:929–943
4. Boyd KE, Farnham PJ (1999) Coexamination of site-specific transcription factor binding and promoter activity in living cells. Mol Cell Biol 19:8393–8399
5. Orlando V, Strutt H, Paro R (1997) Analysis of chromatin structure by in vivo formaldehyde cross-linking. Methods (San Diego, CA) 11: 205–214
6. Lagha M, Kormish JD, Rocancourt D et al (2008) Pax3 regulation of FGF signaling affects the progression of embryonic progenitor cells into the myogenic program. Genes Dev 22: 1828–1837
7. Parrizas M, Maestro MA, Boj SF et al (2001) Hepatic nuclear factor 1-alpha directs nucleosomal hyperacetylation to its tissue-specific transcriptional targets. Mol Cell Biol 21: 3234–3243
8. Havis E, Anselme I, Schneider-Maunoury S (2006) Whole embryo chromatin immunoprecipitation protocol for the in vivo study of zebrafish development. BioTechniques 40:34, 36, 38 passim
9. Lokmane L, Heliot C, Garcia-Villalba P, Fabre M, Cereghini S (2010) vHNF1 functions in distinct regulatory circuits to control ureteric bud branching and early nephrogenesis. Development (Cambridge, UK) 137:347–357
10. Stock JK, Giadrossi S, Casanova M et al (2007) Ring1-mediated ubiquitination of H2A restrains poised RNA polymerase II at bivalent genes in mouse ES cells. Nat Cell Biol 9: 1428–1435
11. Haring M, Offermann S, Danker T et al (2007) Chromatin immunoprecipitation: optimization, quantitative analysis and data normalization. Plant Methods 3:11
12. Verdeguer F, Le Corre S, Fischer E et al (2010) A mitotic transcriptional switch in polycystic kidney disease. Nat Med 16:106–110
13. Livak KJ, Schmittgen TD (2001) Analysis of relative gene expression data using real-time quantitative PCR and the 2 (-Delta Delta C(T)) method. Methods (San Diego, CA) 25: 402–408

Part V

Manipulating Gene Expression in Developing and Adult Kidney

Chapter 26

siRNA-Mediated RNA Interference in Embryonic Kidney Organ Culture

Jamie A. Davies and Mathieu Unbekandt

Abstract

In principle, treatment of embryonic kidneys growing in organ culture with short interfering RNA (siRNA) offers a powerful means of investigating molecular function quickly and cheaply. Experiments using this approach have yielded significant new data, but they have also highlighted important limitations. Here, we briefly describe the published successes and limitations and present detailed instructions for two methods of siRNA treatment. The first method applies siRNA to intact cultured kidneys; this method is the quicker and easier of the two, but it is the one most affected by problems of siRNA uptake by certain renal tissues. The second method reduces kidney rudiments to a suspension of single cells, applies siRNA at that stage, when the cells are highly accessible, and then reaggregates the kidney; this method is more time-consuming but suffers less from problems of limited uptake. As well as proving instructions for the methods, we provide a brief discussion of necessary controls.

Key words: Short interfering RNA, RNA interference, Knockdown, Metanephros, Renal, Screening, Functional genomics, Tubulogenesis, WT1, Tor, hAFSC

1. Introduction

When Elbashir et al. (1, 2) announced that the expression of specific genes could be knocked down in wild-type mammalian cells by short interfering RNAs (siRNAs), researchers envisaged a revolution in studies of mammalian development. In principle, there was a quick and cheap alternative to expensive and time-consuming production of conditional transgenic knockout mice. For the kidney field, in particular, it suggested a method for high-throughput screening based on widely used renal organ culture systems.

Early attempts to apply siRNA technology to metanephric organ cultures worked well and led to the discovery of novel information about molecular functions of fibronectin in branching

Odyssé Michos (ed.), *Kidney Development: Methods and Protocols*, Methods in Molecular Biology, vol. 886,
DOI 10.1007/978-1-61779-851-1_26, © Springer Science+Business Media, LLC 2012

morphogenesis and WT1 in metanephrogenic mesenchyme (3, 4). They therefore gave cause for optimism. Even these early papers had, though, drawn attention to limitations of the method, particularly for achieving strong knockdown in already-formed epithelia, because of poor diffusion of siRNAs through a basement membrane (4). Our own attempts to apply the technology to further targets, together with anecdotal accounts of the attempts of others, have suggested that it is best suited to targeting molecules for which absolute amount is important (such as fibronectin and WT1), and less suited for those for which even a small amount is enough for a tissue to develop normally. Careful studies of the spread of fluorescently labeled siRNAs in cultured organs also indicated that the cap mesenchyme compartment of the kidney is, like already-formed tubules, somewhat resistant to siRNA uptake (5). For these reasons, application of the technique to intact cultured organs has been rather limited, although siRNA has been used very successfully in simple renal cell culture systems, e.g., ref. 6. Nevertheless, where its use is appropriate (e.g., to target a molecule, the absolute amount of which is important and/or which is expressed in loose mesenchyme), application of siRNA to cultured kidneys continues to be a useful technique (7–12): for this reason, the whole organ method is described in this chapter.

Recently, we have applied siRNAs to our renal disaggregation and reaggregation method (13), described elsewhere in this volume, to take advantage of the fact that suspensions of single cells are highly accessible to exogenous agents. We have used this both to knock down gene expression in all cells of a culture (13), and also to make mosaics of knocked-down cells and normal host cells, to test the cell autonomy of a knockdown phenotype (13, 14). It is too early to know whether this technique will be taken up widely but, because it seems to us to be promising, this second technique is described here too.

2. Materials

2.1. Materials Common to Both Methods

1. siRNAs targeting the mRNA encoding the protein of interest and also control siRNAs (see Note 1).
2. A primary antibody against the target protein, suitable for both immuno-staining and Western blotting (or two antibodies, one for each purpose), a primary antibody against a housekeeping protein (e.g., GAPDH) suitable for Western blotting, and appropriate secondary antibodies.
3. 5 μm Polycarbonate filters (Millipore).
4. Stainless steel Trowell grids to support filters at the surface of medium. A simple version can be made by cutting fine stainless

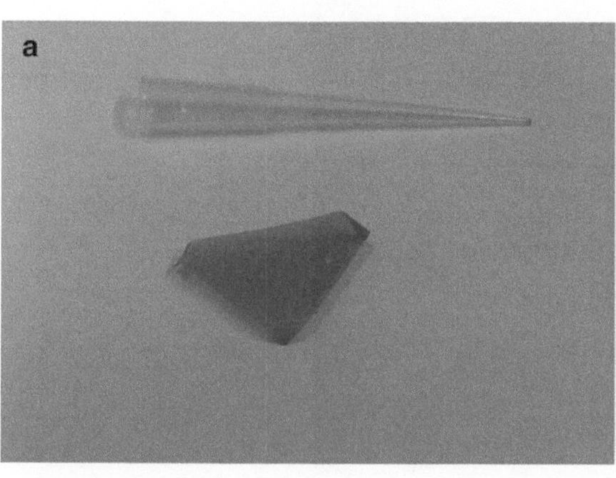

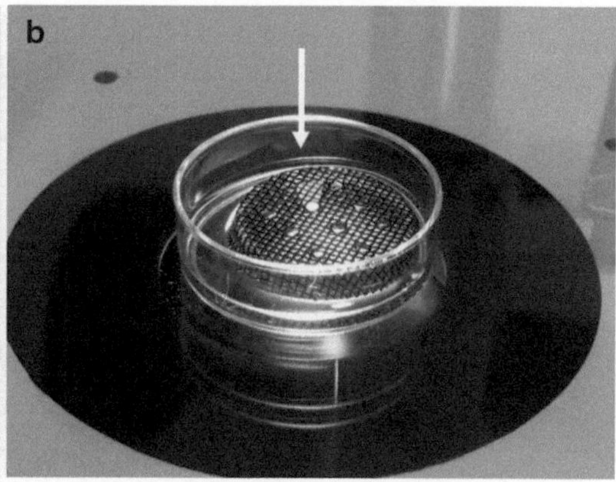

Fig. 1. Hardware of the culture system. (**a**) Simple Trowell culture grid, made by bending a triangle of fine stainless steel mesh as explained in Subheading 2.1: the Gilson tip is present just to indicate scale. (**b**) Other form of Trowell grid described in the main text, with a filter and medium in position (*arrow*—the kidney rudiment on the filter is too small and colorless to discern in this photograph). The grid could take up to about 12 filters, although only one is shown here.

steel mesh into triangles about 1.5 cm per side and bending the corners down to make "legs" about 1–2 mm high (they need to be low to avoid a need for large amounts of expensive siRNA-containing medium). An example can be seen in Fig. 1a. More durable examples can be made by cutting circles of coarser mesh and bending their outer 2 mm or so down to make a circular platform. Clear areas that allow tissues to be seen without pieces of metal grid in the way can be created by forcing a pointed scissor blade into the mesh and turning it. An example of a grid made this way can be seen in Fig. 1b.

5. A high-quality dissecting microscope, such as the Zeiss Stemi-2000 (other excellent microscopes are available, but second-rate ones can make these experiments very difficult to perform. Economies made here tend to be false ones).

2.2. Extra Materials for the Intact Kidney Method

1. Serum-Free Culture Medium (SFCM): Richter's Modified Improved MEM with 10 μg/ml iron-loaded transferrin. Avoid adding antibiotics (see Note 2).
2. A suitable transfection system (see Note 2): the method described below is designed for use with oligofectamine (Invitrogen).

2.3. Extra Materials for the Reaggregate Method

1. Dissecting medium: Eagle's Minimum Essential Medium (DMEM).
2. Kidney culture medium (KCM): Eagle's Minimum Essential Medium with 10% fetal calf serum and 1× penicillin/streptomycin.
3. Trypsin-EDTA 10× made up at 1× in phosphate buffered saline (PBS) itself made from tablets.

4. Glycyl-H1152 dihydrochloride (Tocris).
5. DMEMCM: advanced DMEM, 10% fetal calf serum but with NO antibiotics (see Note 5).
6. DMEMCM, 1.25 μM glycyl-H1152.
7. A suitable transfection system, the method described here uses Lipofectamine 2000 (Invitrogen).
8. Microcentrifuge.
9. 3.5 mm Petri dishes.
10. 40 μm cell strainer.
11. Hemocytometer.

3. Methods

Before work starts, careful attention should be paid to controls (see Note 1).

3.1. The Intact Kidney Method

1. Begin by dissecting metanephric rudiments from E10.5 to E11.5 mouse embryos. It is assumed that anyone reading this chapter is already capable of this dissection, but a detailed guide to one technique is the subject of a chapter in an earlier volume (15). See Note 3 about dissection quality.
2. Transfer the rudiments to SFCM (defined in Subheading 2.2) and allow them to equilibrate in a 37°C, 5% CO_2 incubator while carrying out the next steps.
3. For each siRNA to be used, including controls, prepare the mix of siRNA and transfection vehicle according to the instructions of the manufacturer of the vehicle (see Note 4). For the oligofectamine system in our original report (4), mix 60 μl of 20 μM siRNA with 500 μl SFCM in a microcentrifuge tube and vortex lightly. Immediately afterwards, take a second tube and mix 30 μl oligofectamine with 120 μl SFCM. Leave both tubes 7 min at room temperature (16–17°C here in Scotland; other countries' rooms tend to be warmer, but the difference is probably not critical). Mix the tubes gently and leave for 25 min at room temperature while performing step 4.
4. Prepare culture filters for later use. Immerse a 5 μm polycarbonate filter in SFCM and cut it into small pieces about 5 mm across using a round-bladed scalpel. (Consider cutting different shapes—squares, triangles, etc.—for use with different siRNAs: this allows all samples to be immunostained in the same tube later, economizing on antibody and eliminating one possible source of variation.)

5. Add 1,290 μl SFCM to each siRNA/oligofectamine mix made at the end of step 3—this makes the "transfection mix".
6. Place Trowell grids in fresh 3 cm Petri dishes, and fill these dishes with the transfection mix until the surface of the grids is just wet. Dip pieces of filter into the bulk transfection mix next to the grid, to make sure that they are soaked in it and not just in plain SFCM, and place them on top of the holes in the grid.
7. Pipette kidney rudiments on to the filters, working as rapidly as possible (Fig. 1b).
8. Very gently, pipette a little transfection mix from the bulk under the grid on to the filters, taking care not to disturb them. This step ensures that the kidneys are in proper contact with the transfection mix, and not still in a private zone of the basic SFCM from which they came (see Note 5).
9. Incubate the cultures for 18–24 h at 37°C, 5% CO_2.
10. Replace the transfection mix, either with fresh SFCM, or with an alternative medium suitable for growing kidneys. Incubate for as many days as desired (see Subheading 3.1, on controls, for the desirability of running a time-course).
11. After the experiment, remove the medium and replace it with fixative, filling the dish from the bottom so that the fix rises to the filters from underneath (this minimizes the risk of samples being washed away before they are fixed to the filters, and allows immunostaining to be performed on the filters themselves). Our routine fix is methanol at –20°C for 10 min.

3.2. Application of siRNA to the Disaggregation/ Reaggregation Method

This method proceeds by an essentially normal disaggregation/ reaggregation culture, as described elsewhere in this volume, but with the addition of a siRNA transfection step at the cell suspension stage. Care needs to be taken about pH (see Note 6).

1. Isolate fresh E11.5 metanephric rudiments by manual dissection in dissecting medium (defined in Subheading 2.3). The number needed will depend on the numbers of controls to be run; assume at least eight rudiments per culture to be set up; the exact number depends on how well cells survive the disaggregation and pipetting processes. Place at least one intact kidney aside in a dish in the incubator for use as a control.
2. Using a pulled Pasteur pipette, transfer the rudiments to a Petri dish containing Trypsin-EDTA solution for 4 min at 37°C, 5% CO_2.
3. Remove the kidneys from the dish containing Trypsin-EDTA and place them in a Petri dish containing DMEMCM to protect the rudiments from further digestion. Leave them in this for 10 min at 37°C.

4. This incubation is a good time to prepare culture filters for later use.

   Place a sheet of 5-μm polycarbonate filter in a Petri dish of DMEMCM + 1.25 μM H1152 and cut it into 5-mm squares.

   Place filter grids in fresh 3-cm Petri dishes, and fill these dishes with DMEMCM + 1.25 μM H1152 until the meniscus just reaches the grid.

   Lay the filter pieces on the grid (across the holes in the mesh if you made them). Keep in the 37°C, 5% CO_2 incubator until needed.

5. Dissociate the organs by placing them in a 0.5-ml tube containing 200 μl of DMEMCM, pipetting them through a yellow Gilson tip, strongly enough to separate the cells without destroying them by shear. Examine samples of the solution to monitor progress in disaggregating the tissue.

6. Filter through the cell strainer. Stain a sample with Trypan Blue to check viability, concentration, and that the cells are in a single-celled suspension.

7. Place the cell suspension in a 10-ml tube containing at least 5 ml of advanced DMEM. Centrifuge the cells at 1,000 rpm for 5 min. Remove the supernatant and dilute the cells in advanced DMEM at a concentration of 2×10^5 cells per 100 μl.

8. Aliquot the bulk cell suspension into lots of 10×10^4 cells (50 μl) in 0.5 ml tubes.

9. Place 0.3 μl of Lipofectamine 2000 (0.5 μl for plasmid transfections) in 25 μl of OPTIMEM, mix gently and leave at room temperature for 5 min.

10. Dilute siRNA in 25 μl of OPTIMEM (0.4–0.6 μg of DNA for plasmid transfections) to obtain a final concentration of 100 nM, the final volume being 100 μl.

11. Mix the Lipofectamine 2000 solution with the siRNA solution and leave at room temperature for 20 min.

12. Place the Lipofectamine 2000/siRNA solution on the 50 μl of kidney cells suspension and mix gently. Incubate at 37°C for 2 h.

13. Mix the cells suspensions and centrifuge them for 2 min at $800 \times g$ to make a pellet.

14. Place dishes containing the filters on the grids, prepared at step 4, on the stage of the dissecting microscope. Transfer the pelleted cells on to filters using a pulled pipette, taking care not to wash them away with excessive medium from the pipette. Use a different dish for each siRNA treatment, since there is a risk of siRNAs leaching from the pellets and cross-contaminating them.

15. Recover the intact kidney left as a control in step 1, and pipette it on to the triangular filter. This kidney will act as a positive control for the basic media, incubator, etc.
16. Incubate for 24 h.
17. Replace the medium either with DMEMCM (no 1.25 μM H1152) or KCM and incubate as long as is desired. Antibiotics can be added to the medium after 24 h of culture.

4. Notes

1. All RNA interference experiments need to be supported by very careful controls. As a minimum, consider the following:
   (a) Cultures with no treatment.
   (b) Cultures treated with siRNA transfection vehicle but no siRNA (to check that the vehicle has no effect).
   (c) Cultures treated with irrelevant and/or scrambled siRNA (to check that siRNA per se has no effect).
   (d) Use of multiple siRNAs targeting different parts of the target mRNA, applied individually (to guard against the possibility of a phenotype being due to "friendly fire" attacks against an unknown additional target mRNA).
   (e) Monitoring of protein knockdown (including establishing its time course), both of the target protein and of a housekeeping protein that ought not be affected (to guard against the possibility of a general depression of protein synthesis).
   (f) Use of both Western blot techniques and immunostaining to monitor expression. (Westerns show the average knockdown, say "90%" but not how it is distributed across the tissue: are all cells knocked down by 90% or are 90% of cells knocked down by 100% while 10% of the cells escape inhibition altogether? Are those 10% clustered or distributed randomly?)
   (g) Where possible, attempt a rescue (relatively easy if your target protein is extracellular).

   Particular applications may require additional controls. In general, experimenters should set their caution level to "paranoid" when planning RNA interference work.
2. Techniques for transfecting siRNAs into cells are evolving all the time, with manufacturers frequently announcing products claimed to be better than their predecessors. The instructions above are written with the transfection vehicles oligofectamine and Lipofectamine 2000 in mind, as we have

greatest experience with them, but experimenters may profit greatly from trying others. Most manufacturers are willing to provide free samples.

3. When dissecting kidney rudiments for the whole-organ siRNA method, take great care to remove extraneous adventitia (i.e., mesenchyme that is not strictly part of the kidney): every unnecessary layer of cells is another obstruction to siRNA's diffusion to the places that you need it to be.
4. Invitrogen, the manufacturer of oligofectamine and Lipofectamine 2000, cautions against using antibiotics which can apparently become more toxic in the presence of oligofectamine and similar reagents (this caution appears in the product manual).
5. Although we have not made a detailed statistical study of this, it is our impression that taking care to ensure that the kidneys and filters are in direct contact with transfection mix from the beginning of the experiment, rather than relying on diffusion to equilibrate them with the bulk transfection mic under the grid over time, reduces variation between replicates.
6. The disaggregation/reaggregation method involves significant micromanipulation of tissues, in open-air, in media that are intended to be buffered against 5% CO_2: pay close attention to the color of the pH indicator in the medium while you work, and change medium if it begins to look significantly more alkaline than equivalent medium in a 5% CO_2 incubator. This is important—pH drift is bad for the cells (but so, alas, are all of the non-CO_2 buffers we have tried in an attempt to obviate the problem).

Acknowledgments

This work was supported by NC3Rs grant G0700480 and EU Star-t-Rek network FP7 223007.

References

1. Elbashir SM, Harborth J, Lendeckel W et al (2001) Duplexes of 21-nucleotide RNAs mediate RNA interference in cultured mammalian cells. Nature 411:494–498
2. Elbashir SM, Lendeckel W, Tuschl T (2001) RNA interference is mediated by 21- and 22-nucleotide RNAs. Genes Dev 15:188–200
3. Sakai T, Larsen M, Yamada KM (2003) Fibronectin requirement in branching morphogenesis. Nature 423:876–881
4. Davies JA, Ladomery M, Hohenstein P et al (2004) Development of an siRNA-based method for repressing specific genes in renal organ culture and its use to show that the Wt1 tumour suppressor is required for nephron differentiation. Hum Mol Genet 13:235–246
5. Lee WC, Berry R, Hohenstein P, Davies J (2008) siRNA as a tool for investigating organogenesis: the pitfalls and the promises. Organogenesis 4:176–181

6. Lee WC, Hough MT, Liu W et al (2010) Dact2 is expressed in the developing ureteric bud/collecting duct system of the kidney and controls morphogenetic behavior of collecting duct cells. Am J Physiol Renal Physiol 299:F740–F751
7. Berry R, Harewood L, Pei L et al (2010) Esrrg functions in early branch generation of the ureteric bud and is essential for normal development of the renal papilla. Hum Mol Genet 20:917–926
8. Li X, Hyink DP, Radbill B et al (2009) Protein kinase-X interacts with Pin-1 and Polycystin-1 during mouse kidney development. Kidney Int 76:54–62
9. Sheng W, Wang G, La Pierre DP et al (2006) Versican mediates mesenchymal–epithelial transition. Mol Biol Cell 17:2009–2020
10. Kim HS, Kim MS, Hancock AL et al (2007) Identification of novel Wilms' tumor suppressor gene target genes implicated in kidney development. J Biol Chem 282:16278–16287
11. Michael L, Sweeney DE, Davies JA (2007) The lectin Dolichos biflorus agglutinin is a sensitive indicator of branching morphogenetic activity in the developing mouse metanephric collecting duct system. J Anat 210:89–97
12. Maeshima A, Vaughn DA, Choi Y, Nigam SK (2006) Activin A is an endogenous inhibitor of ureteric bud outgrowth from the Wolffian duct. Dev Biol 295:473–485
13. Unbekandt M, Davies JA (2009) Dissociation of embryonic kidneys followed by reaggregation allows the formation of renal tissues. Kidney Int 77:407–416
14. Siegel N, Rosner M, Unbekandt M et al (2010) Contribution of human amniotic fluid stem cells to renal tissue formation depends on mTOR. Hum Mol Genet 19:3320–3331
15. Davies JA (2010) The embryonic kidney: isolation, organ culture, immunostaining and RNA interference. Methods Mol Biol 633:57–69

Chapter 27

Morpholino-Mediated Gene Knockdown in Mammalian Organ Culture

Alda Tufro

Abstract

We examined the role of semaphorin3a in ureteric bud (UB) branching morphogenesis using mouse metanephric organ culture [Tufro et al. (Mech Dev 125:558–568, 2008)]. In vitro UB injection of *Sema3a* antisense morpholino resulted in increased branching morphogenesis. Cellular and tissue uptake of oligonucleotides was facilitated by a peptide-mediated method. Our findings were validated by in vitro translation and in Sema3a null mice. This chapter describes a method to perfuse the UB lumen with fluorescein-labeled oligonucleotides bound to a peptide carrier.

Key words: Metanephric organ culture, Ureteric bud perfusion, Peptide–morpholino-mediated gene knockdown

1. Introduction

Branching morphogenesis of the ureteric bud (UB) is essential for kidney development (1). Mutations that alter ureteric bud branching result in renal agenesis, hypoplasia, multiple or dysplastic kidneys (1, 2). UB branching requires reciprocal signals to and from the surrounding mesenchyme and stroma (1, 2). Given the multitude of non-cell autonomous signals involved, and the very specific time and spatial constraints of UB branching development, it is necessary to timely examine UB branching in metanephric organ culture or embryonic kidneys.

Gene knockdown through RNA interference or translation inhibition are useful approaches to elucidate gene function (3). However, poor cellular uptake of nucleic acids and degradation by nucleases are major limitations of these technologies (3–5). Viral and nonviral strategies have been used to overcome this in cell culture and in vivo. Lipid-mediated nucleic acid transfection can be achieved in cell lines, but is not efficient in vivo or in organ culture.

Odyssé Michos (ed.), *Kidney Development: Methods and Protocols*, Methods in Molecular Biology, vol. 886, DOI 10.1007/978-1-61779-851-1_27, © Springer Science+Business Media, LLC 2012

Peptide-mediated cell uptake of macromolecules, including oligonucleotides, proteins, and peptides has also been reported (5, 6). Cell-penetrating peptides are either covalently coupled or form noncovalent complexes with plasmid DNA or oligonucleotides. We used a 27 residues translocator peptide, called ΔMPG, consisting of an internalization domain derived from the fusion sequence of HIV protein gp41, a nuclear localization domain derived from the NLS of SV-40 large T antigen, and a spacer domain in between them (6). This peptide is stable at physiologic pH and in the presence of serum, and the peptide–oligonucleotide complex dissociates rapidly after it crosses the cell membrane (7). Morpholinos are oligonucleotides modified by nonionic phosphorodiamidate linking morpholine rings that replace deoxyriboses moieties, to prevent degradation by nucleases (3). Antisense morpholinos are widely used to achieve gene knockdown by injection into Xenopus oocytes and zebrafish blastocysts (3). Their use in mammalian cells has been limited by poor cell uptake.

We developed a method to achieve sema3a gene knockdown in mouse metanephric organ culture using a cell-penetrating peptide–morpholino complex microinjected into the UB lumen in vitro (8). This method may also be used to deliver plasmid cDNA into the UB. This chapter describes the protocols used for peptide–morpholino-mediated knockdown and mouse UB microperfusion.

2. Materials

2.1. Organ Culture

1. Defined serum-free organ culture medium is DMEM/F12 without phenol red, supplemented with 10 mM Hepes, 5 mg/ml insulin, 5 mg/ml transferrin, 2.8 nM selenium (Gibco, #41400), 25 ng/ml PGE1 (Sigma, #P7527), 32 pg/ml T3 (Sigma, T5516), 50 U/ml penicillin, and 50 U/ml mycostatin (see Note 1).
2. Organ culture filters are Millicell-CM Biopore PTFE (Millipore).
3. Organ culture dishes and glass bottom culture dishes (MatTek Corp., #P35GC-1.5-10-C).

2.2. Morpholino Oligonucleotides and Peptide Carrier

1. Fluorescein-labeled *Sema3a* antisense morpholino (Genetools, LLC) is 5′-aggcaatcccagtgaaccagcccat-3′-carboxyfluorescein. Control morpholinos are 5 bp-mismatched morpholinos.
2. Translocator peptide ΔMPG (GALFLGFLGAAGSTMGAWS QPKSKRKV) (6).

2.3. Microperfusion System

1. Injectman NI2 micromanipulator/Femtojet semiautomated microperfusion system (Eppendorf).
2. Glass microcapillary needles (Femtotips II, Eppendorf).

2.4. Imaging

1. Phase microscope (IX81, Olympus).
2. Confocal microscope (Fluoview300, Olympus).

3. Methods

3.1. Metanephric Organ Culture

1. Kidneys are excised from E11.5 mouse embryos by microdissection (see Note 2).
2. Left and right kidneys are placed on separate organ culture filters inside glass bottom culture dishes (see Note 3).

3.2. Preparation of Peptide–Morpholino Complexes

1. Preparation of MPG solution:
   (a) Remove ΔMPG vial from freezer and leave closed at room temperature for 30 min.
   (b) Resuspend in sterile water at 1 mg/ml (0.35 M), vortex briefly.
   (c) Aliquot to avoid repeated freeze–thaw cycles. Stock solution is kept at −20 or −80°C.
2. Preparation of morpholino solutions:
   (a) Oligos are delivered as sterile, salt-free, lyophilized solid in glass vials.
   (b) Make stock solution to 1 mM in distilled water (see Note 4).
   (c) Keep stock solutions at −20°C.
3. Preparation of peptide–morpholino complexes:
   1. Mix morpholinos (1 nmol/μl) with ΔMPG peptide at 1:5–1:10 molar ratio.
   2. Incubate at 37°C for 30 min.
   3. Microinject peptide–morpholino complexes (1 nmol/μl), or add to organ culture medium to final morpholino concentration of 10 μM (see Note 5).

3.3. Ureteric Bud Injection

1. Place organ culture filter with freshly microdissected E11.5 kidney on a glass bottom culture dish with culture media.
2. Place the dish on the microinjection workstation mounted on the microscope and take picture of explant (×10) on phase.
3. Program Femtojet parameters for injection time 2–30 s, injection pressure 50–200 hPa.
4. Fill microcapillary with oligonucleotide–peptide mix in micromanipulator holder and place at 30–60° angle in desired location.
5. Program the injection level (*Z*-axis) on the Injectman, or place it on “standby” to inject manually.

6. Activate the joystick key to inject (see Note 6).
7. Take confocal picture of explant (×10) post injection to visualize fluorescein in UB lumen.

3.4. Metanephric Organ Culture

1. Place filters with injected explant in organ culture dish in incubator at 37°C, 5% CO_2.
2. Change media daily and monitor branching by phase microscopy live.
3. After 48–72 h fix explants in 10% buffered formalin for lectin or immunostaining, or harvest explants in lysis buffer for RNA or protein analysis.

4. Notes

1. The organ culture chambers should be filled with enough defined medium to bathe but not submerge the embryonic kidneys, and distilled water used to fill the outside compartment to prevent explant drying.
2. Care should be taken during microdissection of embryonic kidneys to remove the entire length of the UB intact, because if it is cut too close to the metanephros the perfusate backleaks immediately.
3. To control for variability among embryos and nontarget effects, microinject antisense morpholino–peptide complex into one UB and the corresponding mismatched morpholino–peptide complex to the contralateral one.
4. Morpholinos can be damaged by DEPC.
5. Additional controls should include ΔMPG peptide alone into one UB, and mismatched morpholino–peptide complex into the contralateral UB, as well as antisense and mismatched morpholinos alone.
6. If the injection "missed" the UB lumen, the microcapillary can be placed at different position and procedure tested again, multiple punctures may cause back-leak and poor perfusion.

References

1. Costantini F, Kopan R (2010) Patterning a complex organ: branching morphogenesis and nephron segmentation in kidney development. Dev Cell 18:698–712
2. Schedl A (2007) Renal abnormalities and their developmental origin. Nat Rev Genet 8:791–802
3. Hardy S, Legagneux V, Audic Y, Paillard L (2010) Reverse genetics in eukaryotes. Biol Cell 102:561–580
4. Xia H, Mao Q, Paulson HL, Davidson BL (2002) siRNA-mediated gene silencing in vitro and in vivo. Nat Biotechnol 20:1006–1010

5. Morris MC, Chaloin L, Heitz F, Divita G (2000) Translocating peptides and proteins and their use for gene delivery. Curr Opin Biotechnol 11:461–466
6. Simeoni F, Morris MC, Heitz F, Divita G (2003) Insight into the mechanism of the peptide-based gene delivery system MPG: implications for delivery of siRNA into mammalian cells. Nucleic Acids Res 31:2717–2724
7. Morris MC, Deshayes S, Heitz F, Divita G (2008) Cell-penetrating peptides: from molecular mechanisms to therapeutics. Biol Cell 100: 201–217
8. Tufro A, Teichman J, Woda C, Villegas G (2008) Semaphorin 3A inhibits ureteric bud branching morphogenesis in vitro. Mech Dev 125:558–568

Chapter 28

Microinjection into the Lumen of the Ureteric Tree

Cristina Cebrián

Abstract

During embryonic kidney development, the ureteric bud (UB) undergoes repetitive branching to generate the entire renal collecting system. Defects in UB branching result in renal malformations, from hypoplastic kidneys to renal agenesis. Mouse genetics has become an invaluable tool to identify gene networks regulating UB branching, and the recent use of embryonic chimeras has provided further insight into the cell-autonomous regulation of this process. However, the generation of these mouse models is often resource- and time-consuming. A simplified alternative to the generation of mouse mutants or chimeras relies on the modification of UB gene expression ex vivo. This chapter describes a simple method for microinjection into the lumen of the ureteric tree of embryonic kidney explants. The mouse embryonic kidney is cultured on an air–medium interface and a thin pulled glass needle is used to access the ureteric tree and deliver the reagent of choice. The applications of the technique are multiple: from simple labeling of the ureteric tree with fluorescent markers to overexpression or downregulation of specific genes by introducing viral vectors, siRNAs, morpholinos, or other agents.

Key words: Embryonic kidney, Ureteric tree, Ureter, Branching morphogenesis, Microinjection, Lumen, Chimeras

1. Introduction

In vertebrates, metanephric kidney development is dependent on sequential and reciprocal interactions between an outgrowth of the Wolffian duct, the UB, and the adjacent metanephric mesenchyme (MM). The UB branches and elongates responding to mesenchyme-derived signals, giving rise to the renal collecting system, while the MM is induced by the UB to epithelialize and differentiate into nephrons (1). With the progression of mouse genetics, a growing number of signaling pathways have been identified to play a key role during renal branching morphogenesis (2, 3). Receptor tyrosine kinase (RTK) activity is required for UB branching, mainly via Ret/GDNF/GFRα signaling pathway (4, 5), with minor roles

Odyssé Michos (ed.), *Kidney Development: Methods and Protocols*, Methods in Molecular Biology, vol. 886,
DOI 10.1007/978-1-61779-851-1_28, © Springer Science+Business Media, LLC 2012

assigned to other RTKs such as FGFR2, EGFR, and Met (6–8). Canonical and noncanonical Wnt signaling also regulates the branching and remodeling of the ureteric tree (9–11), as do BMP and TGFβ family members (12–14). Downstream of these pathways a myriad of targets genes are activated or up regulated, in order to coordinate the specific cell behaviors that result in epithelial branching.

A constantly growing number of mouse models are available to study kidney development, from conventional knockouts and gain of function models to inducible and/or tissue-specific gene targeting (15). Recently, the study of embryonic chimeras, in which only a subset of cells is genetically altered to knockout specific target genes, has become a powerful tool in further understanding the regulation of UB branching (16, 17). However, generation of these mouse models involves targeting of Embryonic Stem (ES) cells, injection of these ES cells into blastocysts, reimplantation into foster mice and–with the exception of the chimera experiments—interbreeding to generate pure lines (18). As an alternative, microinjection of viral particles into the ureteric tree provides a simplified model to study ex vivo the effect of overexpression or downregulation of the genes of interest in UB branching.

This chapter describes a simple protocol to microinject a reagent into the lumen of the ureteric tree. Microinjection is far from a novel technique. The oldest published records of microinjection into eukaryotic organisms date from the 1920s, when Robert Chambers devised a microinjection apparatus and used it to test the permeability of starfish eggs (19, 20). Nearly a century later, microinjection has become a routinely used approach to study the development of many model organisms, including Xenopus, zebrafish, and chick, and has revolutionized modern genetics with the generation of mutant mice. The overall idea behind microinjection has not changed much since Chambers' early experiments but, fortunately for us, the tools to perform it have improved significantly. The needles can be purchased or custom-made with a pipette puller, micromanipulators allow for subtle orientation and movement of the needle, and microinjectors generate a wide range of pressures to release the right amount of fluid.

The following protocol outlines a basic approach to microinjection into the lumen of the ureteric tree, and this same protocol can be used to microinject other branching organs, provided they have a lumen and can be cultured on a membrane. As to the reagent of choice, from visible and fluorescent markers to fluorescent beads and mRNA- or shRNA- expressing lentiviruses, what to inject into the branching organ is only limited by the researcher's needs and imagination.

2. Materials

1. Embryonic kidneys. Consider embryonic day 0.5 (E0.5) the morning on which a vaginal plug is observed.
2. Equipment:
   (a) Dissecting stereoscope.
   (b) Micropipette puller.
   (c) Inverted microscope, optional (see Note 1).
   (d) Micromanipulator.
   (e) Microinjector.
   (f) Cell culture incubator at 37°C, 5% CO_2.
3. Consumables:
   (a) Glass capillary tubing (see Note 2).
   (b) 25- and 50-μL disposable micropipettes with wire plunger.
   (c) 3.5-cm tissue culture plates.
   (d) Low profile filter membranes.
   (e) 0.4 μm pore size polyester membrane inserts.
4. Reagents:
   (a) 1× Phosphate-Buffered Saline (PBS), sterile.
   (b) Kidney culture media: Dulbecco's Modified Eagle's Medium (DMEM), High Glucose with HEPES (25 mM), supplemented with Fetal Bovine Serum (10%), Sodium Pyruvate (1 mM), L-glutamine (2 mM), and Penicillin/Streptomycin (50 u/mL).
   (c) Reagent of choice to be injected into the ureteric tree (see Note 3).

3. Methods

Isolate the kidney rudiments from E11.5 to E13.5 embryos in sterile 1× PBS (see Note 4).

3.1. Plating of the Kidney Explants

1. Add 1 mL of prewarmed kidney culture medium to a 3.5-cm plate and place a low profile filter insert inside the plate. Do not add the medium on top of the filter as prewetting the filter's surface may compromise tissue adhesion.
2. Label the plastic edge of the filter with permanent marker indicating the position of the first specimen as a reference.

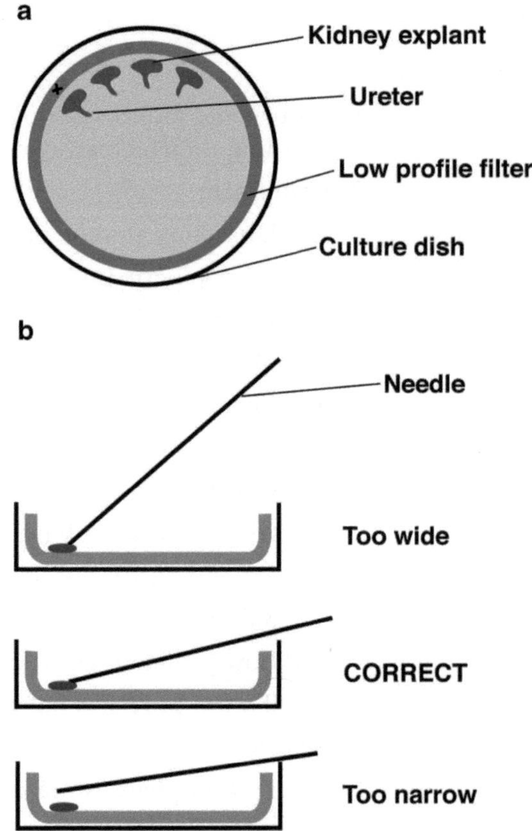

Fig. 1. Diagram of the culture plate. (**a**) *From above*. Positioning of the explants in the periphery of the filter with the ureters facing the inside of the plate. (**b**) *Lateral view* during injection. The needle should be positioned at the right angle.

3. Transfer the isolated kidney rudiments to the filter, one kidney at a time, using a 25–50-μL Wiretrol plunger and pipette. Position the explants on the filter following the circular pattern described in Fig. 1a. This distribution will allow the injection to take place at a narrower angle. Very carefully, orient the kidneys so the ureter faces the inside of the circumference (see Fig. 1a and Note 5).
4. Transfer the kidneys to an incubator at 37 C and 5% CO_2 for at least 1 h (see Note 6).

3.2. Needle Preparation

1. Using an automatic pipette puller, pull a few more needles than you will need for the experiment. It is always advisable to have an excess of microinjection needles so that if one breaks or gets clogged, it can be quickly replaced.
2. The conditions for needle pulling will change depending on the characteristics of the glass tubing used and the fluid to inject, and will need to be adjusted accordingly. If a pipette

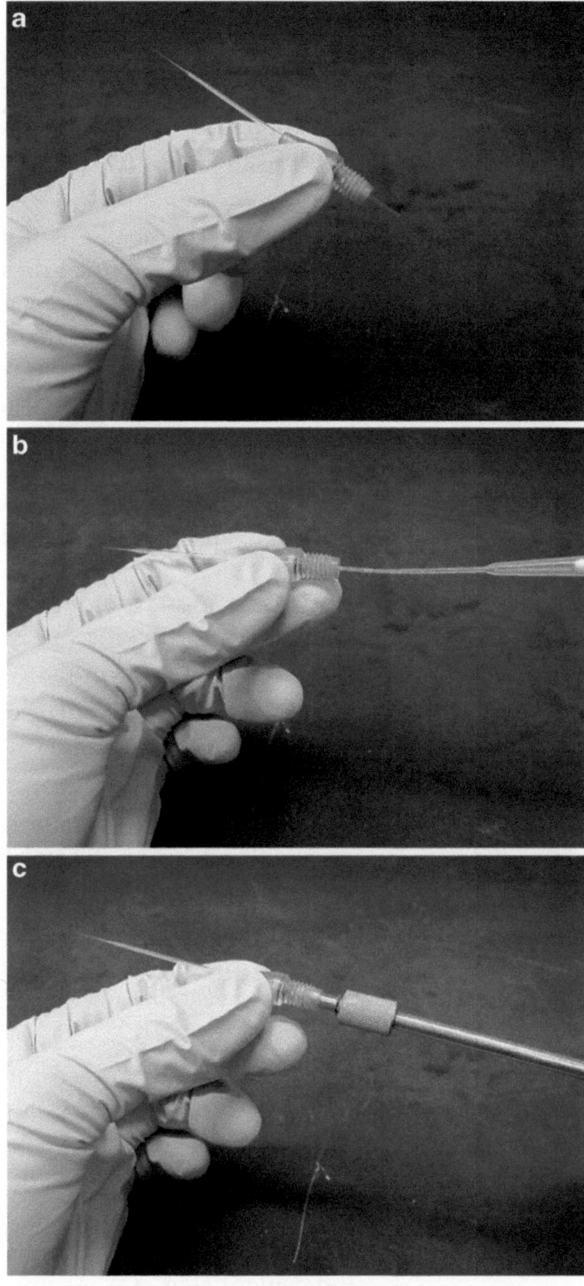

Fig. 2. Preassembling (**a**) loading (**b**) and assembling (**c**) of the needle.

puller is not available, micropipettes can be purchased from commercial sources. The goal is to obtain a needle tip with an inner diameter between 0.5 and 1.5 μm (see Note 7).

3. Assemble the needle in the microinjector grip head as shown in Fig. 2a. Skip this step if using commercial micropipettes that do not use a grip head but are directly screwed into the capillary holder.

4. Back-fill the needle from the rear (wide end) with the desired reagent using a fine tip plastic pipette (Fig. 2b and see Note 8). 2 μL is enough for up to 20 injections.
5. Assemble the needle by screwing the grip head in the capillary holder and mount the holder on the micromanipulator (Fig. 2c).
6. Check that the needle is not blocked by performing a high-pressure release. A small drop of fluid should be released and migrate up the needle, indicating that the needle is not blocked and that it has the right diameter. If there is no release of fluid or if the drop appears but is reabsorbed back in the needle, this indicates that the tip is either blocked or too narrow. If so, disassemble the needle and under the dissecting scope use fine forceps to snap off a very small piece of the tip. If the drop is too big, this indicates that the opening at the tip of the needle is too big and that the needle should be replaced.

3.3. Microinjection into the Ureter

1. Position the plate containing the kidney explants on the stereoscope or microscope stage and confirm that the epithelium of the ureter is evident.
2. Using the micromanipulator, adjust the angle of the injection; aim for the narrower angle allowed without hitting the edge of the plate (Fig. 1b).
3. Position the tip of the needle on top of the kidney to be injected and lower the needle until it is visible through the microscope.
4. Keeping the epithelium of the ureter in focus, lower the needle to sit to the side of the ureter—not on top of it, but close. Slowly lower the needle until it touches the mesenchyme around the ureter.
5. Move the needle toward the ureter. The needle should push the epithelium first and eventually penetrate it (see Note 9 and Fig. 3a, b).
6. Once the needle tip is inside the ureter, use the microinjector to release a small volume. A distinctive change in contrast should be observed, with the lumen of the epithelium becoming evident (Fig. 3c). At this point, the pressure for the microinjector can be increased to release a larger volume at once. Alternatively, injecting pressure can be kept constant while performing multiple releases. At the end of a successful injection, the lumen of the entire collecting tree should be evident (Fig. 3d).
7. Raise the needle and turn the plate to inject the next kidney. Keep record of the direction (clockwise or counterclockwise) and the outcome of each injection.

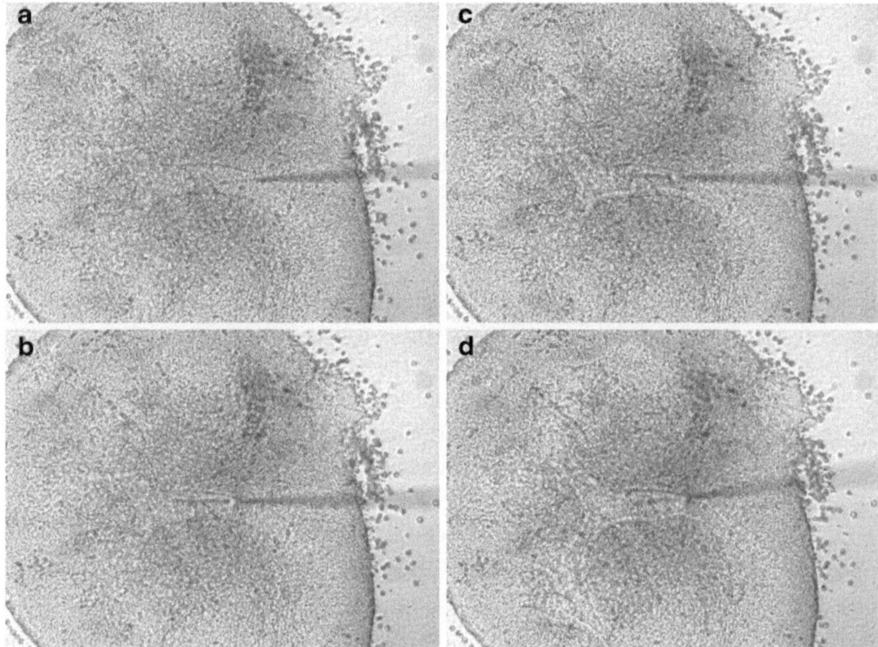

Fig. 3. A successful microinjection into the ureteric tree. (**a**) The ureter epithelium should oppose some resistance to penetration. (**b**) The needle has penetrated the ureter. (**c**) The release of a small volume generates a change in contrast in the lumen. (**d**) Upon completion most of the ureteric tree should have a filled lumen.

3.4. Culture and Imaging of the Injected Kidneys

1. When all the kidneys are injected transfer them to a polyester membrane filter using a disposable pipette with wire plunger. The kidneys should detach easily just by adding some medium on top of the tissue.
2. There is no need to keep a circular pattern, just make sure that the kidneys are well spaced so that they will not overlap during culture.
3. Culture the kidneys at 37°C, 5% CO_2, either in a conventional incubator or—for live imaging—in the culture chamber of a photomicroscope.
4. Image the kidneys at given intervals for as long as 5–7 days after injection.
5. These cultures are suitable for in situ hybridization, LacZ staining or immunolabeling if needed.

4. Notes

1. Traditionally, micromanipulators are set up on an inverted microscope, often on an antivibration table. While this is the standard procedure for blastocyst injection, explant microinjection can be performed on a standard stereoscope without further stabilization.

2. We use thin-wall glass capillary tubing made of borosilicate, with an internal filament to facilitate back filling. Outside diameter is 1.0 μm and inside diameter is 0.78 μm.

3. Keep in mind that the total volume injected per kidney explant will between approximately 0.2 and 2 nL. Therefore, your reagent of choice should be concentrated enough to exert an effect within these low volume ranges.

4. Best results are obtained with embryos between E11.5 and E13.5. We have been able to microinject Wolffian ducts from E10.5 embryos but, at those stages, the optical contrast between the WD and the surrounding mesenchyme is often poor. The optimal embryonic stages for microinjection are after E11.5, when the UB has already branched and the ureter has begun to differentiate so the contrast between the epithelia and the mesenchyme is excellent. At the other end of the spectrum, explants from embryos older than E13.5 are usually too large and their branching pattern is less informative.

5. Fine-tipped plastic pipettes (give an example of the manufacturer and catalog number) are ideal for orienting the kidney rudiments, small enough to manipulate the tissue and soft enough to avoid damaging the membrane.

6. The kidneys should be allowed to sit and flatten a bit on the membrane before injection. This will prevent the tissue from sliding on the membrane during the injection and it may increase the contrast between the ureter and the mesenchyme. If needed, this incubation period can be extended; the injection can be performed 1–2 days after starting the kidney culture.

7. Obtaining the right size needle is an empirical process; the goal, to generate a tip that will be fine enough to penetrate the ureter (instead of just pushing it) and, at the same time, wide enough to release the appropriate amount of fluid. A tip too fine can always be snapped to a bigger size; alternatively, settings on the needle puller can be adjusted to vary the size of the opening.

8. Exercise caution and follow the appropriate safety guidelines when the agent to be injected is toxic or biohazardous. Discard all waste appropriately and disinfect the needle holder with 70% Ethanol and/or diluted bleach between uses.

9. If the epithelium remains undisturbed when the needle is moved, it is likely that the needle is not at the level of the epithelium, but above or below it. Raise the needle until it no longer touches the tissue and start again. If the needle pushes the ureter but cannot penetrate, this suggests that the needle tip is too big. Replace the needle and start again. If the kidney sticks to the needle, it is because the tissue is slightly dry; add a drop of medium on top of each kidney and start again.

References

1. Saxén L (1987) Organogenesis of the kidney. Cambridge University Press, Cambridge (Cambridgeshire), NY
2. Bouchard M (2004) Transcriptional control of kidney development. Differentiation 72: 295–306
3. Bridgewater D, Rosenblum ND (2009) Stimulatory and inhibitory signaling molecules that regulate renal branching morphogenesis. Pediatr Nephrol 24:1611–1619
4. Costantini F, Shakya R (2006) GDNF/Ret signaling and the development of the kidney. Bioessays 28:117–127
5. Song R, El-Dahr SS, Yosypiv IV (2011) Receptor tyrosine kinases in kidney development. J Signal Transduct 869281
6. Bates CM (2011) Role of fibroblast growth factor receptor signaling in kidney development. Am J Physiol Renal Physiol 301: F245–F251
7. Ishibe S, Karihaloo A, Ma H et al (2009) Met and the epidermal growth factor receptor act cooperatively to regulate final nephron number and maintain collecting duct morphology. Development 136:337–345
8. Zhang Z, Pascuet E, Hueber PA et al (2010) Targeted inactivation of EGF receptor inhibits renal collecting duct development and function. J Am Soc Nephrol 21: 573–578
9. Bridgewater D, Cox B, Cain J et al (2008) Canonical WNT/beta-catenin signaling is required for ureteric branching. Dev Biol 317:83–94
10. Iglesias DM, Hueber PA, Chu L et al (2007) Canonical WNT signaling during kidney development. Am J Physiol Renal Physiol 293: F494–F500
11. Karner CM, Chirumamilla R, Aoki S et al (2009) Wnt9b signaling regulates planar cell polarity and kidney tubule morphogenesis. Nat Genet 41:793–799
12. Bush KT, Sakurai H, Steer DL et al (2004) TGF-beta superfamily members modulate growth, branching, shaping, and patterning of the ureteric bud. Dev Biol 266:285–298
13. Cain JE, Bertram JF (2006) Ureteric branching morphogenesis in BMP4 heterozygous mutant mice. J Anat 209:745–755
14. Oxburgh L, Chu GC, Michael SK, Robertson EJ (2004) TGFbeta superfamily signals are required for morphogenesis of the kidney mesenchyme progenitor population. Development 131:4593–4605
15. Ly JP, Onay T, Quaggin SE (2011) Mouse models to study kidney development, function and disease. Curr Opin Nephrol Hypertens 20:382–390
16. Chi X, Michos O, Shakya R et al (2009) Ret-dependent cell rearrangements in the Wolffian duct epithelium initiate ureteric bud morphogenesis. Dev Cell 17:199–209
17. Kuure S, Chi X, Lu B, Costantini F (2010) The transcription factors Etv4 and Etv5 mediate formation of the ureteric bud tip domain during kidney development. Development 137: 1975–1979
18. Hogan B, Costantini F, Lacy E (1986) Manipulating the mouse embryo: a laboratory manual. Cold Spring Harbor Laboratory, Cold Spring Harbor, NY
19. Chambers R (1921) A simple micro-injection apparatus made of steel. Science 54:552–553
20. Chambers R (1922) A micro injection study on the permeability of the starfish egg. J Gen Physiol 5:189–193

Chapter 29

Renal Delivery of Adenovirus and Antisense Oligonucleotides in Rats by Retrograde Renal Vein Injection

Guadalupe Ortiz-Muñoz, Beñat Mallavia, Oscar Lopez-Franco, Purificacion Hernandez-Vargas, Jesus Egido, and Carmen Gomez-Guerrero

Abstract

Renal gene therapy may offer new strategies to treat diseases of native and transplanted kidneys. Several experimental techniques have been developed using viral, nonviral, and cellular vectors, although the effectiveness of such techniques varies widely depending upon the vector used, type of injection, species, and experimental model of renal disease. Here, we describe an optimized technique for renal delivery of DNA in rodents by retrograde renal vein injection as it is currently applied in our laboratory for adenovirus and nonviral vectors. This is an effective gene transfer method with lasting effect on gene expression in the kidney that modulates renal disease in rodents without any apparent harmful effect, thus having a potential therapeutic value for future clinical applications.

Key words: Adenovirus, Antisense oligonucleotides, Kidney, Rat, Retrograde, Renal vein, Injection, DNA delivery

1. Introduction

Kidney-targeted gene therapy has been a realistic purpose, although the only clinical trials against renal disease have focused on renal cancer. At the experimental level, increasing evidence demonstrates that gene therapy is a powerful strategy targeting renal disease in rodents, both in native and transplanted kidneys (1).

Adenovirus is one of the most efficient viral vectors for in vivo transfection. Adenoviral and adeno-associated vectors have a number of advantages as gene delivery agents, including high titers, ability to transduce efficiently nondividing and dividing cells, and relative stable expression. However, major drawbacks still remain,

Odyssé Michos (ed.), *Kidney Development: Methods and Protocols*, Methods in Molecular Biology, vol. 886, DOI 10.1007/978-1-61779-851-1_29, © Springer Science+Business Media, LLC 2012

such as immunogenicity after repeated injection, nonspecific inflammatory responses due to the viral particle (adenovirus) and difficulty of construction (adeno-associated), that limit the widespread development for clinical application (2).

Nonviral vectors are an attractive alternative to adenovirus that continues to be of interest because of their safety and low immunogenicity. Several reports described different formulations of cationic lipids and polymers as good vehicles for delivery in vivo of plasmid DNA, siRNA and antisense oligonucleotides (ODN) (3). These lipid- and polymer-based vectors can associate with DNA and form complexes (which are termed lipoplexes and polyplexes, respectively), therefore avoiding the lysosomal degradation of DNA, thus increasing DNA stability and transfection efficiency without proinflammatory effects (4, 5). The effectiveness of these nonviral vectors has been demonstrated in different animal models after intracerebral injection, kidney perfusion, lung instillation, or systemic delivery (6–10).

The kidney is a well-differentiated organ with specialized compartments composed of glomeruli, tubules, interstitium, and vasculature. Different methods for gene transfer have been experimentally described to target specific renal structures (1, 11), and the variable effectiveness of such techniques has been reported in different animal models of renal disease (12–16).

In this protocol, we describe the process for gene transfer into the kidney of rats by retrograde renal vein injection, as we have previously used for successful transfer of DNA and antisense ODN into glomerular and tubular cells in vivo. We applied this technique for evaluating in vivo the biological activity of suppressors of cytokine signaling (SOCS) family in different animal models. Adenovirus was selected as gene delivery vector for overexpressing specific SOCS1 and SOCS3 genes (17), while antisense ODN complexed with the cationic polymer polyethylenimine (PEI) was used to inhibit individual SOCS gene expression (18, 19). In fact, renal delivery of SOCS expressing adenovirus into diabetic rats decreased renal injury and improved renal function (17). Furthermore, antisense ODN targeting SOCS3 effectively inhibited renal SOCS expression and exacerbated renal damage in rats induced by angiotensin II infusion (18).

2. Materials

2.1. Adenovirus Purification and Titration

1. Our recombinant adenoviruses are driven by the cytomegalovirus promoter and contain different expression genes (17): green fluorescence protein (Ad-GFP), SOCS1 (Ad-S1), and SOCS3 (Ad-S3). Empty adenovirus encoding no transgene (Ad-null) is used as negative control.

2. Human embryonic kidney 293 cells (HEK293, ATCC # CRL-1573) are cultured in DMEM medium supplemented with 10% fetal calf serum (FCS), 100 U/mL penicillin, 100 μg/mL streptomycin, and 1 mM sodium pyruvate (complete culture medium).
3. Cell culture flasks (150 cm^2), 24-multiwell plates, and plastic pipettes.
4. Cell lysis reagent (1,1,2-Trichlorotrifluoroethane, Sigma Chemical) and kits for adenovirus isolation (AdEasy Virus Purification Kit, Agilent Biotech) and titration (Adeno-X Rapid Titer Kit, BD Biosciences Clontech-Takara).

2.2. Reagents for Antisense Oligonucleotides Transfection

1. Antisense ODN and the respective controls (sense and scramble) are synthesized and purified (Metabion; Marinsried, Germany). For initial experiments, it is recommended to synthesize fluorescence labeled ODN to test transfection efficiency and tissue distribution. ODN are resuspended in sterile water to obtain 10 μg/μL stock solutions. Aliquots are stable for several months when stored a −20°C.
2. Cationic polymer transfection reagent: Linear polyethylenimine (PEI) reagent 150 mM in sterile apyrogenic water (in vivo jetPEI, Qbiogene, Montreal, Canada) is stable for 1 year at −20°C. Let the PEI solution thaw to room temperature before use. This transfection reagent increases the stability of unmodified ODN in plasma (see Note 1), enhances their uptake, and protects against nuclease degradation (4, 5).
3. Glucose 5% (w/v) solution in sterile water and stored at 4°C.

2.3. Materials for Surgical Procedure

All the following materials should be sterile.

1. Solutions: isotonic saline solution (0.9%), anesthetics (ketamine, xylazine, isoflurane), and antiseptics (chlorhexidine and 70% Ethanol).
2. Surgical instruments: microdissecting forceps (curved and straight), scissors, scissor-handle forceps, and scalpel.
3. Others: intravenous catheters (Abbocath 24-gauge × 19 mm cannula; Venisystems), 24-gauge needles and 1-mL syringes, suture (absorbable and nonabsorbable), surgical sheets, gloves, adhesive tape, gauzes, and masks.

3. Methods

The present protocol illustrates the surgical procedure for an animal survival surgery and the following steps should be taken to insure a safe and successful technique. We describe a method of gene transfer (using adenoviral and nonviral vectors) on 250–300 g rats by retrograde injection into the renal vein; nevertheless, it could be necessary to introduce some modifications in terms of volume injections to apply to animals of different body weights according to their kidney size.

3.1. Adenovirus Preparation

3.1.1. Biosafety

Adenoviruses are pathogens that can cause respiratory infection, gastroenteritis, and conjunctivitis, and must be treated with respect and considered as a biohazard agent. Manipulations should be conducted in a Biosafety Level 2 laboratory. The requirements include the use of laminar flow hoods, especially when concentrated viruses are used, the establishment of proper procedures for decontamination and disposal of liquid and solid waste, and the disinfection (Virkon 1% solution) of contaminated surfaces and equipment after each use. Separate biosafety cabinets and incubators should be used for infected and noninfected cell cultures, if possible. Common sense precautions should be observed at all times.

3.1.2. Adenovirus Propagation

The deletion or inactivation of early genes E1A and E1B is a common characteristic among adenoviral vectors. Activation of these genes is necessary and essential for viral replication. E1A and E1B functions must be provided by the HEK 293 cells in order to propagate adenoviral vectors.

1. Prepare a HEK 293 monolayer cell culture seeding up to $3–4 \times 10^6$ viable cells into a 150-cm^2 tissue culture flasks containing 25 mL of complete culture medium.
2. Wait until 90–100% confluent monolayer cell at the time of infection. Usually, 25–30 tissue culture flasks ($\sim 15 \times 10^6$ cells/flask) are enough to have a high adenovirus titer.
3. Remove the medium from each flask and replace it with 30 mL of complete culture medium containing adenovirus, at a final multiplicity of infection (MOI) of 2–5 ifu/cell (see Note 2).
4. Usually within 5–7 days post-infection, virus-induced cytopathic effects will be apparent under the microscope. Most of infected cells will rounded up and about half of the cells will be detached or can be removed by a mild tap of the flask. Harvest adenovirus pooling the cell suspensions using a pipette and transfer the cells to 50-mL sterile conical centrifuge tubes and centrifuge $250 \times g$ for 10 min.
5. Remove supernatants, resuspend all the precipitates in 5–10 mL fresh medium and collect up to a single tube.
6. Add one equivalent volume (5–10 mL) of sterile cell lysis reagent (1,1,2-trichlorotrifluoroethane) to the cell suspension and mix briefly.
7. Centrifuge $690 \times g$ for 15 min to pellet the debris. Collect the upper phase (red color) and store at −80°C until purification.

3.1.3. Adenovirus Isolation

1. In the biosafety hood, thaw adenovirus stock (5–10 mL) on ice. Add benzoase nuclease (1 μL/mL, provided in the purification kit) to remove contaminating DNA and incubate at 37°C for 30 min.
2. Filter the solution through a 0.45-μm filter connected to a syringe. Mix the filtered solution with 10× loading buffer slowly while agitating to achieve a final 1× buffer concentration.
3. Prepare the Sartobind filter provided by flushing 10 mL sterile PBS through a sterile syringe and maintain it constantly hydrated.
4. Pass sample solution with adenovirus, very slowly through the Sartobind filter (optimal rate is 10 mL/min). Wash the filter with the same volume of washing buffer, avoiding air bubbles during the process (see Note 3).
5. Add 5 mL elution buffer, fill the filter containing bound adenovirus, and incubate for 5 min at room temperature. Then pass drop-by-drop the remaining buffer through the filter (optimal rate of 10 mL/min) and collect the eluted adenovirus in a sterile tube. Aliquot in small volumes in order to avoid any unnecessary freezing and thawing, and store the adenovirus stock at –80°C until use (see Note 4).

3.1.4. Adenovirus Titration

This method for virus titration uses specific monoclonal antibody directed against the adenoviral hexon protein and detection with anti-mouse secondary antibody linked to horseradish peroxidase, using a commercial kit.

1. Seed HEK 293 cells in a 24-multiwell plate ($5–10 \times 10^5$ cell/well) and incubate overnight in complete culture medium to reach 80–90% confluency.
2. Prepare serial tenfold dilutions of adenovirus stock. Typically, a range of 10^{-2} to 10^{-8} is recommended. Add 200 μL of the serially diluted adenovirus dropwise to each duplicate well of the 24-multiwell plate. After 1 h incubation at 37°C, remove adenovirus, replace fresh medium and incubate for additional 48–72 h (until evidence of morphological cell changes).
3. Aspirate the medium from each well and allow cells to dry for 5 min. Fix cells with 1 mL ice-cold methanol for 10 min at –20°C.
4. Wash cells and incubate with anti-hexon antibody (1/1,000 dilution in PBS-1% BSA) at 37°C for 1 h. Then aspirate primary antibody, gently rinse wells and incubate with secondary antibody (1/500 dilution in PBS-1% BSA). After 1 h at 37°C, remove secondary antibody, wash the cells with PBS and develop reaction product with DAB solution.
5. Count ten fields of brown cells using a microscope (20× objective) and calculate the mean number of positive cells per well.

Select wells with optimal count 5–50 positive cells/field and discard those with higher titers. Calculate infectious adenovirus units (ifu) as follows:

$$\text{ifu/mL} = \frac{\text{mean positive cell number} \times 255}{\text{volume virus(mL)} \times \text{dilution factor}},$$

where 255 is the number of ×20 fields per well in a 24-multiwell plate.

The adenovirus can now be used for in vivo gene transfer experiments. We typically use a dose of $1\text{–}5 \times 10^9$ ifu/rat (diluted in 200 μL sterile PBS) for retrograde kidney injection.

3.2. Preparation of PEI/ODN Complexes

The following protocol is given for iv injection of 200 μg of antisense ODN (25-mer) complexed with PEI 150 mM at N/P = 5 (see Note 5).

1. Dilute 20 μL of ODN (200 μg) into 200 μL of 5% glucose in a 1.5-mL microtube. Mix well and spin down briefly.
2. Dilute 20 μL of PEI reagent into 200 μL of 5% glucose in a 1.5-mL microtube. Mix well and spin down briefly.
3. Add at once the PEI solution to the ODN solution (important: do not reverse the order of addition). Mix well the solution immediately and spin down briefly. Incubate PEI/ODN complexes at room temperature for 15 min before injection into the animals.

3.3. Injection of Adenovirus or PEI/ODN Complexes into the Renal Vein

3.3.1. Preparing Animal for Surgery

All protocols using live animals must be approved by an Institutional animal care and must follow officially approved procedures for the care and use of laboratory animals. Furthermore, experimental animals treated with adenovirus should be handled and disposed using recommended animal biosafety levels.

1. Anesthetize rats with a 1:2 proportion of xylazine and ketamine (see Note 6). Prepare a fresh solution by combining 1 mL of 20 mg/mL xylazine and 2 mL of 50 mg/mL ketamine, and dose at 0.1 mL/100 g of body weight.
2. Carefully shave the abdomen or any areas required using electric clippers, remove excess of hair and cleanse this area with chlorhexidine solution and 70% Ethanol.
3. Place the rat supine on a clean surgical area on a homeothermic table to maintain constant body temperature during surgery and fix the animal with tape strips.
4. Drape the animal with a sterile surgical sheet with an access hole to the abdomen.

3.3.2. Performing Aseptic Surgery

1. Using surgical scissors or scalpel, perform 3–4 cm incision in the medial section of the abdomen and access to the left kidney.
2. In order to expose a good view of the left renal vein, move the organs covering them with prewarmed saline solution.
3. Remove fat around the renal vein and spread muscles bluntly and pull aside, until see a full vein length. This step often caused bleeding issues by tearing of the vein and needed to be performed carefully.
4. Elevate the vein with a curved microdissecting forceps and insert a couple of sterile thread sutures (3-0) underneath the vein in such a way that it straddled the vein and keep it exposed.
5. Place the thread sutures distally 0.3 cm between each other. Raising both sutures upward allow you to clamp the vein and provide a good exposure. The puncture is made between the two threads with the sharp tip of a 24-gauge intravenous catheter. Immediately prior to injection, you should relax the suture nearest to the kidney.
6. Extract the inner needle of the catheter and connect the outer catheter to a 1 mL syringe containing 200 μL saline solution to perfuse the kidney. Then inject the DNA preparation (adenovirus or PEI/ODN complexes) slow but steady. Injection volume should not exceed 500 μL.
7. Raise the two sutures in order to clamp the vein and remove the catheter. Incubate the solution less than 7 min to avoid ischemic effects.
8. Release the sutures and be sure that the flow is restored and kidney become to its natural color (see Note 7).
9. Carefully remove the threads and suture the abdominal incision using absorbable material for inner layers and nonabsorbable material for the skin. Evaluate incisions every 2–3 days until healing. Survival is usually greater than 95%.

Monitor biological effects after the desired time period in kidneys extracted from anesthetized animals. The retroinjection is able to increase gene transfer to the targeted kidney, and modulation of target gene is stable for at least 4 weeks after renal delivery without apparent histological abnormalities.

In general, transduction efficiency is determined by quantitative PCR, Western blot and immunohistochemistry in renal tissue. Noninfused right kidney can be used as negative control to compare with the left transfected kidney. However, a minor collateral transgene expression in right kidney and other distant organs should also be expected.

Renal specific expression of target transgene in rats injected with recombinant adenovirus (Ad-S1/S3 in our case) should be assayed in comparison with rats injected with empty adenovirus encoding no transgene (Ad-null). Additionally, injection of adenovirus containing a reporter gene (Ad-GFP) is recommended in preliminary studies to confirm transgene expression and analyze distribution in renal structures by immunofluorescence microscopy. In our experiments, GFP expression was observed in more than 70% of total glomeruli and most tubular cells after 7 days of transfection.

For in vivo antisense therapy, the use of FITC-conjugated ODN is advisable in the initial experiments to validate the gene transfer method and to assess the kinetics of PEI/ODN complexes distribution (see Note 8) in the transfected kidney by immunofluorescence microscopy. Furthermore, additional groups of study should also be included: sense ODN (do not inhibit gene transcription), scramble ODN (unspecific), and transfection vehicle (PEI in 5% glucose).

4. Notes

1. The jetPEI solution is able to interact with anionic ODN but not with uncharged ODN such as methylphosphonate or phosphorothioate ODN.
2. Multiplicity of infection (MOI) is the ratio of infectious adenovirus units (ifu) to cells. Optimal ratio ranges from 3 to 10, with a minimum of 1 ifu/cell. The optimal MOI for adenovirus propagation is also linked to the time after infection that is best for virus harvest.
3. Air trapped in the Sartobind filter unit may reduce viral titer.
4. The virus infectivity can decrease by 10 times per cycle of freezing and thawing.
5. The N/P ratio (N, moles of nitrogen residues in PEI; P, moles of phosphate groups in DNA) indicates the ionic balance of the PEI/ODN complexes. Commercial PEI contains 150 mM monomer nitrogen, while 1 μg DNA contains 3 nmoles of anionic phosphate. N/P ratio ranges from 4 to 10. The optimal N/P ratio in the range from 4 to 10 should be determined for each application. In our lab, N/P = 5 gave the best transfection results.
6. General anesthesia induction in a chamber containing a 5% isoflurane/oxygen mixture can be an alternative approach.
7. Hemostasis is usually seen at the injected site after applying pressure for 5–10 s.
8. For low transfection level of antisense ODN, it is suggested to optimize either the ODN amount (maximal 400 μg) or the PEI/ODN ratio.

Acknowledgments

The authors have been granted by Spanish Ministry of Science (SAF2005/05857, SAF2007/63648, and SAF2009/11794), Ministry of Health (Instituto de Salud Carlos III, Red RECAVA RD06/0014/0035) and Comunidad de Madrid (S2006/GEN-0247).

References

1. Isaka Y (2006) Gene therapy targeting kidney diseases: routes and vehicles. Clin Exp Nephrol 10:229–235
2. Appledorn DM, Seregin S, Amalfitano A (2008) Adenovirus vectors for renal-targeted gene delivery. Contrib Nephrol 159:47–62
3. Lien YH, Lai LW (2003) Renal gene transfer: nonviral approaches. Mol Biotechnol 24: 283–294
4. Akinc A, Thomas M, Klibanov AM, Langer R (2005) Exploring polyethylenimine-mediated DNA transfection and the proton sponge hypothesis. J Gene Med 7:657–663
5. Bonnet ME, Erbacher P, Bolcato-Bellemin AL (2008) Systemic delivery of DNA or siRNA mediated by linear polyethylenimine (L-PEI) does not induce an inflammatory response. Pharm Res 25:2972–2982
6. Zou SM, Erbacher P, Remy JS, Behr JP (2000) Systemic linear polyethylenimine (L-PEI)-mediated gene delivery in the mouse. J Gene Med 2:128–134
7. Boletta A, Benigni A, Lutz J et al (1997) Nonviral gene delivery to the rat kidney with polyethylenimine. Hum Gene Ther 8:1243–1251
8. Ferrari S, Moro E, Pettenazzo A et al (1997) ExGen 500 is an efficient vector for gene delivery to lung epithelial cells in vitro and in vivo. Gene Ther 4:1100–1106
9. Boussif O, Lezoualc'h F, Zanta MA et al (1995) A versatile vector for gene and oligonucleotide transfer into cells in culture and in vivo: polyethylenimine. Proc Natl Acad Sci USA 92: 7297–7301
10. Wang S, Ma N, Gao SJ, Yu H, Leong KW (2001) Transgene expression in the brain stem effected by intramuscular injection of polyethylenimine/DNA complexes. Mol Ther 3:658–664
11. van der Wouden EA, Sandovici M, Henning RH, de Zeeuw D, Deelman LE (2004) Approaches and methods in gene therapy for kidney disease. J Pharmacol Toxicol Methods 50:13–24
12. Fujishiro J, Takeda S, Takeno Y et al (2005) Gene transfer to the rat kidney in vivo and ex vivo using an adenovirus vector: factors influencing transgene expression. Nephrol Dial Transplant 20:1385–1391
13. Bledsoe G, Shen B, Yao Y et al (2006) Reversal of renal fibrosis, inflammation, and glomerular hypertrophy by kallikrein gene delivery. Hum Gene Ther 17:545–555
14. Gong N, Dong C, Chen Z et al (2006) Adenovirus-mediated antisense-ERK2 gene therapy attenuates chronic allograft nephropathy. Transplant Proc 38:3228–3230
15. Sandovici M, Henning RH, van Goor H et al (2008) Systemic gene therapy with interleukin-13 attenuates renal ischemia-reperfusion injury. Kidney Int 73:1364–1373
16. Zhang Z, Wu F, Zheng F, Li H (2010) Adenovirus-mediated decorin gene transfection has therapeutic effects in a streptozocin-induced diabetic rat model. Nephron Exp Nephrol 116:e11–e21
17. Ortiz-Muñoz G, Lopez-Parra V, Lopez-Franco O et al (2010) Suppressors of cytokine signaling abrogate diabetic nephropathy. J Am Soc Nephrol 21:763–772
18. Hernández-Vargas P, López-Franco O, Sanjuán G et al (2005) Suppressors of cytokine signaling regulate angiotensin II-activated Janus kinase-signal transducers and activators of transcription pathway in renal cells. J Am Soc Nephrol 16:1673–1683
19. Ortiz-Muñoz G, Martin-Ventura JL, Hernandez-Vargas P et al (2009) Suppressors of cytokine signaling modulate JAK/STAT-mediated cell responses during atherosclerosis. Arterioscler Thromb Vasc Biol 29:525–531

Part VI

Analyzing Functional Defects of the Kidney and Urinary Tract

Chapter 30

Estimating Total Nephron Number in the Adult Kidney Using the Physical Disector/Fractionator Combination

Luise A. Cullen-McEwen, Rebecca N. Douglas-Denton, and John F. Bertram

Abstract

Nephron number has emerged as a useful parameter for assessing the roles of specific genes and feto-maternal environmental factors in kidney development. Nephron number is also of clinical interest due to increasing evidence suggesting that low nephron number is associated with increased risk for developing chronic adult disease, including cardiovascular and renal disease. The physical disector/fractionator combination is considered the gold standard method for estimating total nephron number in kidneys. Here we describe the use of this method to estimate total nephron number in mouse and rat kidneys, and variations to the method required to estimate nephron number in larger species, including human.

Key words: Nephron number, Glomerulus, Unbiased stereology, Disector

1. Introduction

The full complement of nephrons in the mammalian permanent kidney (metanephros) is reached at the end of nephrogenesis, approximately 36 weeks gestation in humans and postnatal day 5–10 in rodents. There is increasing evidence that the feto-maternal environment as well as numerous genes regulate kidney development, including nephrogenesis, and so it is perhaps no surprise that total nephron (glomerular) number (N_{glom}) in humans varies widely. Indeed, estimates of N_{glom} range from several hundred thousand to more than two million per kidney (1, 2). In humans, nephron number is directly correlated with birth weight (3), varies between races (4), is lower in females (5), decreases with age (5–8), and is inversely correlated with mean glomerular volume (V_{glom}) (2, 6).

Odyssé Michos (ed.), *Kidney Development: Methods and Protocols*, Methods in Molecular Biology, vol. 886, DOI 10.1007/978-1-61779-851-1_30, © Springer Science+Business Media, LLC 2012

While N_{glom} in specific animal species varies over a much narrower range than that seen in humans, again perturbations to the feto-maternal environment (9–11) as well as gene mutations (12–14) can alter N_{glom}.

While N_{glom} estimates provide an objective index of the efficiency of kidney development and nephrogenesis, this parameter is also of interest because of reports associating low N_{glom} with elevated blood pressure and reduced renal function. Most of this evidence has come from animal studies (1, 15), although the relatively few human studies tend to support these hypotheses (4–7, 16–20). Thus, if nephrogenesis is suboptimal for any reason, the resulting permanent nephron deficit may influence adult kidney structure and function, contributing to the development of adult disease.

The gold standard method of estimating N_{glom} involves the use of the disector principle (21) to sample glomeruli. These sampled glomeruli are then counted (N_{glom}) in order to estimate the total numbers of nephrons. Importantly, the disector samples three-dimensional particles (such as glomeruli) in three-dimensional space (the cortex or kidney) with equal probability. In other words, all glomeruli have the same chance of being sampled, and subsequently counted. There is no assumption of size, size variability, shape, or location of the glomeruli in the kidney making the disector principle unbiased because all glomeruli (nephrons) have an identical chance of being sampled and counted. This is important given the increasing evidence of wide variation of glomerular volume both within and between kidneys (22, 23), and the role of glomerular hypertrophy in many disease settings (4, 17, 24–35). The most common design-based method for estimating N_{glom} is the physical disector/fractionator combination, in which physical disectors are used to count glomeruli in a known fraction of the kidney. This sampling fraction is obtained through a series of sub-sampling steps. Firstly, slicing devices are often used to obtain macroscopic kidney slices, and a known fraction of these slices (usually 1 in 2 or 3) are embedded and exhaustively serially sectioned. During sectioning, a known fraction of the sections is collected and mounted on glass slides. Then, a known fraction of the area of these sections is used for glomerular counting. Finally, simple algebra is used to estimate the number of glomeruli in the whole kidney. When combined with stereological point counting on these same sections, we also obtain estimates of total kidney volume (V_{kid}), V_{glom}, mean renal corpuscle volume (V_{corp}), the total volume of all glomeruli in the kidney ($V_{glom\ (total)}$) and the total volume of all renal corpuscles in the kidney ($V_{corp\ (total)}$).

The physical disector/fractionator combination has been used to estimate N_{glom} in a range of species including human (7, 16), mouse (10, 12–14, 24, 36, 37), rat, (9, 11) and sheep (38–40). The method provides accurate (unbiased) and precise (low variance) estimates. Below we describe how to estimate N_{glom} in small (mouse, rat) and large (sheep, pig, human) kidneys using the physical disector/fractionator combination.

2. Materials

1. Fine-tipped forceps.
2. Fixative. We use 10% neutral buffered formalin (100 mL formalin, 900 mL tap water), 4 g of sodium dihydrogen phosphate, monohydrate ($NaH_2PO_4 \cdot H_2O$), and 6 g disodium hydrogen phosphate, anhydrous (Na_2HPO_4).
3. Single-edge razor blades or an appropriately sized razor blade slicing device with double-edge cutting blades and dividers of known spacing (e.g., 1 mm) (Fig. 1).
4. 70% Ethanol.
5. Glycolmethacrylate medium (provided in a kit) such as Polaron Embedding Medium (Bio-Rad Polaron Instruments) or Technovit 7100 kit (Heraeus Kulzer GmbH).
6. Backing mold medium (provided in a kit) such as Technovit 3040 kit (Heraeus Kulzer GmbH).
7. Digital micrometer with precision of 1 μm, example Mitutoyo.
8. Microtome such as Leica RM 2265 for sectioning glycol-methacrylate blocks.
9. Glass knife maker such as LKB 2078 Histo Knifemaker.

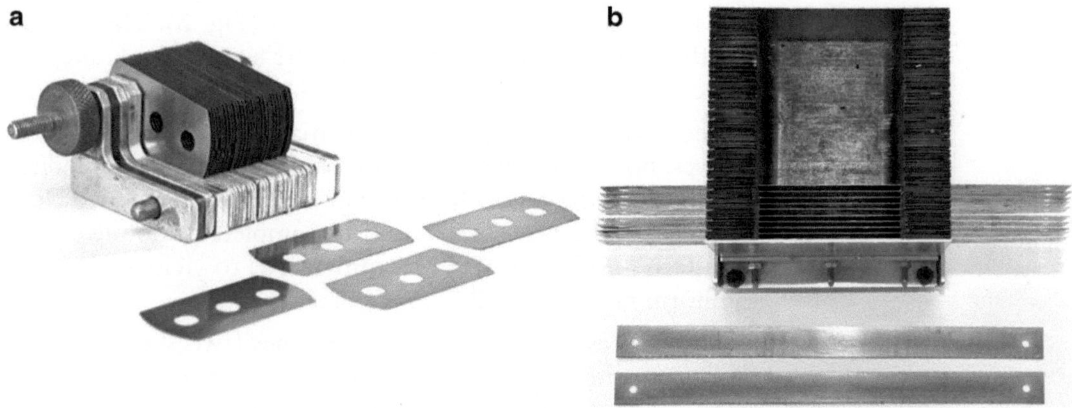

Fig. 1. Razor blade slicing devices. (**a**) Slicing device and double-edge razor blades used to slice kidneys from small animals such as mouse and rat. Each blade is separated by 1 mm dividers, but this can be varied. (**b**) Slicing device and blades used to slice human kidneys and kidneys from large animals such as sheep and pig. Each blade here is separated by 1-mm dividers, but this can be varied. The blades shown here are 30 cm long. The cavity in the slicing device has dimensions of 14 cm (length) × 9 cm (width) × 6 cm (depth).

10. 6-mm thick glass knives (made from strips of 406 mm × 25.4 mm × 6 mm glass).
11. PAS staining:
    - 1% periodic acid (1 g periodic acid dissolved in 100 mL distilled water).
    - Distilled water.
    - Schiffs Reagent.
    - Tap water.
    - Hematoxylin.
    - Scott's tap water.
    - Xylene.
    - DPX mounting medium.
12. 22 × 40-mm glass coverslips.
13. Microfiche reader or alternative (see Note 1).
14. Physical disector setup as shown in Fig. 2 or alternative system (see Note 2).

3. Methods

3.1. Estimating Total Glomerular Number (N_{glom}) in Small Animals (Mouse and Rat)

1. Decapsulate the kidney with fine-tipped forceps. Take care to not damage the kidney with the forceps, as nicks to the cortex will produce artifacts in the tissue section.
2. Immersion or perfusion fix the kidney (see Note 3).
3. Slice the kidney. Small kidneys are sliced into two halves. Larger kidneys are sliced using a razor blade or a razor blade slicing device (Fig. 1) into evenly spaced slices (Fig. 3). The position of the first slice must be random. The size of the kidney will determine slice thickness (see Note 4).
4. Select tissue slices. In the case of smaller kidneys cut into two halves, both halves are used (entire kidney). With larger kidneys often every second or third slice in order is selected (see Notes 4 and 5). The first slice should be sampled randomly (use of random number table is recommended) to yield a systematic uniform random (SUR) sample of slices.
5. Transfer specimen slices to capped tubes (two slices per tube) for processing.
6. Process tissue slices to glycolmethacrylate (GMA). We use Technovit 7100. Paraffin can be used (see Note 6).
    - Dehydrate specimens through a series of graded ethanol solutions: 70% ethanol for 1 h, 100% Ethanol for 3 × 1 h and 100% butanol for 1 × 1 h. Replace butanol and leave overnight.

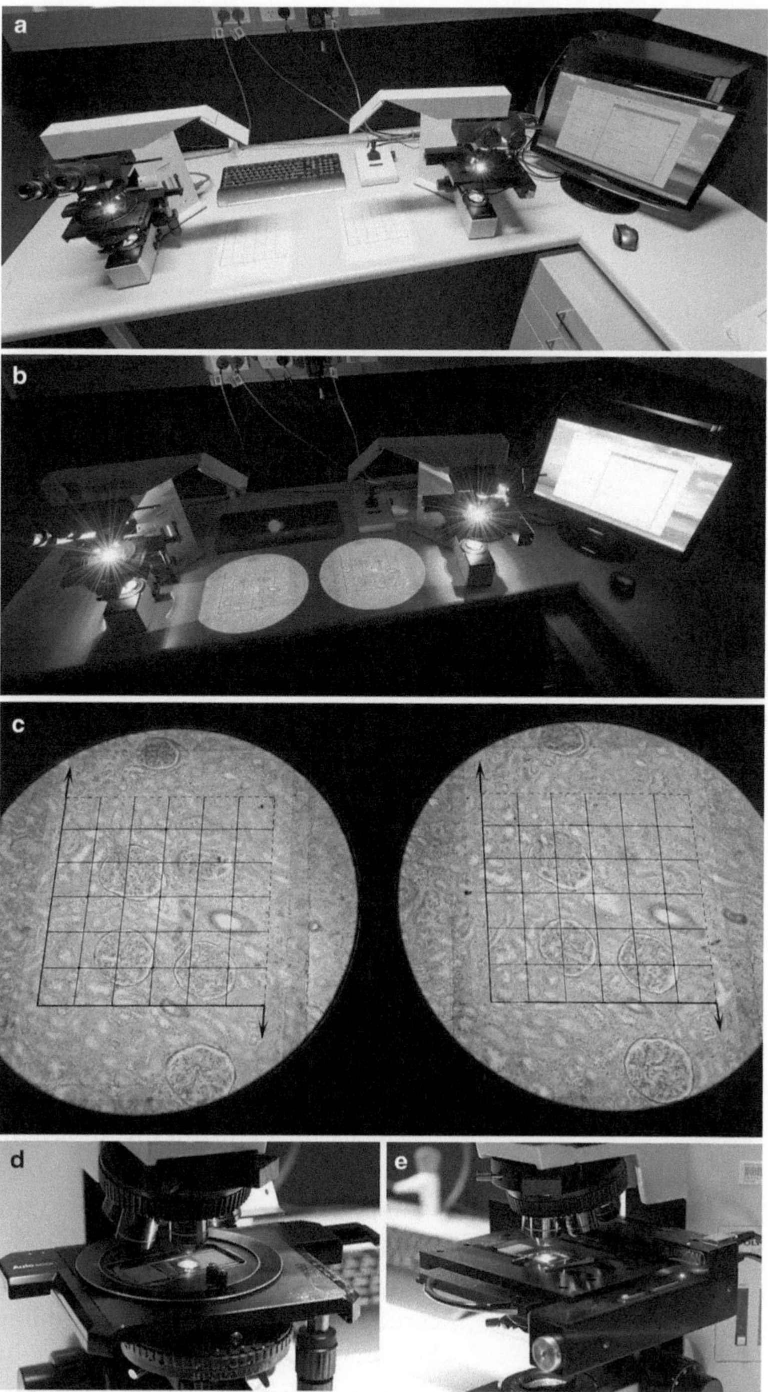

Fig. 2. Physical disector setup (**a**). The physical disector setup in our laboratory consists of two microscopes (Olympus BX50) fitted with projection arms. The left-hand microscope is fitted with a rotating stage (**d**) and the right-hand microscope is fitted with an Autoscan Pty. Ltd. automated stage (**e**) connected to a computer with Autoscan software. Images are projected in a semidarkened room (**b**). The field of view of the left-hand microscope is manually aligned to match the projected image of the right-hand microscope (fitted with the automatic stage), to produce identical regions from paired sections for counting (**c**). Note the unbiased counting frame in (**c**).

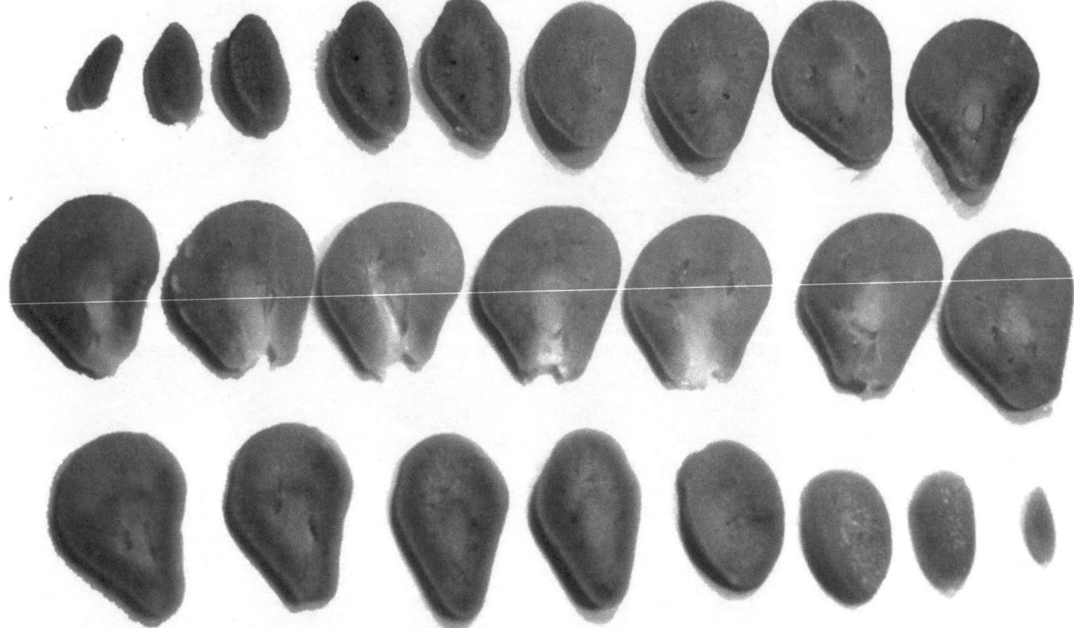

Fig. 3. Slicing the rat kidney. A razor blade slicing device is used to slice rat kidneys into 1-mm slices. All 24 slices from an adult rat kidney are shown.

- Prepare infiltration solution: dissolve 1 g of hardener I in 100 mL of base liquid, stir until dissolved (approximately 30 min) (see Note 7).
- Infiltrate specimens in a sufficient amount of prepared solution overnight.
- To embed tissue prepare embedding solution: add 1 mL of hardener II into 15 mL of infiltration solution and stir slowly to avoid air bubbles. Pour 1–3 mL of the solution into Histoform mold S or Q, place the infiltrated specimens into embedding mold and position cut surface to base of mold (see Note 8).
- Fill mold with embedding solution and leave to polymerize overnight.

7. Mount the embedded blocks onto a microtome chuck. The cured specimen in the embedding mold Histoform S or Histoform Q is mounted with the help of Technovit 3040.
   - Mix Technovit 3040 in a volume ratio of 2 parts powder to 1 part liquid to obtain a viscous liquid (see Note 9).
   - Pour Technovit 3040 into the recess of the embedding mold Histoform S or Histoform Q to a level of about 2 mm above the base of the mold. After about 10 min the block with the fixed specimen can be removed from the mold.

8. Measure the distance from the base of the chuck to the block face using a micrometer (this measurement will later be used to calculate mean section thickness).
9. Sectioning.
   - We use a Leica RM2265 microtome that can cut glycol-methacrylate sections ranging in thickness from 2 to >30 μm.
   - Place chuck into clamp of microtome fitted with a glass knife.
   - Exhaustively section at a nominal thickness of 20 μm (see Note 10), collecting every 10th and 11th section with the first section chosen at random in the interval 1–10 (with use of a random number table).
   - Record number of sections cut.
   - Float every 10th and 11th section on cold water and mount on separate glass slides in similar orientation (see Note 11).
   - Dry slides and sections on hot plate to flatten and adhere sections to slides.
10. Remeasure the distance from the base of the chuck to the block face with the micrometer. Using the starting and final block thickness, and the number of sections cut, calculate mean section thickness.
11. Stain every 10th and 11th section with periodic acid Schiff (PAS).
    - Place sections in 1% periodic acid for 30 min.
    - Wash sections briefly in distilled water.
    - Place sections in Schiff's reagent for 30 min.
    - Wash sections under running tap water for 3–4 min (until the water turns bright pink in color).
    - Place sections in hematoxylin for 30 min.
    - Wash sections under running tap water for 3–4 min (until the water runs clear).
    - Place sections in Scott's tap water for 3–4 min.
    - Wash sections briefly in tap water.
    - Allow sections to dry before clearing in xylene and coverslipping.
12. Identify those sections that contain complete kidney sections. Complete sections are defined as those sections with a complete tissue face. Estimate the area of these complete sections as well as the area of incomplete sections (see Note 12). The relative areas of complete and incomplete sections are used to estimate the fraction of the kidney used for glomerular counting.
13. Estimate the area of sections using point counting. We place every 10th histological slide in a microfiche reader and project

the section at a final magnification of approximately 25× onto a 2×2 cm orthogonal grid with an area per point of 0.64 mm^2 (mouse) or 3×3 cm orthogonal grid with an area per point of 1.44 mm^2 (rat) (see Note 13). Count the number of grid points (defined as intersections between stereological test grid lines) overlying projected kidney section.

14. Estimate kidney volume (V_{kid}) using the Cavalieri principle (41–44) using the following formula:

$$V_{kid} = \sum P \times a(p) \times t \times \frac{1}{f},$$

where, V_{kid} is kidney volume, ΣP is the total number of grid points (P) counted on complete and incomplete sections, $a(p)$ is the area associated with each grid point (1.44 mm^2) (see Note 13), t is section thickness (nominally 0.02 mm), and $\frac{1}{f}$ is the reciprocal of the section sampling fraction 1/(1/10) or 10.

15. Count glomeruli using physical disectors (Fig. 2a). We project the section pairs at approximately 150× side by side onto a table in a semidarkened room using two microscopes modified for projection (Fig. 2b). Identical regions in the section pairs must be examined (Fig. 2c). These regions should be sampled in a systematic uniform random manner. This is achieved with the aid of a microscope fitted with a rotatable stage to enable section alignment and examination of identical regions of tissue (Fig. 2d). A motorized stage is fitted to the other microscope to enable uniform systematic sampling (Fig. 2e). Place the 10th section (reference section) on the microscope fitted with the automated stage. Place the 11th section (look-up section) on the microscope with the rotatable stage.

16. The motorized stage is programmed to step across the kidney section (usually at 1,200×1,200 μm steps). Place a 2×2 cm grid within an unbiased counting frame (45) over each field of view (Fig. 4a).

17. For each field of view count grid points overlying kidney tissue (P_{kid}), glomerular tuft (P_{glom}), and renal corpuscle (P_{corp}) (see Note 14). Count only those glomeruli sampled by the unbiased counting frame (i.e., not overlying exclusion lines) in the field of view of the 10th section (reference section) that are not present in the 11th section (look-up section). Then count those glomeruli sampled by the unbiased counting frame in the 11th section that are not present in the 10th section, to double the efficiency of the technique (Fig. 4b, c). Repeat this process for each complete pair of sections (see Note 15). To estimate the number of glomeruli in a kidney with suitable

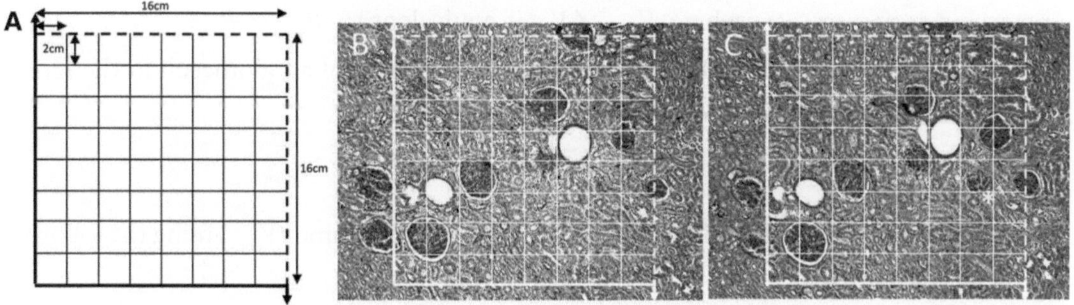

Fig. 4. (**a**) 2 × 2 cm grid with unbiased counting frame. For each field of view, count grid points overlying kidney tissue (P_{kid}), glomerular tufts (P_{glom}), and renal corpuscles (P_{corp}). Count glomeruli sampled by the unbiased counting frame (i.e., completely contained within the frame or touching the inclusion lines (*dashed lines*) but not the exclusion lines (*solid lines*) in the field of view of the 10th section (reference section, **c**) that are not present in the 11th section (look-up section, **b**)). Then count those glomeruli sampled in the 11th section not present in the 10th section. *Asterisk* represents a glomerulus present in the 10th (reference) section (**c**) but not present in the 11th (look-up) section (**b**)—this is the only glomerulus counted in this field.

precision, we aim to count approximately 200 glomeruli on 10–15 section pairs.

18. Calculate total nephron number (N_{glom}) using the following equation:

$$N_{glom} = 1 / \text{SliceSF} \times 1 / \text{SSF} \times P_s / P_f \times \frac{1}{(2f_a)} \times Q^-$$

where, 1/SliceSF is the reciprocal of the slice sampling fraction. If the entire kidney is embedded then 1/SliceSF is 1. If every second slice is selected then 1/SliceSF is 1/(1/2) or 2 etc., 1/SSF is the reciprocal of the section sampling fraction, $1/(1/10)$ or 10, P_s is the number of grid points overlying all kidney sections (complete and incomplete), P_f is the number of grid points overlying complete kidney sections that were used to count glomeruli, $\frac{1}{2f_a}$ is the inverse fraction of the total section area used to count glomeruli. 2 refers to the fact that we use disectors to count in both directions (See step 17).

The fractional section area (f_a) is calculated as follows:

$$f_a = \frac{P_{kid} \times a(p) \text{associated with the physical disectors}}{P_f \times a(p) \text{associated with the microfiche}},$$

Q^- is the actual number of glomeruli counted

19. Calculate mean glomerular volume (V_{glom}) using the following equation:

$$V_{glom} = \frac{V_{glom} / V_{kid}}{N_{glom} / V_{kid}},$$

where V_{glom} / V_{kid} is equivalent to P_{glom} / P_{kid}.

20. Calculate the combined volume of all glomeruli in the kidney ($V_{glom(total)}$) using:

$$V_{glom(total)} = V_{glom} \times N_{glom}.$$

21. Calculate mean renal corpuscle volume (V_{corp}) using the following formula:

$$V_{corp} = \frac{V_{corp} / V_{kid}}{N_{glom} / V_{kid}},$$

where V_{corp} / V_{kid} is equivalent to P_{corp} / P_{kid}.

22. Calculate the combined volume of all renal corpuscles in the kidney ($V_{corp(total)}$) using:

$$V_{corp\,(total)} = V_{corp} \times N_{glom}.$$

3.2. Estimating Total Glomerular Number (N_{glom}) in Humans and Large Animals (e.g., Sheep and Pig)

1. Obtain fresh kidney weight.
2. Perfusion fix the kidney.
3. Immersion fix the kidney in 10% formalin (with two changes of fresh 10% formalin after 24 and 48 h).
4. Carefully decapsulate the kidney with forceps, remove as much fat and vessels/ureter as possible.
5. Weigh the kidney (post-perfusion weight).
6. Sampling:
   - Slice kidney into halves. It is preferable to slice larger kidneys prior to immersion fixation to ensure adequate tissue preservation.
   - Slice one half into 4-mm slices using the device shown in Fig. 1b.
   - Sample 1 in 4 of these 4-mm slices, and weigh the sampled slices (this weight will be divided by post-perfusion kidney weight to obtain a weight fraction to be used as the first sampling fraction) (Fig. 5a). Use of the weight fraction as described is strictly not an unbiased approach, but was used by us to reduce variance. For a completely unbiased estimate, the fractions of slices sampled should be used.
   - Remove the majority of the renal medulla, being careful not to cut too close to the arcuate vessels where glomeruli can be located (Fig. 5b) (see Note 16).
   - Cut the sampled 4-mm slices into smaller pieces of approximately equal size of 1 cm × 1 cm × 4 mm (Fig. 5c).

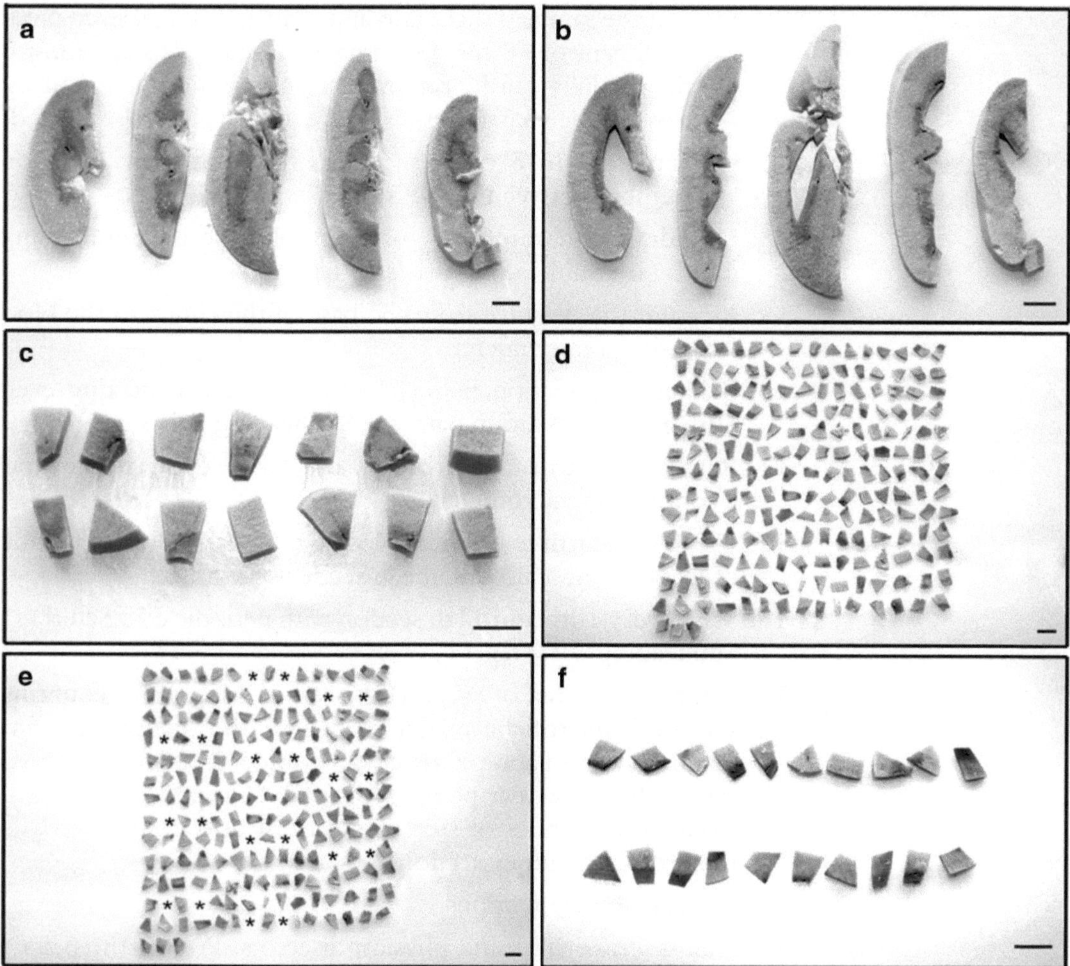

Fig. 5. Sampling the human kidney. Kidneys are first sliced in half and one half is further sliced into 4-mm slices. One in four of these 4-mm slices is selected (**a**). The majority of the renal medulla is removed (**b**) and the sampled 4-mm slices are cut into smaller pieces of approximately equal size (1 cm × 1 cm × 4 mm) (**c**). Each 4-mm piece is sliced into 1-mm pieces (**d**). Then, with a random start two sets of 1 in 20 of these pieces are selected (*asterisk*) (**e**) to obtain two samples of 10 pieces of tissue (**f**). These sampled pieces are embedded in GMA and used for glomerular counting. Scale bars = 1 cm.

- Cut the sampled 1 cm × 1 cm × 4 mm pieces into 1 cm × 1 cm × 1 mm pieces (Fig. 5d).
- Sample 1 in 20 of these pieces (Fig. 5e). Preferably collect two individual samples (see Note 17). The first piece for each sample must be selected randomly in the interval 1–20 (use of random number table is recommended), to yield two systematic uniform random samples (Fig. 5f) (see Note 18).

7. Sampling smaller kidneys (fetal sheep/pig):
    - Cut the kidney into quarters.
    - Slice each quarter into 1-mm slices.
    - Sample 1 in 4 of these slices.

- Cut the sampled slices into approximately equal sized pieces of dimensions 6 mm × 6 mm × 1 mm (at this stage most of the medulla can be removed, being careful not to cut too close to the arcuate vessels where glomeruli can be located).
- Sample 1 in 5 of these pieces (starting with a random number between 1 and 5).

8. Dehydrate, infiltrate, and embed sampled pieces in embedding molds (see Subheading 3.1, step 6).
9. Measure the distance from the base of the chuck to the block face using a micrometer.
10. Exhaustively section tissue blocks at 20 μm collecting every 10th and 11th section pair (see Subheading 3.1, step 9).
11. Remeasure the distance from the base of the chuck to the block face with the micrometer.
12. Using the starting and final block thicknesses and the number of sections cut, calculate mean section thickness.
13. Stain every 10th and 11th section with periodic acid Schiff (see Subheading 3.1, step 11)
14. Estimate the area of every 10th section using point counting. We use a microfiche reader to project the section at a final magnification of approximately 25× onto a 3 × 3 cm orthogonal grid with an area per point ($a(p)$) of 1.44 mm^2 (see Note 13). Count the number of stereological test grid points overlying the projected kidney sections.
15. Select complete sections.
16. Count glomeruli using physical disectors. Project the pairs of complete sections at approximately 150× (human and adult sheep/pig) or 300× (fetal sheep/pig) side by side onto a table in a semidarkened room using two microscopes modified for projection (Fig. 2b). Identical regions in the section pairs must be examined. The motorized stage is programmed to step across the kidney section (usually at a 1,600 μm × 1,600 μm steps). Place a stereological test grid with an unbiased counting frame (45) over each field of view (Fig. 6a).

Fig. 6. Rules for counting glomeruli in tissue with natural and artificial borders (the use of P_f). A stereological test grid with 3 cm × 3 cm squares (**a**) is first used to count P_{kid}, P_{glom} and, P_{corp}. P_f is counted as the number of central grid points (*open circles*) overlying kidney on a 6 cm × 6 cm grid within the unbiased counting frame (**b**). If the entire unbiased counting frame is covered with tissue then all nine points are counted (**b**). If the unbiased counting frame overlies a natural border of the kidney, then only those central points overlying kidney tissue are counted (**c**; seven central points are counted). If the unbiased counting frame overlies an unnatural or artificial border of the kidney (such as a cut border made by a scalpel or razor blade) (**d**), then only those central points associated with an area (6 cm × 6 cm) that is completely filled by kidney tissue are counted (**d**; three points are counted). When counting glomeruli sampled by the unbiased counting frame in the field of view of the reference section that are not present in the look-up section (and vice versa), glomeruli should only be counted if they are completely within the 6 cm × 6 cm area associated with a counted central point (P_f) and are not overlying exclusion

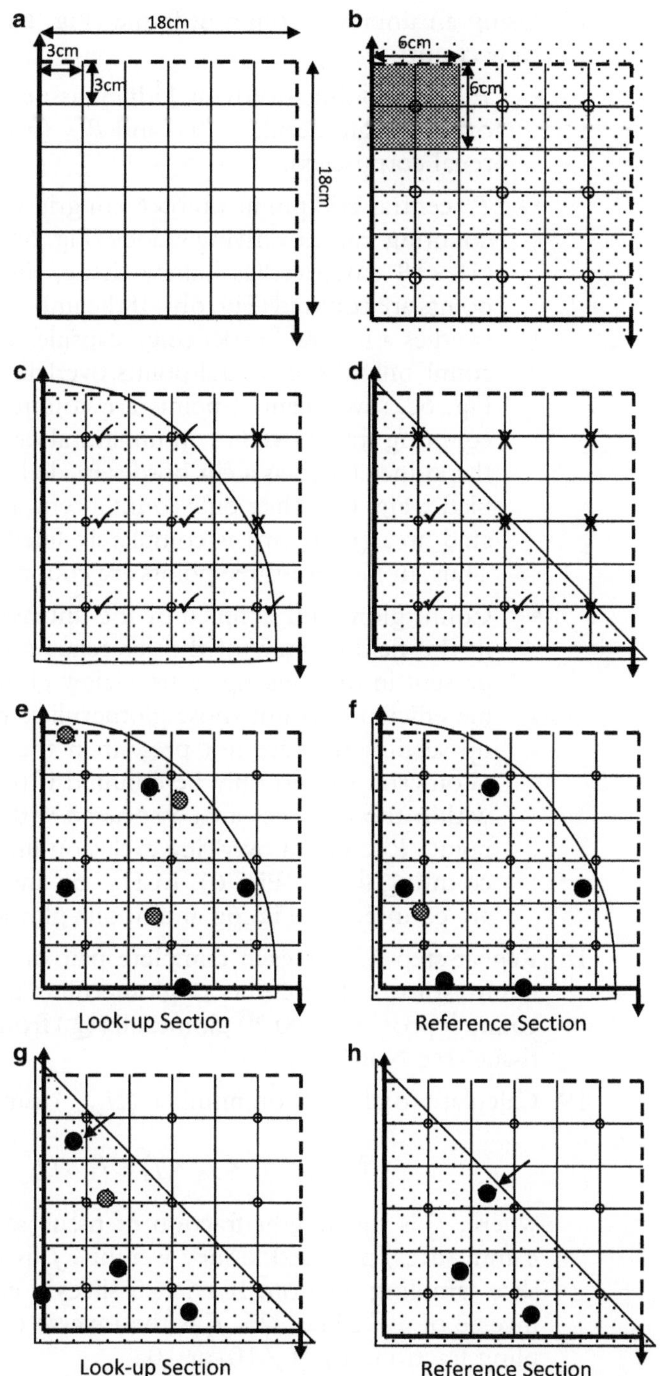

Fig. 6. (continued) lines of the unbiased counting frame. (**e**) and (**f**) show an example of a reference and look-up section with a natural border present. Four glomeruli would be counted (*shaded circles*)—the one glomerulus present in the reference section (**f**) that is no longer present in the look-up section (**e**), and the three glomeruli present in the look-up section that are not present in the reference section (**e**). (**g**) and (**h**) show an example of a reference and look-up section with an artificial border present. One glomerulus (*shaded circle*) would be counted—the glomerulus seen in (**g**) that is absent in (**h**). In both cases (**e** and **f**; **g** and **h**) *black circles* represent glomeruli that are not counted, i.e., are present in both the reference and look-up sections, or present in one section only but overlying exclusion (*solid*) lines, or are located within the area associated with a P_f that has not been counted (the glomeruli indicated by *arrows* in **g** and **h**).

17. Using an unbiased counting frame (Fig. 6a) for each field of view count:
    - P_{kid} (grid points overlying kidney tissue), P_{glom} (grid points overlying glomerular tufts) and P_{corp} (grid points overlying renal corpuscles).
    - P_f: central grid points on 6×6 cm grid within the unbiased counting frame overlying kidney (Fig. 6b). If the entire grid (18×18 cm) overlies kidney tissue, then all nine central points are counted (Fig. 6b). If the unbiased counting frame overlies a natural border (e.g., capsule) of the kidney, then count only those central points overlying kidney tissue. In Fig. 6c, seven central points are counted. If the unbiased counting frame overlies an unnatural or artificial border of the kidney (such as a cut border made by a scalpel or razor blade; Fig. 6d), then only count a central point if its associated area (6×6 cm) is completely filled by kidney tissue. Thus, in Fig. 6d, three points are counted (see Note 19).
    - Count glomeruli sampled by the unbiased counting frame in the field of view of the reference section that are not present in the look-up section (new glomerulus). To double efficiency, count those glomeruli sampled in the look-up section that are not present in the reference section. Glomeruli should only be counted if they are completely within the 6×6 cm area associated with a counted central point (P_f) and not overlying exclusion lines of the unbiased counting frame (Fig. 6). In Fig. 6e and f, four glomeruli are counted. In Fig. 6g and h, one glomerulus is counted.
18. Repeat step 17 for each complete pair of sections. To accurately estimate the number of glomeruli in a human kidney we count approximately 120 glomeruli (Q^-) from 8 to 15 pieces of tissue (see Note 20).
19. Calculate total nephron number (N_{glom}) using:

$$N_{glom} = f_1 \times f_2 \times f_3 \times f_a \times Q^-$$

where, f_1 is the weight fraction of tissue sampled (weight of 4-mm slices/perfused kidney weight). f_2 is the inverse of the slice sampling fraction. If 1 in 25 slices is embedded f_2 is the inverse of $1/25$ i.e., 25, f_3 is the inverse of the section sampling fraction, $1/(1/10)$ or 10,

$$f_a \text{ is } \frac{(P_s \times a(p))}{(2 \times P_f \times a(p))},$$

$P_s \times a(p)$, is the sum of points overlying all kidney sections on microfiche (complete and incomplete) multiplied by the area associated with each grid point (microfiche), $P_f \times a(p)$ is the sum of points overlying complete kidney sections that were used to count glomeruli multiplied by the area associated with each grid point (physical disector), and Q^- is the actual number of glomeruli counted.

20. Estimate kidney volume (V_{kid}) (see Note 16) using the Cavalieri principle:

$$V_{kid} = f_1 \times f_2 \times f_3 \times \sum P_s \times a(p) \times T,$$

where, f_1 is the weight fraction of tissue sampled, f_2 is the inverse of the slice sampling fraction, f_3 is the inverse of the section sampling fraction, ΣP_s is the total number of points counted on every 10th complete section using the microfiche, $a(p)$ is the area associated with each grid point (1.44 mm^2), and T is section thickness (nominally 0.02 mm).

21. Calculate mean glomerular volume (V_{glom}) as described in Subheading 3.1, step 19.
22. Calculate the combined volume of all glomeruli in the kidney ($V_{glom\ (total)}$) as described in Subheading 3.1, step 20.
23. Calculate mean renal corpuscle volume (V_{corp}) as described in Subheading 3.1, step 21.
24. Calculate the combined volume of all renal corpuscles in the kidney ($V_{corp\ (total)}$) as described in Subheading 3.1, step 22.

4. Notes

1. An alternative to a microfiche reader is to use a smaller grid size and a 2–4× lens fitted to a projection microscope.
2. An alternative to projection microscopes is the use of commercially available systems such as CASTGrid (Olympus) or Stereo Investigator (MicroBrightField Inc.) whereby the two fields are shown on a split-computer screen.
3. V_{glom} estimates will be influenced by perfusion pressure, fixative, the tissue processing schedule, and embedding medium. The shrinkage artifact can be significant.
4. Small kidneys such as in the mouse can be sliced into two halves through the hilus. The entire kidney is processed, embedded, and sectioned. Larger kidneys such as rat kidneys should be sliced using the razor blade slicing device into 1-mm slices.
5. A minimum of eight to ten 1-mm slices sampled uniformly (evenly through the kidney) are required.
6. N_{glom} estimates obtained using the physical disector/fractionator combination are not affected by the dimensional changes associated with fixation, processing, and sectioning. This is a

major advantage of this technique. However, V_{glom} estimates can be markedly affected. Dimensional changes are greater in paraffin than glycolmethacrylate embedded tissue. Also, alignment of microscopic fields in paraffin sections is much more difficult than in GMA sections, due to variable section compression (during sectioning) and expansion (on the water bath).

7. At 4°C the infiltration solution remains stable for approximately 4 weeks.
8. Time of workability at room temperature (23°C) is approx. 5–7 min. At 23°C the specimens will cure within approximately 2 h.
9. It is recommended that the liquid be placed into the container first followed by half the required powder and mixed thoroughly. Then add second half of powder and mix for a further 40 s. Let set for 15–20 s and stir again for 20 s. Do not mix with a beating movement to avoid air bubbles in the resin dough. To avoid excess heat caused by polymerization do not mix more than 30 g (20 g powder/10 g liquid).
10. 20-μm sections provide a reasonable number of glomeruli that are present in one section (reference section) but absent in the adjacent section (look-up section) and are therefore countable with the disector principle.
11. Ensure that sections do not flip over (i.e., are mounted upside down)—if this happens, the necessary section alignment required for the disector technique is impossible.
12. Incomplete sections are not used for glomerular counting because of the mechanical damage observed at artificial edges where glomeruli may have been lost or damaged.
13. Area per point $a(p)$ calculation: $a(p) = [\text{grid size (mm)/magnification}]^2 = (30/25)^2 = 1.2^2 = 1.44\ \text{mm}^2$.
14. A grid point represents the area associated with one 2 × 2 cm square. To count grid points, count the top right hand point of the 2 × 2 cm square only. Note that the unbiased counting frame in Fig. 4 contains 64 squares and 64 grid points.
15. 10–15 pairs of sections are required for a precise estimate of N_{glom}. If more section pairs are available select every second or third complete pair for analysis.
16. The majority of the medulla is removed to minimize sampling medulla when using the physical disectors. Removal of medullary tissue reduces time spent scanning tissue without glomeruli. However, it is important to note that estimates of V_{kid} are actually estimates of V_{cortex}.
17. The sampling fraction can change depending on the number and size of the pieces. We aim to have a minimum of 8 and a maximum of 15 pieces of tissue for analysis from each kidney.

18. Two samples are collected, one for initial use and the second as a backup if required.
19. P_f accounts for the presence of artificial edges created from tissue sampling and the possible loss or damage of glomeruli near these edges.
20. From each piece of tissue, a minimum of two complete section pairs is typically required to obtain an adequate Q^- and therefore a precise estimate of N_{glom}. It is important to count glomeruli in all sampled tissue and to not stop counting glomeruli when total Q^- exceeds 120.

References

1. Hoy WE, Ingelfinger JR, Hallan S et al (2010) The early development of the kidney and implications for adult health. J Dev Orig Health Dis 1:216–233
2. Puelles VG, Hoy WE, Hughson MD et al (2011) Glomerular number and size variability and risk for kidney disease. Curr Opin Nephrol Hypertens 20:7–15
3. Hughson MD, Douglas-Denton R, Bertram JF et al (2006) Hypertension, glomerular number, and birth weight in African Americans and white subjects in the southeastern United States. Kidney Int 69:671–678
4. Hoy WE, Hughson MD, Singh GR et al (2006) Reduced nephron number and glomerulomegaly in Australian aborigines: a group at high risk for renal disease and hypertension. Kidney Int 70:104–110
5. Hoy WE, Bertram JF, Douglas-Denton R et al (2008) Nephron number, glomerular volume, renal disease and hypertension. Curr Opin Nephrol Hypertens 17:258–265
6. Hoy WE, Douglas-Denton RN, Hughson MD et al (2003) A stereological study of glomerular number and volume: preliminary findings in a multiracial study of kidneys at autopsy. Kidney Int 83:S31–S37
7. McNamara BJ, Diouf B, Hughson MD et al (2008) Renal pathology, glomerular number and volume in a West African urban community. Nephrol Dial Transplant 23:2576–2585
8. Nyengaard JR, Bendtsen TF (1992) Glomerular number and size in relation to age, kidney weight, and body surface in normal man. Anat Rec 232:194–201
9. Gray SP, Denton KM, Cullen-McEwen LA et al (2010) Prenatal exposure to alcohol reduces nephron number and raises blood pressure in progeny. J Am Soc Nephrol 21:1891–1902
10. Hoppe CC, Evans RG, Moritz KM et al (2007) Combined prenatal and postnatal protein restriction influences adult kidney structure, function, and arterial pressure. Am J Physiol Regul Integr Comp Physiol 292:R462–R469
11. Singh RR, Cullen-McEwen LA, Kett MM et al (2007) Prenatal corticosterone exposure results in altered AT1/AT2, nephron deficit and hypertension in the rat offspring. J Physiol 579:503–513
12. Cullen-McEwen LA, Drago J, Bertram JF (2001) Nephron endowment in glial cell line-derived neurotrophic factor (GDNF) heterozygous mice. Kidney Int 60:31–36
13. Sims-Lucas S, Cullen-McEwen L, Eswarakumar VP et al (2009) Deletion of Frs2α from the ureteric epithelium causes renal hypoplasia. Am J Physiol Renal Physiol 297:F1208–F1219
14. Walker KA, Sims-Lucas S, Caruana G et al (2011) Betaglycan is required for the establishment of nephron endowment in the mouse. PLoS One 6:e18723
15. Moritz KM, Singh RR, Probyn ME et al (2009) Developmental programming of a reduced nephron endowment: more than just a baby's birth weight. Am J Physiol Renal Physiol 296:F1–F9
16. Douglas-Denton RN, McNamara BJ, Hoy WE et al (2006) Does nephron number matter in the development of kidney disease? Ethn Dis 16:40–45
17. Hughson M, Farris AB III, Douglas-Denton R et al (2003) Glomerular number and size in autopsy kidneys: the relationship to birth weight. Kidney Int 63:2113–2122
18. Keller G, Zimmer G, Mall G et al (2003) Nephron number in patients with primary hypertension. N Engl J Med 348:101–108
19. McNamara BJ, Diouf B, Douglas-Denton RN et al (2010) A comparison of nephron number,

glomerular volume and kidney weight in Senegalese Africans and African Americans. Nephrol Dial Transplant 25:1514–1520
20. McNamara BJ, Diouf B, Hughson MD et al (2009) Associations between age, body size and nephron number with individual glomerular volumes in urban West African males. Nephrol Dial Transplant 24:1500–1506
21. Sterio D (1984) The unbiased estimation of number and sizes of arbitrary particles using the disector. J Microsc 134:127–136
22. Samuel T, Hoy WE, Douglas-Denton R et al (2005) Determinants of glomerular volume in different cortical zones of the human kidney. J Am Soc Nephrol 16:3102–3109
23. Zimanyi MA, Hoy WE, Douglas-Denton RN et al (2009) Nephron number and individual glomerular volumes in male Caucasian and African American subjects. Nephrol Dial Transplant 24:2428–2433
24. Cullen-McEwen LA, Kett MM, Dowling J et al (2003) Nephron number, renal function, and arterial pressure in aged GDNF heterozygous mice. Hypertension 41:335–340
25. Shweta A, Cullen-McEwen LA, Kett MM et al (2009) Glomerular surface area is normalized in mice born with a nephron deficit: no role for AT1 receptors. Am J Physiol Renal Physiol 296:F583–F589
26. Chen HM, Liu ZH, Zeng CH et al (2006) Podocyte lesions in patients with obesity-related glomerulopathy. Am J Kidney Dis 48:772–779
27. Cho M, Hong E, Lee T et al (2007) Pathophysiology of minimal change nephrotic syndrome and focal segmental glomerulosclerosis. Nephrology (Carlton) 12:S11–S14
28. Fogo A (2000) Glomerular hypertension, abnormal glomerular growth, and progression of renal diseases. Kidney Int Suppl 75: S15–S21
29. Hall JE, Brands MW, Henegar JR (1999) Mechanisms of hypertension and kidney disease in obesity. Ann N Y Acad Sci 892: 91–107
30. Lemley K (2003) A basis for accelerated progression of diabetic nephropathy in Pima Indians. Kidney Int Suppl 83:S38–S42
31. Lemley K (2008) Diabetes and chronic kidney disease: lessons from the Pima Indians. Pediatr Nephrol 23:1933–1940
32. Shen WW, Chen HM, Chen H et al (2010) Obesity-related glomerulopathy: body mass index and proteinuria. Clin J Am Soc Nephrol 5:1401–1409
33. Suzuki H, Tokuriki T, Saito K et al (2005) Glomerular hyperfiltration and hypertrophy in the rat hypoplastic kidney as a model of oligomeganephronic disease. Nephrol Dial Transplant 20:1362–1369
34. Vats AN, Costello B, Mauer M (2003) Glomerular structural factors in progression of congenital nephrotic syndrome. Pediatr Nephrol 18:234–240
35. Zhu WW, Chen HP, Ge YC et al (2009) Ultrastructural changes in the glomerular filtration barrier and occurrence of proteinuria in Chinese patients with type 2 diabetic nephropathy. Diabetes Res Clin Pract 86:199–207
36. David FS, Cullen-McEwen L, Wu XS et al (2010) Regulation of kidney development by Shp2: an unbiased stereological analysis. Anat Rec 293:2147–2153
37. Dickinson H, Walker DW, Cullen-McEwen L et al (2005) The spiny mouse (Acomys cahirinus) completes nephrogenesis before birth. Am J Physiol Renal Physiol 289:F273–F279
38. Moritz KM, Johnson K, Douglas-Denton R et al (2002) Maternal glucocorticoid treatment programs alterations in the renin-angiotensin system of the ovine fetal kidney. Endocrinology 143:4455–4463
39. Wintour EM, Moritz KM, Johnson K et al (2003) Reduced nephron number in adult sheep, hypertensive as a result of prenatal glucocorticoid treatment. J Physiol 549:929–935
40. Mitchell E, Louey S, Cock M et al (2004) Nephron endowment and filtration surface area in the kidney after growth restriction of fetal sheep. Pediatr Res 55:769–773
41. Gundersen HJ, Bagger P, Bendtsen TF et al (1988) The new stereological tools: disector, fractionator, nucleator and end point sampled intercepts and their use in pathological research and diagnosis. Acta Pathol Microbiol Immunol Scand 96:857–881
42. Gundersen HJG, Bendtsen TF, Korbo L et al (1988) Some new, simple and efficient and stereological methods and their use in pathological research and diagnosis. Acta Pathol Microbiol Immunol Scand 96:379–394
43. Gundersen H, Jensen E (1987) The efficiency of systematic sampling in stereology and its prediction. J Microsc 147:229–263
44. Bertram J (1995) Analyzing renal glomeruli with the new stereology. Int Rev Cytol 161:111–172
45. Gundersen H (1977) Notes on the estimation of the numerical density of arbitrary profiles: the edge effect. J Microsc 111:219

Chapter 31

Assessing Urinary Tract Defects in Mice: Methods to Detect the Presence of Vesicoureteric Reflux and Urinary Tract Obstruction

Inga J. Murawski, Christine L. Watt, and Indra R. Gupta

Abstract

Congenital Anomalies of the Kidney and Urinary Tract (CAKUT) encompass a spectrum of kidney and urinary tract disorders. Here, we describe two assays that can be used to determine if a mouse has vesicoureteric reflux (VUR) or urinary tract obstruction, two urinary tract defects observed in CAKUT. To test for VUR, dye is injected into the mouse bladder and then monitored to determine if it passes retrogradely from the bladder towards the kidneys, indicating the presence of VUR. To test for urinary tract obstruction, the renal pelvis is microinjected with dye and its passage along the urinary tract is monitored to determine if there is evidence of impaired flow along the tract. These methods will facilitate the analysis of CAKUT phenotypes in the mouse.

Key words: Vesicoureteric reflux, Urinary tract obstruction, Intravesical ureter, Mouse

1. Introduction

In both humans and mice, the kidneys and ureter develop from the ureteric bud, an epithelial structure that emerges from the caudal end of the mesonephric duct and interacts with the surrounding mesenchyme (1, 2). The ureter further differentiates into three distinct layers: the urothelium, a specialized epithelial layer impermeable to urine, the lamina propria, a vascularized layer of connective tissue, and a smooth muscle layer necessary for ureteral peristalsis (2, 3). At the junction with the kidney, the ureter becomes enlarged and forms the renal pelvis and the ureteropelvic junction (UPJ). Akin to the ureter, the renal pelvis contains connective tissue and smooth muscle layers (4, 5). At the junction with the bladder, the developing ureter undergoes complex cellular and morphologic

Odyssé Michos (ed.), *Kidney Development: Methods and Protocols*, Methods in Molecular Biology, vol. 886, DOI 10.1007/978-1-61779-851-1_31, © Springer Science+Business Media, LLC 2012

rearrangements such that it separates from the mesonephric duct and acquires an independent insertion through the bladder wall (1, 6). The insertion site is referred to as the ureterovesical junction (UVJ) and it functions as a one-way valve that prevents the retrograde flow of urine from the bladder towards the kidneys. A number of components of the UVJ are essential to prevent vesicoureteric reflux (VUR) or the retrograde flow of urine, including an adequate length of the intravesical ureter, an oblique angle of ureter entry into the bladder wall, a well-formed ureter and bladder muscle layer that compress the ureteral orifice during voiding, and a correctly positioned ureteric orifice within the bladder (3, 7).

When the kidneys and the urinary tracts do not develop properly, a number of defects can arise and are commonly known as Congenital Anomalies of the Kidney and Urinary Tract (CAKUT). CAKUT accounts for 20–30% of all malformations identified in the newborn period (8) and encompasses a spectrum of abnormalities in both humans and in mice including renal agenesis, renal hypo/dysplasia, urinary tract obstruction, ureteroceles, duplex urinary tracts, ectopic ureters, and VUR. Importantly, more than one of these phenotypes can be observed in the same individual (or mouse), demonstrating the need for a careful assessment of the kidneys and urinary tracts (9).

VUR is one of the most common congenital urinary tract defects, with a reported incidence as high as 1%, and it arises from a defect in the formation of the UVJ (3, 10, 11). Urinary tract obstruction refers to a blockage in the flow of urine along the ureters and can be subclassified into anatomical or functional obstruction (3). Anatomical obstruction is a physical blockage that can occur at the UPJ, the UVJ, or the urethra and results in dilation of the urinary tract above the site of obstruction. Functional obstruction is obstruction without structural hindrance and can be caused by defective peristalsis due to a deficiency in the smooth muscle layer, neural innervation of the smooth muscle layer or from an aberrant increase in connective tissue surrounding the ureter (3, 12, 13).

In humans, VUR is diagnosed by a voiding cystourethrogram (VCUG), an invasive test that requires catheterization via the urethra, filling of the bladder with a radiopaque solution, and repeated X-ray images of the urinary tract to determine whether the contrast flows retrogradely from the bladder into the ureter or renal pelvis (14–16). Urinary tract obstruction is typically diagnosed in humans using a diuresis renogram: an isotope, MAG3 or DTPA, is injected intravenously, taken up by the kidneys and its excretion into the urine is monitored over time. Urinary tract obstruction is suspected if there is a delay in filling of the kidney or excretion of the isotope as well as dilation of the ureter proximal to the site of obstruction (3). Another test for urinary tract obstruction is a nephrostogram in which a tube is inserted into the renal pelvis and contrast is injected. Obstruction is suspected if the contrast agent is retained in the pelvis or ureter and/or if there is evidence of an anatomical narrowing (3).

Mouse models have been extensively used to study the genetic and developmental origins of CAKUT. A number of assays have been developed to assess for VUR in both live and euthanized mice (9, 17–22). Most of these methods involve the injection of dye into the mouse bladder to determine whether the dye flows retrogradely towards the kidneys (17–19). The dye can be either injected manually with a syringe or the needle can be attached to a column of dye that is raised vertically to increase bladder pressure along a gradient (9, 19, 23). A variation to this method includes clamping the urethra closed with forceps or sutures to create bladder outlet obstruction and to determine if reflux can be induced when bladder pressure is increased. This variation results in VUR in all animals but functional differences in the competence of the UVJ can be assessed by examining the pressure at which VUR occurs (17, 18). More recently, another variation of the method relies on injecting microbubbles into the bladder of anesthetized mice and tracking their passage retrogradely into the kidneys using ultrasound technology (20).

In this chapter, we describe the most commonly used VUR assay in mice that uses a column of dye to exert hydrostatic pressure in the absence of bladder outlet obstruction. This assay can be easily performed on embryonic, postnatal or adult mice. The mice are euthanized and VUR is assayed immediately postmortem. We also describe an assay to measure the length of the intravesical ureter and to test for urinary tract obstruction. The length of the intravescial ureter is an important determinant of UVJ competence, and short intravesical ureters in mice are correlated with an increased incidence of VUR (22). For this method, dye is microinjected into the pelvis of a newborn kidney and outlines the morphology of the urinary tract. In addition to visualizing the intravesical ureter, dilation of the ureter can be observed, and urinary tract obstruction can be identified and localized to the UPJ, UVJ, or elsewhere in the urinary tract.

2. Materials

2.1. Dissection of Newborn Mice for VUR and Intravesical Ureter Assays

1. Ice.
2. Disposable petri dishes.
3. Dissecting forceps (such as Dumont #5 Straight Tip Forceps–Rustless Dumoxel).
4. Fine dissecting scissors (such as Sar-Med or Delicate Scissors 4½).
5. Capsulotomy scissors (Miltex Vannas 3¼ in., curved, extra delicate 18-1622) if performing intravesical ureter assay only (optional).

6. Surgical blade (Bard-Parker no.22 Stainless Steel Surgical Blade—single use).
7. Dissecting microscope equipped with a camera.
8. Software to measure lengths and planar surface areas (such as SPOT v.3.5.9) (optional if kidney phenotype is desired).
9. 70% ethanol.
10. 4% paraformaldehyde in phosphate buffered saline (PBS).
11. Microfuge tubes (1.5 mL).
12. Beaker.
13. Scale.
14. Plastic wrap.

2.2. Material for VUR Assay

1. IV tubing that is at least 185 cm in length (Microbore Fat Emulsion Extension Set, 74 in. tubing).
2. 60-mL syringe.
3. Methylene blue (diluted to 1 mg/mL in 1× sterile PBS).
4. Timer.
5. Needle (26-gauge 3/8 intradermal bevel needle–Precision Glide).

2.3. Materials for Intravesical Ureter Assay

1. Glass microinjection needle (from a 1×90 mm glass capillary tube (Narishige) in a vertical pipette puller (Kopf–model 270)).
2. Micromanipulator (such as Narishige model MM3).
3. Thin tubing such as that from an EZ Set Winged Needle package with the needle removed (Becton Dickinson–27-gauge 3/8 in. with 12 in. tubing).
4. 1-mL syringe (Becton Dickinson "tuberculin slip tip").
5. 1% fast green diluted in 1× sterile PBS.

3. Methods

3.1. Dissection of Newborn Mice for VUR and Intravesical Ureter Assays

1. Place newborn mice in a petri dish on ice wait approximately 20 min for mice to become hypothermic.
2. Weigh newborn mice on scale to record body weights.
3. Newborn mice are sacrificed by decapitation (see Note 1).
4. Collect tails or other tissue if genotyping is required.
5. A midline incision is made from the thorax and abdominal cavity using fine dissecting scissors to expose the ribcage and underlying organs. Ensure that the bladder is not punctured at this time.

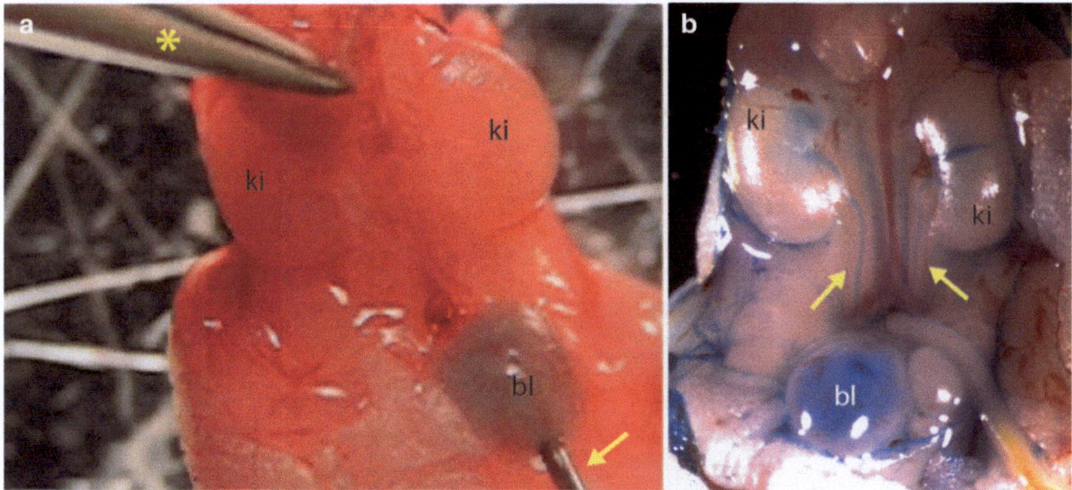

Fig. 1. Vesicoureteric reflux assay. (**a**) A midline incision is made from the neck down to the bladder to expose the thorax and the abdomen. Excess tissue is removed to expose the kidneys (ki), ureter (ur), and bladder (bl). Using forceps (*star*), the mouse is held in place and the needle (*arrow*) is inserted into the bladder as shown. (**b**) Once the bladder is needled, the column of dye is raised at specific intervals and the rate of dye flowing into the bladder is determined by the pressure exerted by the column of dye. When VUR is present, the dye can be seen flowing up the ureters (*arrows*) into the renal pelvis. The hydrostatic pressure at which VUR is observed is recorded and is represented by the height of the column of methylene blue in relation to the level of the mouse. For the mouse shown, VUR was noted at 60 cm for the left ureter and 90 cm for the right ureter.

6. Two additional incisions are made from the midline out towards each hind limb to expose the kidneys and the urinary tract.
7. Remove excess tissue above the kidneys using the forceps and disposable surgical blade.
8. Record the gender of the mouse if desired.
9. Remove any excess tissue such that all that remains are the hind limbs, spine, kidneys, and urinary tract (Fig. 1a).
10. If performing the VUR assay, go to Subheading 3.2.
11. If performing the intravesical ureter assay, dissect the bladder, ureters, and kidneys intact from the body cavity en bloc by gently lifting the bladder and freeing the tissue from the rest of the body using fine dissecting scissors or capsulotomy scissors (Fig. 2a).

3.2. Screening Newborn Mice for VUR

1. The assay is performed using a dissecting microscope equipped with a digital camera for photographs (see Note 2).
2. Set up pre-designated markers on the wall adjacent to the microscope to record the height of the column of dye that induces VUR (see Note 3).
3. Ensure that the IV tubing has the 60-mL syringe attached at one end, with the 26-gauge 3/8 needle attached to the opposite end.

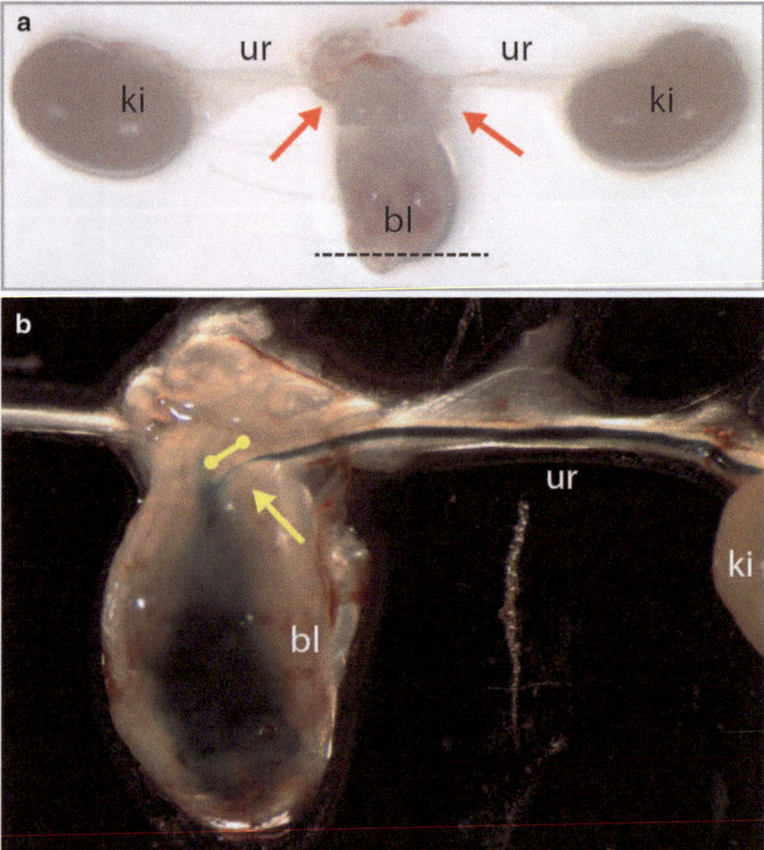

Fig. 2. Intravesical ureter length assay. (**a**) When performing the intravesical ureter assay, the bladder (bl), ureters (ur), and kidneys (ki) are removed en bloc from the body cavity and placed on a petri dish such that the kidneys and ureters are at a 90° angle to the bladder (*arrows*). The lower end of the bladder is cut (*dashed line*) to allow the dye to exit the bladder freely during the assay. (**b**) Using the micromanipulator, the glass microinjection needle is inserted into the renal pelvis. A gentle push on the syringe head is sufficient to allow for a few drops of dye to flow out of the needle into the renal pelvis. The dye will flow naturally from the renal pelvis down the ureters and into the bladder (see dye in figure). The dye clearly outlines the ureter and the intravesical ureter (*arrow*). The distance between the bladder periphery and the ureteral orifice (site of dye exit) is defined as the intravesical ureter length (*line and arrow*). Dilation of the ureter or obstruction can also be detected with this assay.

4. Fill the 60-mL syringe with methylene blue dye (see Note 4).
5. Place the mouse on the base of the dissecting microscope and dissect it carefully to expose the kidneys and the urinary tract as described above.
6. While holding the bladder firmly with forceps, needle the bladder with the 26-gauge 3/8 needle while looking through the eyepieces (ensure that the bladder is not double-needled) (Fig. 1a and see Note 5).
7. Start the timer for 30 s and begin raising the syringe vertically.

8. Raise the syringe filled with dye vertically from 30 cm to 150 cm by 30 cm/5 s intervals, once a final height of 150 cm is reached, maintain for 10 s (see Note 6). Lower the column of dye before removing the needle from the bladder to avoid excess dye on the specimen.
9. Record the height of the column when dye is seen exiting the urethra. This is the voiding pressure (see Note 7).
10. Record the height of the column when dye is seen going up the left and right ureters. This is the VUR pressure (see Note 8).
11. If a phenotypic examination of the kidneys is desired, proceed with Note 9.
12. Place kidneys and bladders in labeled microfuge tube filled with 4% PFA, if desired. Store specimens at 4°C.
13. Clean scissors, forceps, and petri dish with 70% Ethanol between each mouse that is tested for VUR.
14. When all mice have been tested, the IV tubing and the 60-mL syringe can be rinsed with dH_2O and reused. All needles and blades are disposed of in designated containers.

3.3. Measuring the Length of the Intravesical Ureter in Newborn Mice

1. The assay is performed on a dissecting microscope equipped with a digital camera for photographs.
2. Fill a 1 mL syringe with 1% fast green in PBS.
3. Obtain a microinjection needle: Use a 1 × 90 mm glass capillary tube in a vertical pipette puller (Kopf—model 270).
4. Attach one end of the 27-gauge tubing to the 1-mL syringe and attach the other end of the tubing to the glass microinjection needle (see Note 10).
5. Fix the glass microinjection needle onto the micromanipulator (Fig. 3) such that the needle can be easily lowered and moved forward to reach the dissecting microscope.
6. Check that when the syringe stopper is pushed gently, drops of dye emerge from the tip of the glass microinjection needle (see Note 11).
7. Dissect one mouse to expose the kidneys and the urinary tract and proceed to gently remove the kidneys and urinary tract intact as described above (Fig. 2a).
8. Place the kidneys and ureters at a 90° angle to the bladder, as shown in Fig. 2a.
9. Photograph the kidneys and record planar surface area measurements if desired.
10. Cut off the lower end of the bladder (Fig. 2—dashed line and see Note 12).
11. Slowly adjust the micromanipulator and insert the glass microinjection needle into the renal pelvis.

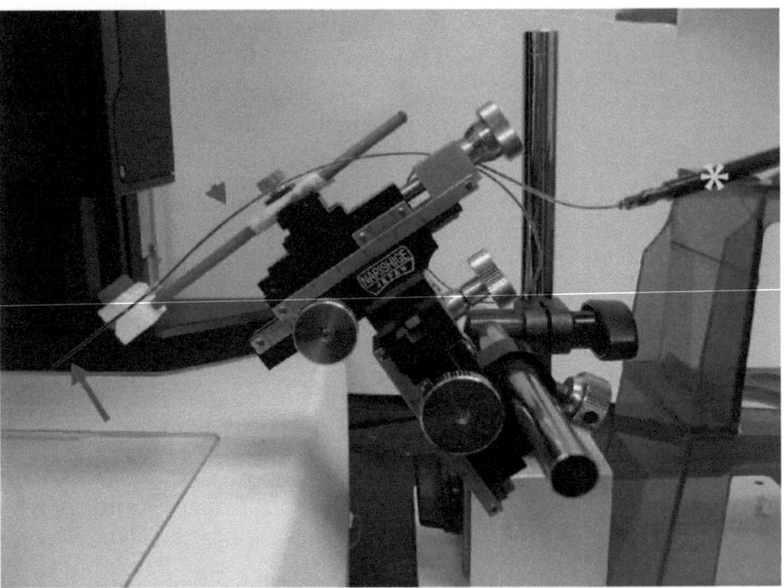

Fig. 3. Micromanipulator used for intravesical ureter length assay. The micromanipulator is set up to hold the glass microinjection needle (*arrow*), which is attached to a syringe (*star*) with thin tubing (*arrowhead*). The micromanipulator controls the glass microinjection needle and can be adjusted to insert the tip of the needle into the renal pelvis.

12. Gently pushes on the syringe head so that a few drop of dye are injected into the renal pelvis. The dye will naturally flow from the renal pelvis, down the ureters, and into the bladder (see Note 13).
13. As the dye is traveling down the ureter, photograph the bladder and the UVJ. The fast green dye clearly outlines the ureter and the intravesical ureter (Fig. 2b).
14. Measure the length of the intravesical ureter, using software such as SPOT. The intravesical ureter length is defined as the distance between the bladder periphery and the site of dye exit.
15. Both kidneys can be injected in the same mouse to record the length of the left and the right intravesical ureter.
16. Record whether obstruction is observed at the UPJ or the UVJ.
17. Record whether the ureter is dilated.
18. Gently remove the kidneys using fine forceps and immediately record their weights.
19. Place kidneys and bladders in labeled microfuge tube filled with 4% PFA, if desired. Store specimens at 4°C.
20. Clean forceps with 70% ethanol between each mouse that is examined.

21. The 27-gauge tubing and the glass microinjection needle can be rinsed with dH_2O and reused.
22. Normally, an individual mouse is screened for VUR or intravesical ureter lengths, but not both simultaneously. See Note 14 for an adaptation of these two methods such that both assays can be performed in the same mouse.
23. See Note 15 for a variation of this assay to screen for ureter patency.

4. Notes

1. Dissect one mouse at a time immediately prior to performing the VUR or the intravesical ureter assay. Please note that the VUR assay is described in newborn mice; however, this method can be used to test embryonic (aged embryonic day 16 and older) as well as adult mice that are euthanized by CO_2 inhalation.
2. The VUR assay is performed with two people. One person needles the bladder and observes whether any dye flows retrogradely from the bladder into the ureters and/or kidneys. The second person raises the column of dye to the desired height. Cover the microscope base with plastic wrap to ensure that any spilled dye does not stain the equipment.
3. Pre-set heights can be marked on the wall adjacent to the dissecting microscope, and serve as a guide during the VUR assay. A ruler is used to measure 5 cm intervals from the base of the microscope. When the syringe filled with dye is raised vertically, the hydrostatic pressure at which VUR is noted is represented by the height of the column of methylene blue relative to the level of the mouse (placed on the microscope base).
4. Insert the syringe stopper to begin the flow of dye out of the needle and then remove the stopper. There is no need to replace the stopper. Raising and lowering the column is sufficient to start or stop the flow of dye as needed for the assay. When the column of dye is not being raised for an assay, rest it on the bench by placing it in a beaker or any other support. When the needle is not being used, ensure that it too is placed within a falcon tube or beaker to ensure that no dye is spilled.
5. Prior to puncturing the bladder wall with the needle, ensure that there are no air bubbles within the needle or the IV tubing. Air bubbles can be avoided by keeping the syringe filled with dye and by keeping it level with the base of the microscope.
6. The column of dye is raised vertically to specific heights relative to the dissecting microscope. As the column is raised, the

hydrostatic pressure increases and the flow of dye increases into the bladder. We have standardized these heights/pressures for use at 30, 60, 90, 120, and 150 cm relative to the microscope. At 150 cm, the dye usually exits quickly from the urethra. We have raised the syringe up to 200 cm and have never induced a bladder to rupture, nor have we been able to induce VUR in control animals at this high pressure. If different height intervals are desired, the VUR assay can be modified accordingly. For instance, the column of dye can be raised by 5 cm intervals every second. This variation is useful if all mice reflux and one wants to distinguish between low and high pressure refluxing mice.

7. The voiding pressure varies between each mouse, but usually occurs between 30 and 60 cm (average 45 cm).
8. Ensure that VUR is recorded separately for left and right ureter/kidney units. Some mice exhibit unilateral VUR while others exhibit bilateral VUR. The individual at the microscope needling the bladder monitors when the dye exits the urethra and when VUR occurs, while the person raising the column of dye monitors the height at which voiding and VUR occurs.
9. To gather information on kidney morphometrics, photograph the kidneys and measure their planar surface areas using software such as SPOT. Gently remove the kidneys using fine forceps and immediately record their weights. Planar surface area and weight measurements are normalized for body weight to account for any differences in gestational age in newborn mice, and to account for any differences in body size in adult mice.
10. Depending on the final thickness of the glass microinjection needle and the opening of the 1 mL syringe, small adjustments with larger tubing may have to be made to ensure that the needle and syringe fit tightly onto the 27-gauge tubing (Fig. 3).
11. When pulling microinjection needles, the tip of the needle may need to be severed with forceps to ensure that the tip of the needle has a beveled edge so that dye can flow freely. The fast green dye may dry and obstruct the tip of the glass microinjection needle. Dipping the end of the needle into a microfuge tube filled with 70% ethanol between injections is usually sufficient to maintain the flow of dye.
12. The lower end of the bladder is removed to ensure that once dye is injected into the renal pelvis, it does not get trapped in the bladder, but flows freely out of the bladder such that the intravesical ureter is not obscured.
13. If there is obstruction at the UPJ or UVJ, the dye will stop flowing at the junction of the ureter and the renal pelvis or at the junction of the ureter and bladder. Dilation of the ureter may also be detected.

14. To test for VUR and measure the length of the intravesical ureter in the same mouse, start with the VUR assay as described. Proceed with carefully dissecting out the bladder/ureter/kidneys en bloc as in the intravesical ureter assay. To continue with the intravesical ureter assay, do not use fast green, but another dye that will show contrast with the methylene blue from the VUR assay. Eosin can be seen in the presence of the methylene blue dye and can be imaged using either light or fluorescent microscopy. Eosin is toxic and flammable. Wear protective gloves and a lab coat when handling.
15. Ureter patency can also be tested in embryonic mice. Dissect the mice as in the VUR assay such that the kidneys, ureters, and bladder remain within the body cavity. Inject fast green dye into the renal pelvis through the glass microinjection needle as in the intravesical ureter assay. If the dye flows down the ureters into the bladder, the ureter is patent.

References

1. Batourina E, Choi C, Paragas N et al (2002) Distal ureter morphogenesis depends on epithelial cell remodeling mediated by vitamin A and Ret. Nat Genet 32:109–115
2. Young B, Heath JW (2000) Wheater's functional histology, 3rd edn. Harcourt Publishers, Edinburgh
3. Campbell M (2002) Campbell's urology, 8th edn. Saunders Harcourt Publishing, Philadelphia
4. David SG, Cebrian C, Vaughan ED Jr, Herzlinger D (2005) c-kit and ureteral peristalsis. J Urol 173:292–295
5. Mendelsohn C (2004) Functional obstruction: the renal pelvis rules. J Clin Invest 113:957–959
6. Batourina E, Tsai S, Lambert S et al (2005) Apoptosis induced by vitamin A signaling is crucial for connecting the ureters to the bladder. Nat Genet 37:1082–1089
7. Tanagho EA, Guthrie TH, Lyon RP (1969) The intravesical ureter in primary reflux. J Urol 101:824–832
8. Schedl A (2007) Renal abnormalities and their developmental origin. Nat Rev Genet 8:791–802
9. Murawski IJ, Myburgh DB, Favor J, Gupta IR (2007) Vesico-ureteric reflux and urinary tract development in the Pax21Neu+/– mouse. Am J Physiol Renal Physiol 293:F1736–F1745
10. Burger RH, Smith C (1971) Hereditary and familial vesicoureteral reflux. J Urol 106: 845–851
11. Chapman CJ, Bailey RR, Janus ED, Abbott GD, Lynn KL (1985) Vesicoureteric reflux: segregation analysis. Am J Med Genet 20:577–584
12. Chen F (2009) Genetic and developmental basis for urinary tract obstruction. Pediatr Nephrol 24:1621–1632
13. Murakumo M, Nonomura K, Yamashita T et al (1997) Structural changes of collagen components and diminution of nerves in congenital ureteropelvic junction obstruction. J Urol 157: 1963–1968
14. Hodson EM, Wheeler DM, Vimalchandra D, Smith GH, Craig JC (2007) Interventions for primary vesicoureteric reflux. Cochrane Database Syst Rev CD001532
15. (1981) Medical versus surgical treatment of primary vesicoureteral reflux: report of the International Reflux Study Committee. Pediatrics 67: 392–400
16. Sengar DP, Rashid A, Wolfish NM (1979) Familial urinary tract anomalies: association with the major histocompatibility complex in man. J Urol 121:194–197
17. Mannen H, Tsuji S, Goto N (1991) Incomplete protection mechanism against vesico-ureteral reflux and hydronephrosis in the inbred mouse strain DDD. Lab Anim 25:156–161
18. Nishimura H, Yerkes E, Hohenfellner K et al (1999) Role of the angiotensin type 2 receptor gene in congenital anomalies of the kidney and urinary tract, CAKUT, of mice and men. Mol Cell 3:1–10
19. Pedersen A, Skjong C, Shawlot W (2005) Lim 1 is required for nephric duct extension and ureteric bud morphogenesis. Dev Biol 288:571–581

20. Paredes J, Sims-Lucas S, Wang H et al (2011) Assessing vesicoureteral reflux in live inbred mice via ultrasound with microbubble contrast agent. Am J Physiol Renal Physiol
21. Hains DS, Sims-Lucas S, Carpenter A et al (2010) High incidence of vesicoureteral reflux in mice with Fgfr2 deletion in kidney mesenchyma. J Urol 183:2077–2084
22. Murawski IJ, Maina RW, Malo D et al (2010) The C3H/HeJ inbred mouse is a model of vesico-ureteric reflux with a susceptibility locus on chromosome 12. Kidney Int 78:269–278
23. Yu OH, Murawski IJ, Myburgh DB, Gupta IR (2004) Overexpression of RET leads to vesicoureteric reflux in mice. Am J Physiol Renal Physiol 287:F1123–F1130

Chapter 32

Ischemia–Reperfusion Injury of the Mouse Kidney

Leif Oxburgh and Mark P. de Caestecker

Abstract

Studies of the complex responses of the kidney to acute injury have yielded important insights into mechanisms of tissue injury and repair. A variety of injury models have contributed to this impressive body of knowledge, but the ischemia–reperfusion (IR) model has perhaps been the most widely used. This chapter contains a detailed method description for IR injury in the mouse together with notes on blood sampling and tissue harvesting. The aim of the chapter is to provide the novice with a step-by-step guide to establishing this procedure in their research program.

Key words: Acute kidney injury, Acute tubular necrosis, Nephron injury, Nephron repair, Kidney fibrosis

1. Introduction

Acute kidney injury (AKI) is associated with diverse clinical conditions including trauma, sepsis, toxicity, and cardiac arrest (1). In the acute phase, functional impairment of the kidney significantly increases mortality in hospitalized patients (2). In surviving patients, AKI predisposes to chronic kidney disease and ultimately end-stage renal disease (3–5). Rodent models have been instrumental in studying the pathobiology of AKI, and diverse methods including sepsis, toxicity, and ischemia have been employed to provoke injury. Ischemia–reperfusion (IR) has been most widely used, and a vast body of knowledge is now available on the response of genetically, pharmacologically, and surgically modified rodents to this highly specific disease model. Significant pathobiological differences have been reported between common forms of human AKI and the rodent IR model, limiting the direct clinical translatability of rodent studies (6). However, despite these limitations, impressive progress has been made in our understanding of the fundamental responses of the kidney to acute injury using this model.

Odyssé Michos (ed.), *Kidney Development: Methods and Protocols*, Methods in Molecular Biology, vol. 886,
DOI 10.1007/978-1-61779-851-1_32, © Springer Science+Business Media, LLC 2012

Although IR injury causes cellular changes throughout the nephron and collecting duct, irreversible damage resulting in apoptotic and necrotic cell death (acute tubular necrosis) is largely restricted to the S3 or straight segment of the proximal tubule (Fig. 1) (7, 8). This remarkably localized cell death results in sloughing of epithelial cells into the tubule lumen and formation of protein casts that block the passage of filtrate through the nephron. Approximately 24 h after the ischemic insult, extensive cell proliferation can be seen in the proximal tubule lumen, and this proliferative response continues until approximately 120 h after the insult (8, 9). Activation of cellular markers of dedifferentiation in tubule epithelial cells occurs concomitantly with this proliferative

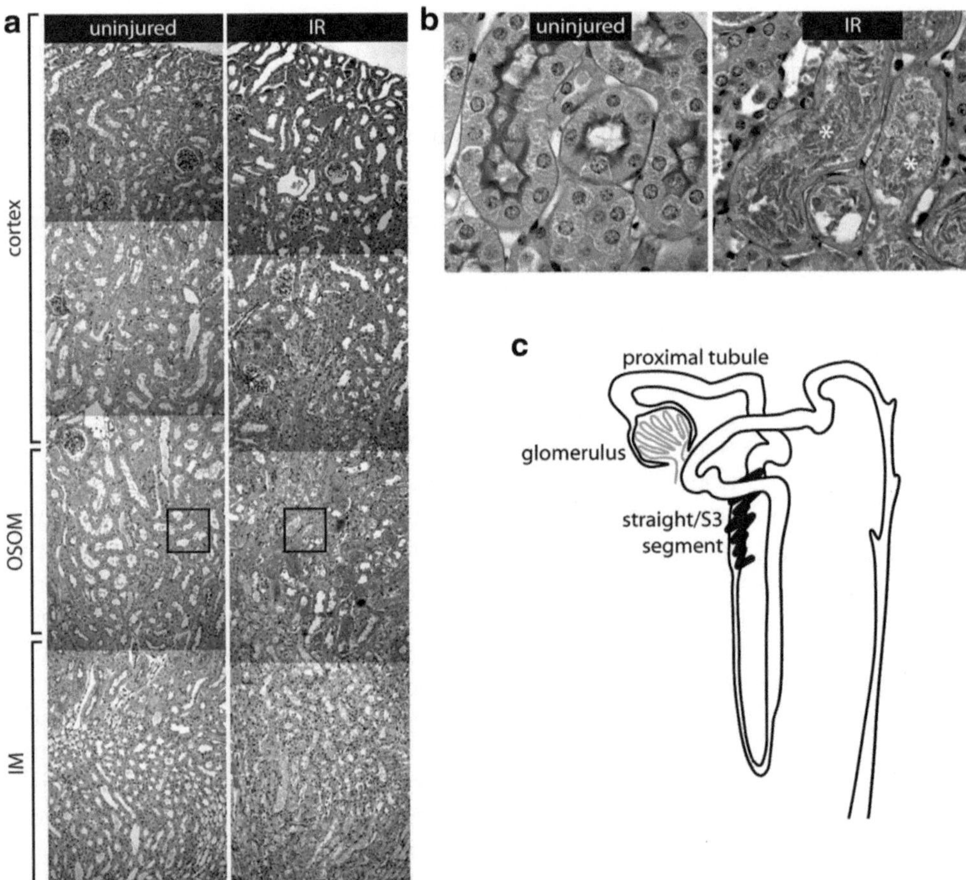

Fig. 1. Kidney injury following transient ischemia. Wild-type ICR mice were subjected to 30 min ischemia and kidneys were harvested after 24 h of perfusion for histological processing and Periodic Acidic Schiff (PAS) histochemical staining. (**a**) Tiled histological images of uninjured control and ischemically injured kidneys show tubule blockage primarily in the outer stripe of the outer medulla (OSOM). *Boxed regions* are enlarged in (**b**). Straight segments of the proximal tubule are highly enriched in the OSOM of the mouse kidney, and IR injury is characteristic in this zone. In the uninjured kidney, intact tubules with strong apical PAS staining are tightly packed. In the IR injured OSOM, many tubules contain protein casts (*asterisks*), and little apical PAS staining can be detected. (**c**) Schematic representation of a nephron indicating showing the straight or S3 segment of the proximal tubule (*black fill*) where the majority of epithelial cell death is seen in the IR injured kidney.

response: for example, Vimentin, Clusterin, and c-Fos are expressed, as is the developmental regulator PAX2 which is normally restricted to the collecting duct epithelium in adults (9, 10). Genetic lineage marking experiments have shown that the cells that repopulate the proximal tubule derive from nephron epithelial cells, rather than neighboring or circulating progenitor cells (11). Using a novel cell labeling approach, Humphreys et al. have shown that sublethally injured proximal tubule epithelial cells are the progenitors for repopulating epithelial cells in this form of injury rather than a specialized progenitor cell population within the nephron (12). Thus, the regenerative process within the nephron is well described, and many groups are currently working toward an understanding of the molecular mechanisms underlying this clinically significant phenomenon.

Depending on the severity of the ischemic insult, acute IR injury can either resolve with regeneration of damaged tubules, or it can progress to chronic kidney disease with interstitial fibrosis (13). Although surviving proximal tubule epithelial cells proliferate comparably in response to diverse degrees of ischemic injury, severe ischemia predisposes to interstitial fibrosis (14). In the bilaterally injured mouse, moderate ischemic injury (30 min in these studies) results in a regenerative response and resolution of injury, whereas severe ischemic injury (32 min) results in a fibrotic outcome. Surprisingly, a different response is seen in unilaterally injured mice in which moderate ischemic injury predisposes to a fibrotic outcome. Removal of the uninjured kidney within the first 48 h after ischemia reverses this effect, suggesting that the fibrotic response may in some way be regulated by signals from the contralateral uninjured kidney during the early phase of recovery. This key difference is important in the interpretation of long-term outcomes of these IR injury models.

In this methods description, we provide a step-by-step procedure for bilateral and unilateral renal ischemia reperfusion. The procedure is in principle quite simple, and the main challenge in developing proficiency with this model is achieving consistency. Minor differences in parameters such as surgery time, body temperature, and hydration profoundly influence the outcome of renal IR, and extensive practice is required to ensure that interpretable data is generated.

2. Materials

1. DC temperature control system (FHC Inc, 40-90-8). Similar systems are available from other vendors of rodent physiology equipment such as Harvard Apparatus and CWE Inc.
2. Heating pad (for postoperative warming) (Braintree Scientific).

3. Scissors:
   (a) 1 pair iris scissors.
   (b) 1 pair dissecting scissors.
4. Forceps:
   (a) 1 pair tissue forceps.
   (b) 1 pair dissecting forceps.
   (c) 2 pairs blunt forceps.
5. 2 Micro clamps (S&T Vascular Clamps, Straight/11mm, Fine Science Tools).
6. Micro clamp holding forceps (S&T CAF4L Clamp Applying Forceps, Fine Science Tools).
7. Needle holder.
8. Absorbable suture material: Ethicon Vicryl 5-0.
9. Nonabsorbable suture material: Ethicon Ethilon 5-0.
10. Weighing scale.
11. Hair clippers.
12. Timer.
13. 1-mL syringes and 26-gauge needles.
14. 0.5-mL insulin syringes.
15. Autoclave and glass bead sterilizer.
16. Betadine.
17. Sterile gauze pads.
18. Surgical drapes.
19. Alcohol wipes.
20. Surgical tape.
21. Sterile gloves.
22. Normal Saline (sterile).
23. Ophthalmic ointment: Dechra Puralube Vet.
24. Buprenorphine: Buprenorphine HCl injection, Bedford Laboratories. (This is a controlled substance, and in the USA its use requires a DEA license).
25. Buprenorphine (working concentration): 0.075 mg/mL diluted in saline.
26. Isoflurane inhalation anesthesia apparatus.

    If ketamine–xylazine injection anesthesia is being used, the following will be required:
27. Ketamine (stock): Ketaset, Fort Dodge. (This is a controlled substance, and in the USA its use requires a DEA license).
28. Xylazine (stock): Xylazine HCl Injection, Teva Animal Health.

29. Atipamezole (stock): Antisedan, Pfizer Animal Health.
30. Ketamine–Xylazine cocktail (working concentration): 21 mg/mL ketamine, 3.2 mg/mL xylazine diluted in saline.
31. Ketamine (working concentration): 16 mg/mL ketamine diluted in saline.
32. Buprenorphine (working concentration): 25 μg/mL diluted in saline.
33. Atipamezole (working concentration): 0.7 μg/mL diluted in saline.

3. Methods

IR surgery requires that you are familiar with the anatomy of the mouse kidney and associated vasculature, which we have illustrated in a simplified form in Fig. 2. The surgical procedure itself can be performed via ventral (laparotomy) or dorsal (retroperitoneal) approaches. We favor the dorsal IR surgery approach because it allows faster recovery times and better survival rates (particularly when you are first learning the procedure). We therefore outline the dorsal IR surgery technique here.

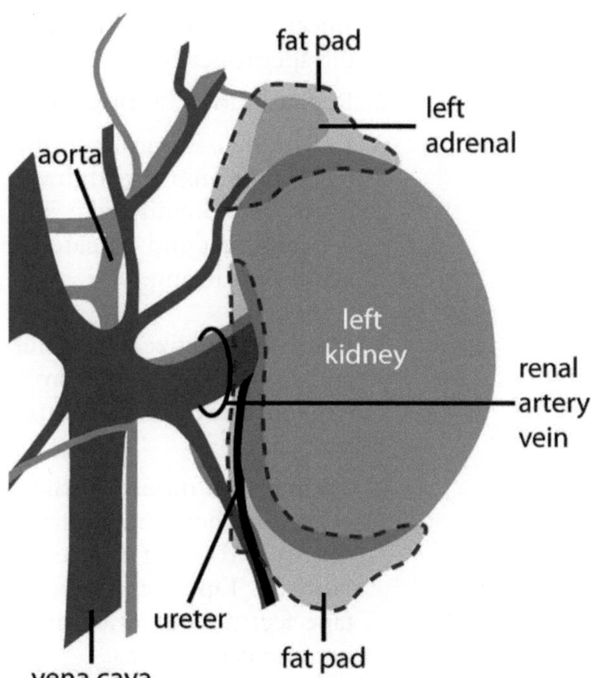

Fig. 2. Ventral image illustrating common anatomy of the mouse kidney.

3.1. Preparation for the Procedure (see Note 1)

1. Sterilize instruments to be used in the procedure by autoclaving. Use a glass bead sterilizer between surgeries after washing the instruments, if you are performing multiple surgeries on different mice. Rinsing in ethanol is not an acceptable method of sterilization.
2. Clean the working area, making sure to separate zones for animal preparation and surgery.
3. Make working solutions of the drugs and warm the saline.
4. Set up the temperature controllers.
5. If mice are operated on in the afternoon, inject 0.5 mL saline subcutaneously 1 h preoperatively (animals will be less well hydrated in the afternoon than the morning).
6. Weigh mice.

3.2. Isoflurane Anesthesia (see Note 2)

1. Administer 15 μL buprenorphine (working solution) per 10 g subcutaneously.
2. Induce surgical anesthesia: wait until mouse breathing rate drops and then make sure that the mouse does not withdraw its limb when a rear paw is pinched. If anesthesia is incomplete increase the percentage of isoflurane.
3. Switch to maintenance of surgical anesthesia and control that the level of anesthesia is maintained by paw pinching.

3.3. Ketamine–Xylazine Anesthesia (See Note 2)

1. Inject 50 μL ketamine–xylazine cocktail per 10 g body weight intraperitoneally.
2. Replace mouse in original cage and do not disturb for 5 min.
3. Ensure that surgical anesthesia is complete by pinching a rear paw. If the animal withdraws, more ketamine–xylazine cocktail must be administered: increments of 25 μL followed by 2–3 min rest and repeated reflex testing are recommended to avoid overdosing.

3.4. Preparation for Surgery

1. Once anesthetized, transfer mouse to the preparation zone and shave entire area from 0.5 cm cranial to the last rib to the base of the tail, and ventrally to expose the entire flank on both sides.
2. Transfer the mouse to the surgical area and place the mouse prone on the temperature control pad (covered with surgical drape) and insert the rectal probe, taping it to the tail (see Note 3). Tape the legs to the surgical surface. Take care not to tape feet directly onto the heating pad, since it can get quite hot and cause burns.
3. Apply ophthalmic lubricating ointment to the eyes to prevent drying.

4. Scrub the exposed skin three times with gauze soaked in betadine, cleaning off each time with alcohol wipes, making sure that stray hairs are cleaned off, and with the last wipe ensure that all of the residual betadine has been removed.
5. Cover surgical field with sterile surgical drape. It will help prevent stray hair from entering the surgical field and provide an area on which to lay sterile instruments during surgery.
6. Allow core temperature to stabilize at 36.5–37°C; this should take approximately 5 min.
7. If you are using ketamine–xylazine anesthesia, inject 20 μL ketamine (working concentration) per 10 g subcutaneously immediately before surgery, to ensure that the duration of surgical anesthesia is sufficient.

3.5. Surgery (See Note 4)

1. Locate the most caudal rib by palpation and locate a reference point approximately 3 mm caudal to the last rib.
2. Using iris scissors and tissue forceps cut a 1.5-cm skin incision running along the midline caudally from the reference point toward the tail.
3. Separate skin and subcutaneous layers over the left and right dorsal sides through this incision by blunt dissection using dissecting scissors and dissecting forceps.
4. Using tissue forceps and iris scissors make a small incision through the left flank muscle and fascia above the kidney and exteriorize the left kidney (see Note 5).
5. Irrigate the kidney with warmed sterile saline.
6. Carefully hold the kidney using blunt forceps while releasing the renal pedicle from surrounding fat tissue using another pair of blunt forceps (Fig. 3a, see Note 6).

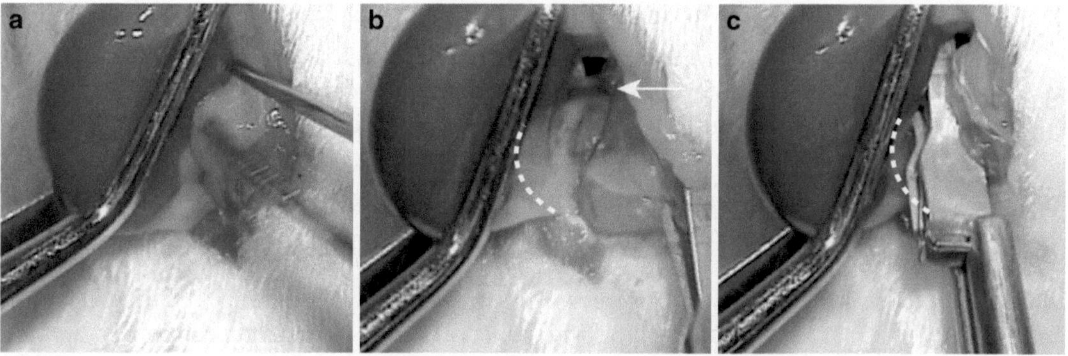

Fig. 3. Exposure and clamping of the mouse kidney vascular sheath. (**a**) The left kidney is held gently using blunt forceps while perinephric fat is carefully removed using forceps. (**b**) Exposed left kidney vascular sheath (*white arrow*) demonstrates large renal vein, and smaller caliber main renal artery lying just above the renal vein. The *white dotted line* marks the expected position of the ureter within the hilar fat pad. (**c**) Applying micro clamp to the left kidney using clamp holder.

7. While holding the kidney up by resting it between the shanks of the forceps, carefully apply the micro clamp to the exposed renal vascular sheath (Fig. 3b, c, see Note 7). Start timer immediately upon application (see Note 8).
8. The kidney should change to a darker color within 1–2 min of clamp application. If there is no color change, the clamp is not properly applied.
9. With the clamp attached, return the kidney carefully into the retroperitoneal space so that it does not dry out.
10. Repeat the procedure for the right kidney, setting a different timer (see Note 9 for unilateral injury).
11. After both kidneys have been clamped, cover the skin incision in saline-soaked gauze to prevent drying.
12. At the end of the ischemic period remove the left kidney from the body cavity and irrigate it with warmed saline. The organ should have a dark purple color. Animals that do not display a marked color change should be excluded from the study.
13. Gently remove the micro clamp. The kidney should return to normal color within a minute or two. Animals that do not display this color change possibly have a vascular rupture or clot and should be excluded from the study.
14. Close the muscle layer using absorbable suture while waiting on timer for the right kidney.
15. Repeat procedure on the right side.
16. Close muscle layer using absorbable suture, and close the skin incision using nonabsorbable suture material.
17. Inject 0.7 mL prewarmed saline subcutaneously to compensate for the loss of body fluid during surgery. If you have already given 0.5 mL preoperatively, only give 0.2 mL.
18. If isoflurane anesthesia was used: inject 30 μL buprenorphine (working solution) per 10 g subcutaneously.
19. If ketamine–xylazine anesthesia was used: inject 45 μL buprenorphine (working solution) per 10 g subcutaneously, and 15 μL atipamezole (working concentration) per 10 g subcutaneously.
20. Place the mouse in a clean cage on a heating pad and monitor until it wakes up.

3.6. Postoperative Care

1. Monitor mice three times daily, injecting 75 μL buprenorphine (working solution) per 10 g subcutaneously at 12 h intervals for the first 48 h. After this time, buprenorphine should only be administered to animals showing signs of pain and discomfort.

4. Notes

1. Mouse numbers for surgery: The procedure description is for a single animal and it is recommended that mice be operated one at a time until a relatively high level of proficiency is attained. At this point surgery can be performed on several animals simultaneously. With experience, batches of five animals can be operated comfortably.
2. Anesthesia: Two alternative methods are given: isoflurane inhalation anesthesia and ketamine–xylazine injection anesthesia. Inhalation anesthesia is preferable for performing single surgeries, since it is rapidly reversible. Because isoflurane does not have analgesic properties, buprenorphine needs to be administered preoperatively. To avoid oversedating the mice, one third the full dose of buprenorphine is given preoperatively and the remaining two third after skin closure. For surgery sessions in which multiple procedures are batched, or in facilities that do not have access to inhalation anesthesia apparatus, ketamine–xylazine injection anesthesia can be used. Atipamezole functions as an antidote to xylazine and speeds recovery from anesthesia. Its use is not essential to the success of the procedure. Despite the general guidelines provided above, dosing may require adjustment for particular strains of animals.
3. Temperature control: The feedback based temperature control system used in this procedure maintains mouse core temperature with a tolerance of approximately 0.5°C throughout surgery. Although it represents a significant investment, this degree of precision is essential to ensure consistent results. Outcomes of IR injury conducted at different body temperatures vary widely (15), and accurate temperature control in small rodents is extremely challenging due to their high surface area to volume ratio.
4. Surgical technique: Sterile technique should be employed as specified by the standards of practice for the institution at which the procedure is being performed. Basic sterile technique includes the use of sterilized instruments, sterile surgical gloves, and the establishment of a sterile zone on which instruments can be placed while they are not in use.
5. Retrieval of the kidney from the retroperitoneal space: consistently locating the kidney in the body cavity of a prone mouse may be the most challenging aspect of this method. To establish a feeling for the location of the organ, practice on recently sacrificed mice placed in a prone position is strongly recommended prior to embarking on surgery. When retrieving the kidney from the body cavity, it is easy to traumatize the organ or

the vascular pedicle by applying too much pressure with the forceps. Therefore sham controls should be included in the experiment in which all steps are performed with the exception of renal pedicle clamping. If histopathology and/or clinical chemistry indicate traumatic damage in sham controls, try using saline soaked cotton tipped applicators instead of forceps to retrieve the kidney.

6. Exposure of the renal vesicle for clamping: note that the two key purposes of this dissection are:
   (a) To separate artery/vein from the lower part of the hilum that includes the ureter (which will not be clamped in this procedure); and
   (b) To remove excess fat which would get in the way of the vessel clamp and reduce compression of the artery and vein. The latter is essential to the success and reproducibility of the experiment. Note also that that the vein is above the artery and is the most prominent (and dark) vessel. The artery has a smaller caliber, is quite difficult to see, looks pinkish and lies just above the vein in a common vascular sheath (Figs. 2 and 3b). Do not attempt to separate artery and vein for mouse IR surgery, since this is technically difficult.
7. Micro clamps: the choice of clamp is critical to the outcome of the procedure, and clamps from different vendors vary in pressure ratings. The micro clamps in this protocol provide relatively low closing pressures of 5–15 g depending on vessel size. This contrasts with other protocols using Roboz Micro Clips, which provide 70 g pressure (note that Roboz Micro Clip Applying Forceps are required to apply these). Anecdotal experience from our laboratories indicates that the latter require substantially shorter ischemia times and induce more severe renal injury. The Fine Science Tools clamps we describe in this protocol exert graduated pressure, so you need to be sure that you apply the clamp each time at the same point, otherwise pressures will differ between kidneys. To a large extent, the efficiency of the clamps also depends on how much perihilar fat and tissue you include with the vessels when you place the clamps, and this is additionally affected by the angle at which the clamps are placed. These clamps come in different sizes: the 3.5 × 1.5 mm clamp in the protocol is recommended for mice weighing 30–38 g. 7.5 × 1.75 mm clamps should be used for larger mice, and 3.5 × 1 mm clamps for smaller mice. Once the optimal method and time for clamping have been established for your mouse strain in your hands, you should not change the brand of clamp, since this will affect the degree of vascular occlusion. Because the compression of the clamps changes with wear, it is recommended that they be renewed every ten procedures.

8. Ischemia times: because of technical variations between operators and facilities, it is not possible to give exact reference times for ischemia. Based on our experience, suggested starting points for calibration of times in the male mouse would be 26 min for moderate injury and 35 min for severe injury.
9. Unilateral injury: the method description for bilateral injury is followed, but only one kidney is clamped. Although the contralateral uninjured kidney provides interesting study material, it cannot substitute for a sham control because it undergoes physiological changes following clamping of the other kidney (16).

IR surgery can be performed on mice of almost any age and size by a skilled surgeon. However, anecdotal experience from our two centers indicates that technical issues limit speed of surgery and consistency of outcomes in obese mice, and that mice under 10 weeks of age have increased perioperative mortality. It is therefore recommended that lean mice around 12 weeks of age be selected for surgery. It is very tempting to perform a pilot experiment using mice of varying ages, genders, and sizes that are not being used for other purposes. This type of experiment is not recommended, especially for the less experienced surgeon, because experimental variation will be too great to draw any robust conclusions. Considering the time, effort, and cost associated with an IR experiment, it is worth breeding a cohort of gender- and age-matched mice specifically for the experiment. The following are some important parameters that should be considered in the selection of animals for an IR experiment.

Sample size. The number of animals required to draw a statistically robust conclusion from an experiment will of course vary depending on the magnitude of the effect and variability of outcomes between animals. The latter is operator dependent: the better the surgical technique and care of the animals, the greater the consistency. As a simple guide we recommend a two-step process in which outcomes of a pilot experiment with five animals per group are used as the basis for a calculation of final group size for the experiment. Quantitative outcomes of the pilot experiment will enable a power analysis from which an appropriate group size can be determined. For a pilot experiment aiming to analyze five animals, surgery on six gender- and age-matched animals is recommended in case an individual mouse has to be excluded at the time of surgery. Note that many studies will require 10–15 mice per group to reliably detect (or exclude) statistically significant differences between groups.

Age. Surgery on young adult mice of 12 weeks age generally results in the most consistent data. As mice age they tend to deposit extensive intra-abdominal fat which makes surgery more difficult and more variable. Fat deposition varies between strains and facilities, and some experimentation may be required to define the best age for IR for a particular series of experiments. Old mice (18–24 months) develop more severe injury and have reduced regenerative capacity compared to younger mice (3 months) (17, 18). For very young mice, the small size of the animal demands a steady hand and perioperative mortality tends to be high.

Strain. In general, strains or stocks with high body fat deposition are more challenging to use for surgery. Furthermore, some intrinsic differences in the response to injury between genetic backgrounds has been reported, with out-bred NIH Swiss mice displaying a more rapid return to baseline blood urea nitrogen values after ischemia than the BALB/c and C57BL/6 inbred strains (19). We have experience in our centers using BALB/c, C57BL/6, 129, FVB, and out-bred CD1 (or ICR) backgrounds. It is unfortunately not possible to prescribe ischemic times for each strain of mouse, since these times are significantly affected by minor technical differences between operators. To avoid confounding genetic influences, it is therefore essential not only to establish sensitivity of the particular strain to IR injury in your own hands but also to restrict comparisons within an experiment to mice of identical genetic background. In the case that animals on mixed and undefined backgrounds are being analyzed, littermates should be used as controls.

Gender. Gender is a major influence on the outcome of IR, with males displaying much greater susceptibility to injury than females. Therefore, it is very important to restrict comparisons within an experiment to a single gender. This gender difference is testosterone-dependent as castration of males decreases their susceptibility to IR injury, and testosterone treatment of females has the inverse effect (20). Surgically, the approach to IR injury in the female using flank incision is slightly more complicated than the male because the ovary must be displaced before the kidney can be accessed. For this reason, it is recommended that male mice be used until a degree of proficiency with the technique has been attained.

Evaluation of renal function by measurement of blood urea nitrogen and/or serum creatinine levels is an important component of most bilateral IR experiments, but care must be taken to limit the influence of blood sampling on the outcome of IR. In unilateral IR, compensation by the uninjured kidney precludes evaluation of function. It is recommended that blood volumes as small as possible be drawn, with a maximum bleed volume for a 30 g mouse of 200 μL (approximately 10% of the blood volume) once a week, which should provide 75–100 μL of serum. Therefore choice and timing of renal function tests (each with different blood volume requirements) using serum samples should be carefully considered. For example, if larger volumes of blood have to be drawn preoperatively, for example for a serum creatinine assay using HPLC (*see* below), these should be taken at least a week before surgery to allow the mouse time to recover from intravascular volume depletion prior to IR surgery.

Blood urea nitrogen (BUN) is the simplest assay that can be performed in-house using one of a number of different commercially available microplate colorimetric assays on as little as 5 μL of serum per sample. Impairment of renal function causes accumulation of circulating BUN, and the level of BUN largely correlates with the severity of renal injury and recovery following bilateral IR injury. The disadvantages of BUN measurements however are twofold:

1. BUN increases in response to dehydration (prerenal renal failure) so that the levels of BUN may be artificially increased if the mouse does not drink sufficiently during the postoperative period.
2. Anecdotally, we have found that the level of BUN does not correlate with the severity of injury following bilateral IR surgery (as verified by serum creatinine levels), when BUN values are substantially higher than 100–120 mg/dL. Therefore, it is of limited value in tracking severity or recovery from severe AKI following bilateral IR surgery.

Serum creatinine provides a more robust measure of renal function that is less affected by the hydration status of the animal that BUN. However, since creatinine is generated from muscle tissue, lower levels of serum creatinine may be generated in older mice that have lower muscle mass. Traditional assays for serum creatinine using the Jaffe reaction accurately measure serum creatinine in rat and human samples using small volumes of serum, but greatly overestimate serum creatinine levels in mice due to the presence of noncreatinine chromogens in mouse serum (21, 22). This effect is particularly pronounced in mice with normal renal function (up to 6× the level of serum creatinine is detected with the Jaffe method compared with the HPLC-method (22)). Serial analyses of creatinine levels using the Jaffe reaction in mice following bilateral IR surgery will thus tend to give a skewed result as renal function improves. Alternative assays for serum creatinine measurement in mice have been described and are available at a number of institutions on fee a basis. The original description of HPLC-based assays for serum creatinine measurement in mice required approximately 25 μL of serum per sample (21). These assays should be performed in duplicate so that approximately 50 μL of serum or 100 μL of blood must be used for each assay. Since the original description, more sensitive HPLC-based assays have been described that can utilize as little as 5 μL of serum per sample (22). In addition, more recently a liquid chromatography mass spectrometry (LC-MS) method has been developed to measure creatinine using small volumes of serum (23). This assay has also been developed for use in mice and is available on a fee basis in certain institutions.

Glomerular filtration rate (GFR): definitive analysis of renal function by measuring GFR can be performed in conscious mice by FITC-inulin clearance studies (24). These studies can be performed relatively inexpensively in-house, but require that the mouse be immobilized, injected with FITC-conjugated inulin and then have serial 20 μL blood samples drawn over a 75 min period (7 × 20 μL blood = 140 μL per assay). FITC-conjugated inulin can then be quantified using a microplate reader fluorometer. As outlined above, since these studies involve drawing a significant amount of blood they should only be performed preoperatively (more than 1 week before surgery) or as a terminal procedure at the end of the study.

The end-point of most IR experiments is analysis of kidney tissue after sacrifice. Quantitative analyses can be based on scoring of pathological change or expression of RNA and/or protein biomarkers. Standardizing an approach for a series of experiments will ensure that appropriate comparisons can be made between animals. The kidney is highly regionalized, and it is possible to entirely miss important changes in the inner medulla if histological sections are prepared from the pole of the kidney.

Tissue preparation: we have developed a standardized approach for harvest of kidneys for these different assays. Since immunofluorescence studies (for example to detect cell proliferation or de-differentiation markers) depend on thorough and uniform fixation of tissue prior to embedding, we perfusion fix one of the kidneys in vivo. For this, the mouse is first anesthetized (using ketamine–xylazine or inhaled isoflurane). The hilum of the left kidney is tied off using nonabsorbable suture material and the pedicle cut distal to the ligature so that the mouse does not exsanguinate. This kidney is prepared as shown in Fig. 4 as it provides RNA, protein,

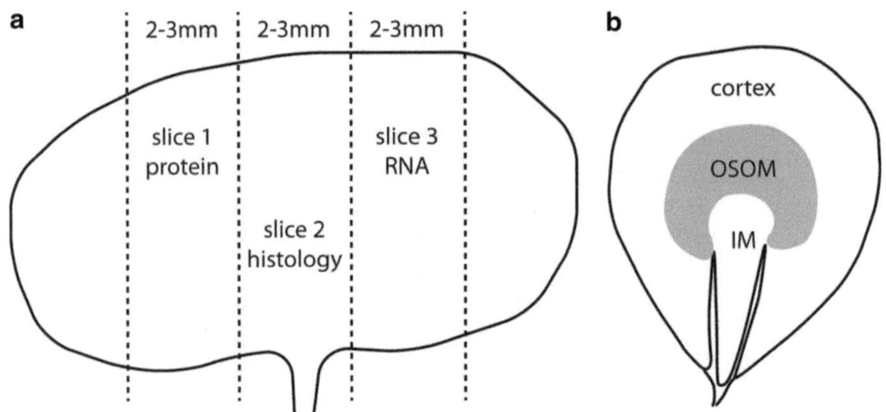

Fig. 4. Schematic representation of a generalized tissue harvest approach. (**a**) Sagittal view of a kidney showing the placement of four incisions with a sharp razor blade or scalpel (*dashed lines*). All three slices will contain tissue from the cortex, outer medulla, and inner medulla. (**b**) Schematic representation of a histological section cut from slice two: cortex, outer stripe of outer medulla (OSOM), and inner medulla (IM) are represented.

and histology with representation of each zone of the kidney. All three samples are seldom required for any one experiment, but banking them provides a great resource for future studies, and can significantly decrease animal usage. Having removed the left kidney, the chest wall is opened and the left ventricle punctured with a 23-gauge butterfly needle and perfused with normal saline at a pressure of 20–30 cm of water while the heart is still beating. Immediately after setting up the infusion, the right ventricle is punctured so allow for replacement of the whole mouse blood volume with saline. This normally requires approximately 10 mL until the returning fluid is clear. Then normal saline is replaced with 10% formalin and perfusion is continued for another 10 mL. The right kidney is then removed, cut horizontally (as shown in Fig. 4), and the central portion fixed for 4 h in 10% formalin before washing in normal saline prior to paraffin embedding. Note that since this procedure requires use of quite large volumes of 10% formalin, it has to be performed in a fume cabinet.

RNA: nucleic acids can be prepared from kidney tissue using standard procedures. Because of the instability of RNA it is advisable to process tissue from each mouse immediately and to avoid storing the tissue sample on ice for extended periods of time. Alternatively, the tissue sample can be snap frozen and stored at –80°C for future use. Tissue from adult animals is generally quite challenging to homogenize for a representative nucleic acid preparation compared to embryonic tissue or cultured cells. Therefore, we either use a manual Dounce homogenizer or an automated Autogen tissue homogenizer for sample preparation. Transcripts of interest can be analyzed by a variety of standard techniques. Two transcripts are particularly noteworthy since they are widely used as quantitative markers of injury in both the unilateral and bilateral IR models: Kidney injury marker 1 (human: KIM1, mouse: Havcrl) (25, 26), and Neutrophil gelatinase-associated lipocalin (human: NGAL, mouse: Lcn2) (27, 28). The Havcrl assay is routinely used in our facilities, and oligonucleotide sequences for qPCR analysis are Havcrl forward, 5′-TCGTGTCACC TATCAGAAGA GC-3′, Havcrl reverse, 5′-ACAATACAGA CCACTGTCAC TC-3′. QPCR analysis is performed on cDNA with iQ SYBR Green SuperMix (BioRad, 170–8880) on a MyiQ real-time detection system (BioRad). Cycling parameters are 95°C for 15 s, 55°C for 45 s.

Protein: standard methods for protein purification can be used with kidney tissue. Tissue dissociation can be challenging, and we freeze tissue immediately in liquid nitrogen, pulverize using a mortar and pestle, and resuspend in SDS-PAGE sample cocktail. Alternatively, use of a Dounce homogenizer is possible.

Histology: in our experience, the main challenge in obtaining good histological material is tissue fixation. We generally work with 10% formalin or 4% paraformaldehyde fixation, as these fixatives allow detection of both protein and RNA. As noted above, perfusion fixed tissue is used for immunohistochemical studies. Moreover, our experience suggests that tissue morphology for histological analysis is best preserved in nonperfused tissue samples, so we use the excised right kidney samples for histochemical analyses. We have found that slicing the tissue as shown in Fig. 4 greatly facilitates penetration of these fixatives, limiting fixation time to approximately 4 h at 4°C. Samples in which whole or half kidneys are fixed using formalin require such long fixation times that the cortex is generally overfixed and the medulla shows signs of postmortem degradation. Alternate fixatives such as Bouin's may improve morphology, especially in larger tissue samples, but because they compromise antigen and RNA detection we avoid using them. Tissue stains of particular interest include Hematoxylin–Eosin (H&E) for general histology, Periodic Acidic Schiff's (PAS) which strongly stains carbohydrates on the surface of proximal tubule epithelial cells and is useful to assess tubular injury (Fig. 1), and Trichrome or Sirus Red, which enable quantitative analysis of collagen deposition.

References

1. Himmelfarb J, Ikizler TA (2007) Acute kidney injury: changing lexicography, definitions, and epidemiology. Kidney Int 71:971–976
2. Palevsky PM, Zhang JH, O'Connor TZ et al (2008) Intensity of renal support in critically ill patients with acute kidney injury. N Engl J Med 359:7–20
3. Lo LJ, Go AS, Chertow GM et al (2009) Dialysis-requiring acute renal failure increases the risk of progressive chronic kidney disease. Kidney Int 76:893–899
4. Lafrance JP, Miller DR (2010) Acute kidney injury associates with increased long-term mortality. J Am Soc Nephrol 21:345–352
5. Ishani A, Xue JL, Himmelfarb J et al (2009) Acute kidney injury increases risk of ESRD among elderly. J Am Soc Nephrol 20: 223–228
6. Heyman SN, Rosenberger C, Rosen S (2010) Experimental ischemia-reperfusion: biases and myths-the proximal vs. distal hypoxic tubular injury debate revisited. Kidney Int 77:9–16
7. Hanley MJ (1980) Isolated nephron segments in a rabbit model of ischemic acute renal failure. Am J Physiol 239:F17–F23
8. Venkatachalam MA, Bernard DB, Donohoe JF, Levinsky NG (1978) Ischemic damage and repair in the rat proximal tubule: differences among the S1, S2, and S3 segments. Kidney Int 14:31–49
9. Witzgall R, Brown D, Schwarz C, Bonventre JV (1994) Localization of proliferating cell nuclear antigen, vimentin, c-Fos, and clusterin in the postischemic kidney. Evidence for a heterogenous genetic response among nephron segments, and a large pool of mitotically active and dedifferentiated cells. J Clin Invest 93:2175–2188
10. Imgrund M, Grone E, Grone H et al (1999) Re-expression of the developmental gene Pax-2 during experimental acute tubular necrosis in mice 1. Kidney Int 56:1423–1431
11. Humphreys BD, Valerius MT, Kobayashi A et al (2008) Intrinsic epithelial cells repair the kidney after injury. Cell Stem Cell 2:284–291
12. Humphreys BD, Czerniak S, Dirocco DP et al (2011) Repair of injured proximal tubule does not involve specialized progenitors. Proc Natl Acad Sci USA 108(22):9226–9231
13. Burne-Taney MJ, Yokota N, Rabb H (2005) Persistent renal and extrarenal immune changes after severe ischemic injury. Kidney Int 67: 1002–1009
14. Yang L, Besschetnova TY, Brooks CR, Shah JV, Bonventre JV (2010) Epithelial cell cycle arrest in G2/M mediates kidney fibrosis after injury. Nat Med 16:535–543, 531p following 143
15. Delbridge MS, Shrestha BM, Raftery AT, El NAM, Haylor JL (2007) The effect of body temperature in a rat model of renal ischemia-reperfusion injury. Transplant Proc 39:2983–2985
16. Lin J, Patel SR, Cheng X et al (2005) Kielin/chordin-like protein, a novel enhancer of BMP

signaling, attenuates renal fibrotic disease. Nat Med 11:387–393

17. Schmitt R, Marlier A, Cantley LG (2008) Zag expression during aging suppresses proliferation after kidney injury. J Am Soc Nephrol 19:2375–2383
18. Schmitt R, Cantley LG (2008) The impact of aging on kidney repair. Am J Physiol Renal Physiol 294:F1265–F1272
19. Burne MJ, Haq M, Matsuse H, Mohapatra S, Rabb H (2000) Genetic susceptibility to renal ischemia reperfusion injury revealed in a murine model. Transplantation 69:1023–1025
20. Park KM, Kim JI, Ahn Y, Bonventre AJ, Bonventre JV (2004) Testosterone is responsible for enhanced susceptibility of males to ischemic renal injury. J Biol Chem 279: 52282–52292
21. Dunn SR, Qi Z, Bottinger EP, Breyer MD, Sharma K (2004) Utility of endogenous creatinine clearance as a measure of renal function in mice. Kidney Int 65:1959–1967
22. Yuen PS, Dunn SR, Miyaji T et al (2004) A simplified method for HPLC determination of creatinine in mouse serum. Am J Physiol Renal Physiol 286:F1116–F1119
23. Hetu PO, Gingras ME, Vinet B (2010) Development and validation of a rapid liquid chromatography isotope dilution tandem mass spectrometry (LC-IDMS/MS) method for serum creatinine. Clin Biochem 43: 1158–1162
24. Qi Z, Whitt I, Mehta A et al (2004) Serial determination of glomerular filtration rate in conscious mice using FITC-inulin clearance. Am J Physiol Renal Physiol 286:F590–F596
25. Kuehn EW, Park KM, Somlo S, Bonventre JV (2002) Kidney injury molecule-1 expression in murine polycystic kidney disease. Am J Physiol Renal Physiol 283:F1326–F1336
26. Ichimura T, Bonventre JV, Bailly V et al (1998) Kidney injury molecule-1 (KIM-1), a putative epithelial cell adhesion molecule containing a novel immunoglobulin domain, is up-regulated in renal cells after injury. J Biol Chem 273:4135–4142
27. Mishra J, Ma Q, Prada A et al (2003) Identification of neutrophil gelatinase-associated lipocalin as a novel early urinary biomarker for ischemic renal injury. J Am Soc Nephrol 14:2534–2543
28. Paragas N, Qiu A, Zhang Q et al (2011) The Ngal reporter mouse detects the response of the kidney to injury in real time. Nat Med 17:216–222

Chapter 33

Variable Partial Unilateral Ureteral Obstruction and Its Release in the Neonatal and Adult Mouse

Barbara A. Thornhill and Robert L. Chevalier

Abstract

Obstructive nephropathy is the most important cause of renal failure in children. Unilateral ureteral obstruction (UUO) in the neonatal mouse provides a useful model to investigate the response of the developing kidney to urine flow obstruction. Creation of reversible variable partial UUO (compared to complete UUO) more closely approximates congenital lesions, and permits the study of recovery following release of the obstruction. Implementation of this technique requires the appropriate optical, surgical, and anesthetic equipment, as well as adaptations appropriate to the very small animals undergoing surgical procedures. Care of the pups must include minimizing trauma to delicate tissues, close monitoring of anesthesia and body temperature, and ensuring acceptance of the pups by the mother. It is important to document the severity and patency of the partial UUO by ureteral measurement and pelvic injection of India ink. Finally, removal of kidneys for histologic examination should be accomplished with gentle handling and processing.

Key words: Ureteral obstruction, Kidney, Neonate, Mouse, Recovery, Remodeling, Fibrosis, Apoptosis

1. Introduction

1.1. Models of Partial Neonatal Ureteral Obstruction

Surgical unilateral ureteral obstruction (UUO) in the rodent has become the most widely used animal model of progressive renal disease and of obstructive nephropathy (1). Because clinical obstructive nephropathy entails partial, rather than complete, urinary tract obstruction, we initially developed a model of variable chronic partial UUO in the neonatal rat (2). The major advantages of the model are the reproducibility of the variable obstruction, the lack of injury to the ureter at the point of stenosis, and the opportunity to make serial measurements over time. This study shows that tubular atrophy and interstitial fibrosis are less severe following 14 days partial UUO than complete UUO (2). Notably, growth

Odyssé Michos (ed.), *Kidney Development: Methods and Protocols*, Methods in Molecular Biology, vol. 886, DOI 10.1007/978-1-61779-851-1_33, © Springer Science+Business Media, LLC 2012

of the obstructed kidney is significantly impaired at a critical degree of ureteral stenosis (approximately 70% reduction in ureteral diameter), such that renal growth is preserved with stenosis less than 60%, but markedly impaired by more severe stenosis (2). Nephrons are progressively lost between 14 and 28 days of partial UUO in the neonatal rat (2), indicating ongoing injury in the presence of persistent obstruction.

1.2. Recovery Following Relief of Obstruction

The severity of renal injury from UUO in the developing kidney is dependent on both the severity of obstruction and the duration of obstruction (2–5). Any delay in surgical relief of obstruction is associated with progressive deterioration of function (6). While surgical relief of complete UUO removes the primary stimulus for ongoing injury, recovery is incomplete, with persistent residual interstitial lesions (4). Five days of complete UUO in the neonatal rat reduces the number of glomeruli by 50% after 1 month of recovery, whereas 2 or 3 days obstruction has a minor impact (7). Although 1 month of recovery following the relief of obstruction attenuates the renal cellular injury, alterations persist in the renal vasculature, tubules, and interstitium, with a persistent reduction in the number of nephrons (4). Although the glomerular filtration rate of the postobstructed kidney is normal at 1 month (indicating hyperfiltration by remaining nephrons) (4), after 1 year following relief of obstruction, glomerular filtration rate is decreased by 80% and proteinuria has developed (8). Notably, glomerular sclerosis, tubular atrophy, and interstitial fibrosis are increased in both hydronephrotic and contralateral kidneys at this time (8). This indicates late progression of the renal lesions. Temporary complete UUO during the period of renal maturation following nephrogenesis also leads to significant renal injury, including a reduction in number of glomeruli (7).

We have subsequently developed a model of surgically induced partial UUO in the neonatal mouse, in which relief after 5 days obstruction results by 21 days in tubular apoptosis, tubular atrophy, formation of atubular glomeruli, and interstitial fibrosis. However, after survival to 42 days, the renal parenchyma of the postobstructed kidney undergoes remarkable remodeling, with virtually complete resolution of tubular atrophy and interstitial fibrosis (9). Compared to sham-operated mice, persistent chronic partial UUO impairs growth of the obstructed kidney and induces compensatory growth of the contralateral kidney. Relief of obstruction normalizes growth of both kidneys, whose weight is not different from that of sham-operated animals. The use of this model of obstructive nephropathy permits the study not only of the cellular response of the obstructed and recovering postobstructed kidney, but also of the adaptation of the contralateral kidney. This is important in view of functional or cellular changes in the contralateral kidney which may mirror those of the obstructed kidney, as in the case of renal vasoconstriction, renin expression, endogenous antioxidant enzymes, or tubular atrophy (10–13). Alternatively, changes in the contralateral kidney may parallel those of the obstructed kidney, as in expression of epidermal growth factor (11), immune modulator genes (14), or kielin/chordin-like protein (KCP), an enhancer of BMP signaling (15). Therefore, while it is tempting to rely on the unobstructed kidney as a control for the obstructed kidney, such findings indicate that sham-operated littermates should be used to account for adaptive changes by the contralateral kidney.

The major procedures described in this chapter include the management of breeding mice and pups, surgical placement of a partial or complete obstruction around one ureter, and release of the obstruction following a period of recovery. The described techniques are performed in an aseptic manner and have been approved by the University of Virginia Institutional Animal Care and Use Committee.

2. Materials

2.1. Equipment

1. Isoflurane vaporizer and flow meter (Stoelting Scientific).
2. Two pressurized oxygen tanks with regulators.
3. Anesthesia scavenger, double armed (Stoelting Scientific).
4. Rodent/feline mask, size small (Stoelting Scientific).
5. Stereomicroscope (Leitz MZ6)–1:6 Zoom, 0.5× objective, 10×121B eyepiece, 9″ working distance (Leica-Microsystems).
6. Light source can be independent or through the microscope.
7. Heated operating surface.
8. Heated postoperative recovery surface.
9. Recovery box for neonatal mice is a lidded pipette tip box with a hole drilled in the lower half to receive tubing from an oxygen tank. This box does not seal tightly, since its purpose is simply to hold the pups in an enriched atmosphere during recovery.

2.2. Instruments

1. One straight iris scissors.
2. Two 45° angle S&T SuperGrip forceps.
3. Two delicate spring action needle holder with lock.
4. One #5 straight or 45° angle Dumont forceps.
5. One McPherson-Vannas scissors (RS-5602) with combined tip width 0.2 or less (Roboz).
6. One laboratory animal microtattoo system (magnifying glass removed).

2.3. Supplies

1. 8-0 Ethilon black monofilament nylon suture (Owens & Minor) (All models).
2. 7-0 Prolene suture (Ethicon) (Owens & Minor)–Pups (All Models).

3. 8-0 Vicryl suture (Ethicon) (Owens & Minor)–Pups (Release Model).
4. 6-0 Prolene suture (Ethicon) (Owens & Minor)–Adults (All Models).
5. 6-0 Vicryl Suture (Ethicon) (Owens & Minor)–Adults (All Models).
6. 0.20 mm Stainless steel wire (SWGX-090-30) (Small Parts, Inc.)–Pups (Partial Model).
7. 0.30 mm Stainless steel wire (SWGX-120-30) (Small Parts, Inc.)–Adults (Partial Model).
8. Opthalmic sponges/Adsorption spears–Pups.
9. 8″ Cotton-tip applicators–Adults.
10. One 30-gauge or 26-gauge ½″ needle for tattooing.
11. Buprenorphine (Buprenex) (Reckitt & Colman Pharmaceutical, Inc.).
12. Bupivacaine (Hospira, Inc).
13. Euthasol solution (Virbac).

3. Methods

3.1. Anesthesia/ Surgical Preparation

1. The anesthesia scavenger used here has two arms. One arm is fixed to the surgery table with tape, so that the head of the mouse is pointed away from the surgeon and the mouse is lying with its left side up. The finger of a sterile glove is cut 2–3 cm long with the tip cut out sufficiently for the mouse's head to fit inside, and is attached to the inner tube of the surgery arm with a small rubber band (Fig. 1).
2. Pre-anesthesia chamber for neonates. The narrow end of a 10 cm plastic funnel is cut off so that it fits over the end of the outside tube of the second arm of the scavenger. This directs escaping anesthesia into the scavenger. A small rodent/feline mask is inserted into the inner tube. Tape can be wrapped around the male end of the mask to ensure a snug fit in the tube. The mask should not be inserted so far into the tube that the bulbous end occludes the vacuum flow through the outer tube. The palm of a latex glove is cut to fit over the wide end of the mask to form a diaphragm. The mouse is inserted into the mask and the rubber mask ring is fixed over the diaphragm to keep it in place. A small slit is made in the center of the diaphragm so that the anesthesia will pass through (Fig. 2).
3. Adult animals may be anesthetized in a standard induction chamber or may be held gently by the scruff of the neck in the open second arm of the scavenger until unconscious.

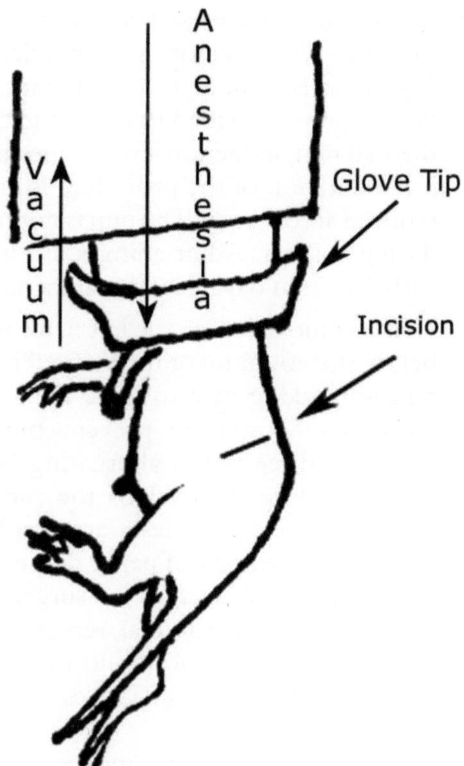

Fig. 1. Detail of placement of mouse head in modified mask, and location of subcostal incision.

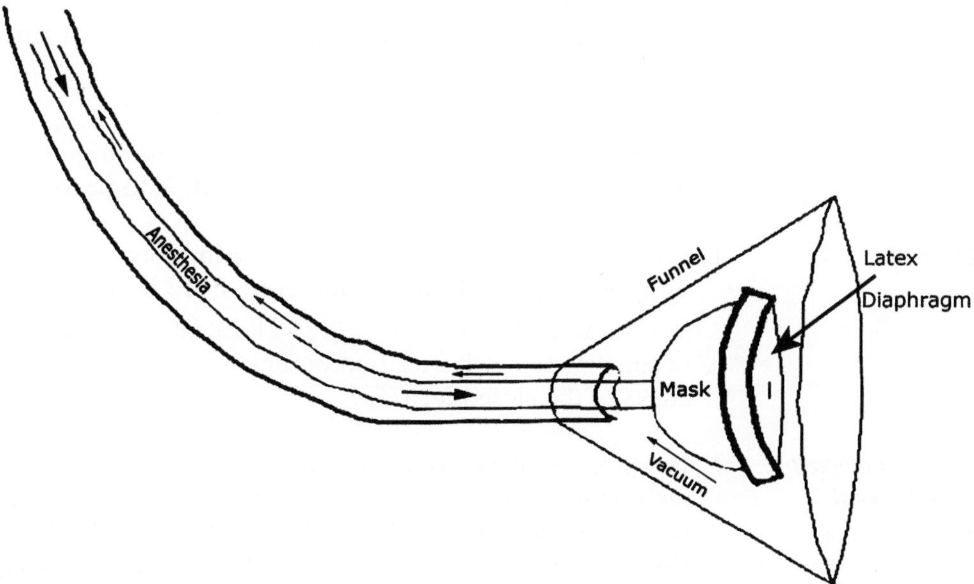

Fig. 2. Detail of customized pre-anesthesia chamber, showing double-lumen tube that supplies anesthetic and scavenges gases; and mask chamber into which the mouse pup is inserted.

4. Animals are anesthetized with isoflurane and oxygen, monitored for toe reflex, color and regular respiration throughout. Anesthesia is induced at 3% isoflurane with 400 mL/min oxygen flow in pups. Provided that the duration of the procedure is less than 10 min, induction level of anesthesia is adequate. However, if the duration of the procedure is longer, anesthesia should be reduced accordingly. The pup is not tied or restrained in any way during surgery. Adult animals are induced with 3% isoflurane with 1 L/min oxygen and maintained at 1–1.5% isoflurane.
5. Hair is removed from the left flank area of the adult animal just below the costal margin. We prefer using a depilatory for hair removal, taking care to leave the solution on the skin for no more than 1 min to prevent burns. The operative site is scrubbed three times, alternating between betadine and 70% alcohol before removal of the mouse to the surgery table. Neonates, being hairless, are scrubbed in situ on a sterile 4.5×4.5 cm section of paper drape, which is changed for each animal (the fresh section for surgery of one animal is used for the prep of the next animal, removed and replaced, etc.). Sterile cotton-tipped applicators allow the surgeon to do this without having to remove sterile gloves.

3.2. Tattoos

1. Tattoos are an easy and inexpensive way to identify neonatal mice. Complete instructions are included with the laboratory animal microtattoo system (see instrument list).
2. Tattoos are applied after induction of anesthesia. The use of the microscope makes the attached magnifying glass unnecessary and somewhat awkward to handle (it is easily removed). Be certain that the foot is completely dried prior to tattooing so that the ink is not diluted.
3. Use a 30-gauge ½ needle for the newborns.
4. Tattoos may be reapplied at the time of release surgery and/or weaning which may be helpful if the study is to be long-term.

3.3. Analgesia

1. Buprenorphine, 0.1–0.2 mg/kg is administered subcutaneously at the time of surgery and every 8–12 h for 1–2 days.
2. Bupivacaine, 0.02–0.05 mL, 0.25% local infiltration at the time of surgery. In newborns, bupivacaine is dripped on the wound edges of the closed incision.

3.4. Surgery: Complete Unilateral Ureteral Obstruction

1. Position pup on its right side and make a 2–4 mm flank skin incision in a line even with the umbilicus as shown in Fig. 1. If the incision is properly placed, there will be a small line of fatty tissue visible on top of the muscle layer. The muscle layer is gently lifted with the forceps and nicked just above the fat line with the iris scissors. A second pair of forceps is then placed

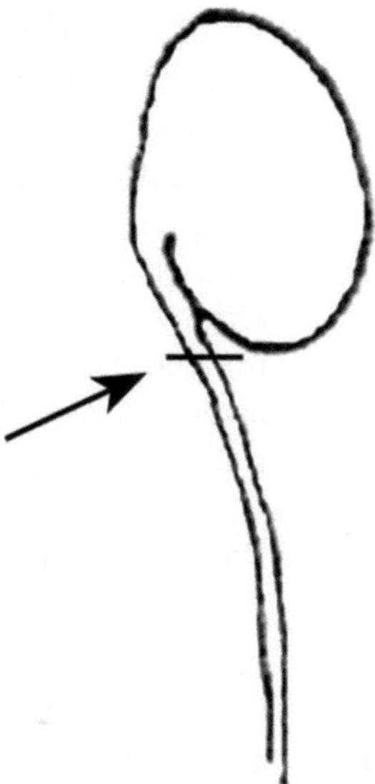

Fig. 3. Location of ureteral ligature in line with lower pole of kidney.

inside the nick and gently spread to increase the size of the opening. This eliminates bleeding at the incision site. A perfectly placed incision will allow visualization of the lower pole of the kidney.

2. Insert an ophthalmic sponge into the incision just below the kidney and hold for several seconds to absorb fluids, and then remove it. Avoid "dabbing". Hold one pair of the 45° forceps closed in the right hand as if they were a spoon and insert under the lower pole of the kidney. Gently lift the kidney with the closed forceps to visualize the ureter at the point of the ureteropelvic junction. Using the left-hand forceps, very gently grasp the ureter and lift. Insert the right-hand forceps under the ureter and spread the tips just enough to pierce the peritoneum. These techniques work best with the SuperGrip forceps because of their atraumatic surface. If using other types of forceps, insert the right-hand tips under the ureter, moving gently from side to side at the same time to free the ureter from attached tissue without grasping it (see Notes 1 and 2).
3. Use the left-hand forceps to place a length of 8-0 nylon suture into the tips of the right-hand forceps and slide the suture back under the ureter (Fig. 3, Arrow indicates ligation site).
4. Tie the suture completely with a surgeons knot. One ligature is sufficient when using nylon or prolene suture.
5. In the case of neonates, close the incision in a single layer with one or two horizontal mattress sutures. The skin acts to support the delicate muscle tissue and prevents tearing.

6. In adults the incision is made about 0.5 cm below the costal margin, first through the skin and then the muscle layer. Lifting the muscle layer as it is incised will prevent damage to the underlying organs. The surgery is performed as above (steps 1–5). Sterile cotton-tip applicators may be substituted for ophthalmic sponges. It is generally not necessary to lift the kidney to visualize the ureteropelvic junction. 6-0 prolene may be used to ligate the ureter. The incision is closed in two layers using 6-0 vicryl for the muscle layer and 6-0 prolene for the skin.

3.5. Surgery: Partial Unilateral Ureteral Obstruction

1. Proceed with steps 1–3 above.
2. Partially tie the surgeon's knot, leaving space between the ureter and the suture. Insert a 2 mm section of steel wire, 0.2 mm diameter in neonates, 0.3 mm in adults, into the space and tighten until the ligature is closed, but not tight. Tie the second portion of the knot closed, but not tight (such that the spaces between the two sections of the knot just disappear). Tighten the third portion of the knot to lock all in place. Trim the ends close (to avoid additional compression of the ureter by the free ends), and slide the wire out of the knot (see Notes 1–3).
3. Close the incision as in steps 5 or 6 above (see Notes 4–7).

3.6. Surgery: Release of Partial Obstruction

1. The partial obstruction described above can be easily released as late as 10 days following the initial surgery. After this time, release can still be performed, but risks increasing difficulty because of adhesion formation at the site of the obstruction.
2. Place the anesthetized pup on its back. Hair is removed with depilatory solution if needed using care that all trace of the solution is removed after 1 min to prevent skin burning and to deter its ingestion by the pup or the mother. The incision is made in a line parallel to and just left of mid-line to expose the ureter with its obstruction.
3. Under high magnification, tissue around the knot of the ligature is gently dissected until the knot can be grasped with #5 Dumont forceps. The knot can either be cut in half with Vannas scissors and the remaining ends teased apart, or the knot can be lifted so that the finer blade of the Vannas scissors can be slipped between the ligature and the ureter and the ligature cut (see Notes 1 and 2).
4. Close the incision in a single layer if the animal is less than 7 days old. If the pup is 7 days or older, close the muscle layer with 8-0 vicryl and the skin layer separately with 7-0 prolene.
5. Adult surgery is performed exactly the same as in neonates using 6-0 vicryl and prolene for the closure.

3.7. Tissue Harvest

1. Animals are euthanized with euthasol solution, 0.05 mL intraperitoneally (IP) in neonates 21 days of age and younger, 0.1 mL IP in older animals. Kidneys may be drop-fixed, perfused or frozen as necessary for histological study by means of standard immersion perfusion or cryopreservation techniques.
2. The kidneys are exposed and hydronephrosis is scored visually under low magnification on a scale of 1–4, as described below:
   (a) Normal in appearance.
   (b) Kidney appears hydronephrotic (i.e. distended), but without obvious translucent areas.
   (c) Kidney is distended with obvious translucent areas, but retains significant remaining parenchyma.
   (d) Very severe hydronephrosis with little if any remaining parenchyma.
3. India ink is injected into the pelvis of the kidney through a catheter made from PE-10 tubing connected to a 30-gauge ½ needle. Clamp the needle into a sturdy, smooth-surfaced needle holder approximately halfway down the needle. Holding the hub in one hand, gently bend the needle back and forth with the needle holder until it breaks leaving cleanly broken ends. Insert the hub end of the needle into one end of the tubing and the needle end into the other, and then attach to a 1 mL syringe. In the case of the neonates, the needle is inserted through the renal parenchyma until the tip is just visible in the pelvis. In adults, the needle may be inserted directly into the pelvis. A small amount of ink is injected into the pelvis. If the ureter is patent, ink will pass through the ureter into the bladder. No matter how carefully the surgery is done, the investigator can expect variation of patency and severity of obstruction within groups (see Notes 8 and 9).
4. Kidneys are excised with ureter, fat and other adhering tissue removed. To avoid histologic damage, capsules are left in place in mice (see Note 10).

4. Notes

1. Bracing the hands on the table will give additional control and assist in damping any hand tremors during surgery.
2. In the neonatal mouse care must be taken to avoid injury to the aorta and vena cava when dissecting out the ureter.
3. These are surprisingly easy techniques when done with the proper instruments and magnification. However, consistency

of technique is vitally important. Each time the ligature is tied, every effort should be made to tie it exactly the same as previously done, and at the same site. Tying the first or second cast of the surgeons knot too tightly will stretch the suture, resulting in excessive stenosis as well as risking damage to ureteral nerves and vessels, thus resulting in loss of peristalsis. Tying the third cast of the knot tightly removes the slack between the first and second casts so that the knot does not loosen and thus cause a loop to droop down onto the ureter, thereby increasing the obstruction. The free ends of the knot should be cut short to avoid compression of the ureter. Placing the partial ligature below the ureteropelvic junction may result in slippage and decreased degree of obstruction, while placing it above this point may cause the ureter to adhere to the kidney as it enlarges, also resulting in more severe obstruction.

4. Because these techniques apply primarily to neonatal mice, some comment is appropriate concerning how the pups are housed. In this laboratory, breeding pairs are maintained in a colony with one male and one female per box under standard housing conditions with standard mouse chow, lighting, and water. The one male/one female breeding arrangement, with the male continuously left with the female, is preferred because the mice appear to do better in family units. Frequently this leads to postpartum breeding. The date of birth is day 0. Surgery is performed on day 1 (~18–36 h following birth). Litters are reduced to 5 or 6 to limit variability in caloric intake. Extra pups can be fostered to females with fewer pups if they are the same age. Parents are removed to a clean cage at the time of surgery. Pups will be returned to the original nest following recovery from anesthesia. Only then are the parents returned to the cage.

5. Occasionally, pups are returned to their parents in apparent good health, and although surgeries went well, all the pups are dead the following morning. Why does this happen? Pups should be allowed to recover in an oxygen-enriched environment for at least 45 min prior to returning to the parents. If the pups are in any way subdued, the parents may not accept them. It is possible that the lingering odor of the exhaled isoflurane produces anxiety in the parents. All pups should be returned to the cage at one time to reduce parental anxiety.

6. Mouse parents as a rule do not disrupt prolene sutures, nor do they seem concerned by miniscule blood smears on the neonates. However, pups should always be handled with gloves. A "nestlet" in the cage with the litter allows the parent to "hide" their pups. It can be transferred with the pups when the cage is changed.

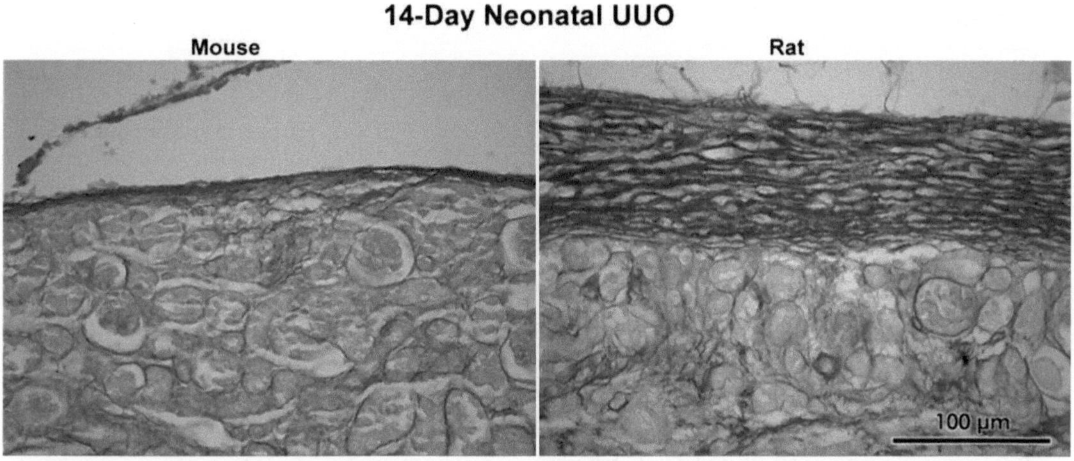

14-Day Neonatal UUO

Mouse

Rat

100 μm

Fig. 4. Histologic sections through capsule and cortex of neonatal mouse and rat kidneys showing relatively thin renal capsule of mouse (darker staining).

7. First-time mothers may be more anxious than older experienced ones. Some strains of mice may be more prone to kill their offspring than others, or may have varying levels of nurturing abilities. Death of the pups occasionally has nothing to do with the surgery.
8. Past studies using the persistent partial obstruction model have shown that 70% of neonates retain ureteral patency after 28 days. However, patency may drop to less than 50% by 42 days. Release of obstruction preserves ureteral patency, however.
9. Ink must not be injected into any kidneys intended for molecular studies.
10. Removal of the renal capsule at the time of harvest exerts undue traction on the underlying cortex. Capsular cells in the mouse, unlike the rat, have been found to be integrated into the cortex of the kidney. Leaving the capsule intact thus protects the architecture of the cortex and also makes sectioning the kidney easier (Fig. 4).

Acknowledgments

We are grateful for the technical assistance and Fig. 4 provided courtesy of Michael Forbes, PhD. Funding has been provided by NIH grant RO1-DK803372 and a Career Enhancement Award from the University of Virginia Children's Hospital.

References

1. Chevalier RL, Forbes MS, Thornhill BA (2009) Ureteral obstruction as a model of renal interstitial fibrosis and obstructive nephropathy. Kidney Int 75:1145–1152
2. Thornhill BA, Burt LA, Chen C et al (2005) Variable chronic partial ureteral obstruction in the neonatal rat: a new model of ureteropelvic junction obstruction. Kidney Int 67:42–52
3. Chevalier RL, Thornhill BA, Wolstenholme JT et al (1999) Unilateral ureteral obstruction in early development alters renal growth: dependence on the duration of obstruction. J Urol 161:309–313
4. Chevalier RL, Kim A, Thornhill BA et al (1999) Recovery following relief of unilateral ureteral obstruction in the neonatal rat. Kidney Int 55: 793–807
5. Shi Y, Pedersen M, Li C et al (2004) Early release of neonatal ureteral obstruction preserves renal function. Am J Physiol 286:F1087–F1099
6. Eskild-Jensen A, Jorgensen TM, Olsen LH et al (2003) Renal function may not be restored when using decreasing differential function as the criterion for surgery in unilateral hydronephrosis. BJU Int 92:779–782
7. Chevalier RL, Thornhill BA, Chang AY et al (2002) Recovery from release of ureteral obstruction in the rat: relationship to nephrogenesis. Kidney Int 61:2033–2043
8. Chevalier RL, Thornhill BA, Chang AY (2000) Unilateral ureteral obstruction in neonatal rats leads to renal insufficiency in adulthood. Kidney Int 58:1987–1995
9. Thornhill BA, Forbes MS, Marcinko ES et al (2007) Glomerulotubular disconnection in neonatal mice after relief of partial ureteral obstruction. Kidney Int 72:1103–1112
10. Chevalier RL, Gomez RA (1988) Response of the renin-angiotensin system to relief of neonatal ureteral obstruction. Am J Physiol 255: F1070–F1077
11. Chung KH, Chevalier RL (1996) Arrested development of the neonatal kidney following chronic ureteral obstruction. J Urol 155:1139–1144
12. Fern RJ, Yesko CM, Thornhill BA et al (1999) Reduced angiotensinogen expression attenuates renal interstitial fibrosis in obstructive nephropathy in mice. J Clin Invest 103: 39–46
13. Kinter M, Wolstenholme JT, Thornhill BA et al (1999) Unilateral ureteral obstruction impairs renal antioxidant enzyme activation during sodium depletion. Kidney Int 55: 1327–1334
14. Silverstein DM, Travis BR, Thornhill BA et al (2003) Altered expression of immune modulator and structural genes in neonatal unilateral ureteral obstruction. Kidney Int 64:25–35
15. Lin J, Patel SR, Cheng X et al (2005) Kielin/chordin-like protein, a novel enhancer of BMP signaling, attenuates renal fibrotic disease. Nat Med 11:387–393

Chapter 34

Urinary Diversion via Cutaneous Vesicostomy in the Megabladder Mouse

Ashley R. Carpenter, Brian Becknell, Daniel A. Hirselj, and Kirk M. McHugh

Abstract

Lower urinary tract obstruction in mice can lead to end-stage renal disease and death. We have developed a surgical technique to create a cutaneous vesicostomy in mice providing an external outlet for drainage of urine, thereby relieving the obstruction and slowing and/or preventing the development of end-stage renal disease and death.

Key words: Bladder, Congenital obstructive nephropathy, Cutaneous vesicostomy, End-stage renal disease, Kidney, Megabladder mouse

1. Introduction

Congenital obstructive nephropathy is the leading cause of end-stage renal disease in children. Despite advanced prenatal screening and surgical intervention, many children with congenital obstructive nephropathy progress to end-stage renal disease. The economic and social impact of congenital obstructive nephropathy is significant, with end-stage renal disease costing over $15 billion annually in the United States (1–3).

The megabladder mouse (*mgb*) represents a unique transgenic mouse model of congenital obstructive nephropathy that develops signs of lower urinary tract obstruction *in utero* secondary to a nonfunctional, overdistended bladder. Male homozygotes (*mgb–/–*) develop early renal insufficiency and rarely survive beyond 5–6 weeks. In contrast, the disease progression in female *mgb–/–* mice appears much less severe with animals frequently living up to a year (4).

Odyssé Michos (ed.), *Kidney Development: Methods and Protocols*, Methods in Molecular Biology, vol. 886, DOI 10.1007/978-1-61779-851-1_34, © Springer Science+Business Media, LLC 2012

In an attempt to extend the life of male *mgb–/–* mice, we performed cutaneous vesicostomy (CV) to relieve the lower urinary tract obstruction before the development of end-stage renal disease. During this surgical procedure, a stoma is formed by anastomosis of the bladder mucosa to the abdominal skin, thereby creating an alternative outlet through the abdominal wall. Urine is drained through the outlet with the help of gravity and ambulation. The procedure extends the life of male *mgb–/–* mice by preventing or slowing any further upper urinary tract deterioration associated with obstruction.

2. Materials

1. Anesthesia station (901808, VetEquip, Inc.).
2. Forane, isoflurane, USP (Baxter).
3. Ophthalmic lubricant (Dechra Veterinary Products).
4. Deltaphase* isothermal pad (39DP, Braintree Scientific, Inc.).
5. Sterile surgical pad/recovery pad.
6. Depilatory cream, Nair®.
7. Sterile cotton swab applicators.
8. 2 × 2 sterile gauze.
9. Sterile water, autoclaved ddH_2O.
10. Chlorhex-Q-Scrub, 2.0% chlorhexidine digluconate (Vedco, Inc.).
11. Chlorhexidine 2% solution (Vedco, Inc.). Dilute 2% chlorhexidine solution to 0.5% chlorhexidine solution: 4 parts of distilled water, 1 part 2% chlorhexidine solution.
12. Graefe forceps, 0.8-mm tips, slight curve.
13. Spring scissors, 6-mm blades, straight.
14. 24-gauge IV catheter (26751, Exel International Medical Products).
15. 10-mL sterile syringe.
16. 15-mL conical tube.
17. Castroviejo needle holder, 14 cm with Lock.
18. 6-0 PDS* II (polydioxanone) Suture, 9.3-mm 3/8c taper needle (Z117H, Ethicon, Inc.).
19. 70% Isopropyl alcohol prep pad (McKesson Corp.).
20. 1-mL sterile syringe with subcutaneous needle.
21. 0.9% sodium chloride injection, USP (Hospira, Inc.).
22. Topical triple antibiotic ointment (0168-0012-09, Nycomed US, Inc.).

3. Methods

Prior to surgery, *mgb–/–* mice are allowed unlimited access to a low-fat diet and water. Male *mgb–/–* animals are generally 21–36 days old at the time of CV, but CV has been performed as early as 17 days. Candidates for CV have bulging flanks due to megabladder. The degree of hydronephrosis may be assessed by ultrasound prior to CV (5). *mgb–/–* animals, particularly males, should be monitored after weaning for signs of dehydration, dyspnea, or general morbidity (hunched appearance, immobility, and ruffled fur), as such moribund animals may not tolerate the procedure and rarely survive past 2 weeks in our experience.

3.1. Preoperative/ Surgical Preparation

1. Anesthesia induction: The mouse is anesthetized with inhaled isoflurane in an induction chamber at a rate of 3.5% isoflurane in 1 liter per minute (L/min) oxygen flow. Ophthalmic lubricant is applied to prevent corneal dehydration prior to the animal being placed supine on a 37°C warmed, sterile surgical pad with the nose placed in a mouse nose cone.
2. Anesthesia maintenance: Anesthesia is sustained with 2.5% isoflurane in 1 L/min oxygen via nose cone, for the remainder of the surgical procedure.
3. Hair removal: A chemical depilatory (Nair®) is used for complete hair removal surrounding the surgical site. Using a sterile swab, depilatory cream is applied to the ventral abdomen for approximately 60 s (Fig. 1a). The abdomen is wiped using sterile gauze to remove the hair and depilatory cream, followed by sterile, water-soaked gauze (see Note 1).
4. The surgical site is cleansed with antimicrobial, 2% chlorhexidine digluconate surgical scrub applied via sterile swab. The chlorhexidine scrub is wiped away with sterile water-soaked gauze. The ventral abdomen is prepped with three consecutive applications of disinfectant, 0.5% chlorhexidine gluconate surgical solution (see Note 2) (Fig. 1b).

3.2. Intraoperative/ Surgical Technique

1. Forceps are used to lift the skin and an 8-mm low transverse abdominal incision is made just lateral to the midline (Fig. 2a).
2. Forceps are use to lift the peritoneum and a 6-mm transverse cut is then made to divide the peritoneum (see Note 3) (Fig.2b, c).
3. To prevent uroperitoneum, a 24-gauge IV catheter is introduced to the bladder (Fig. 2d).
4. The stylet is removed leaving the plastic IV catheter sleeve in place (Fig. 3a). A 10-mL sterile syringe is attached to the IV

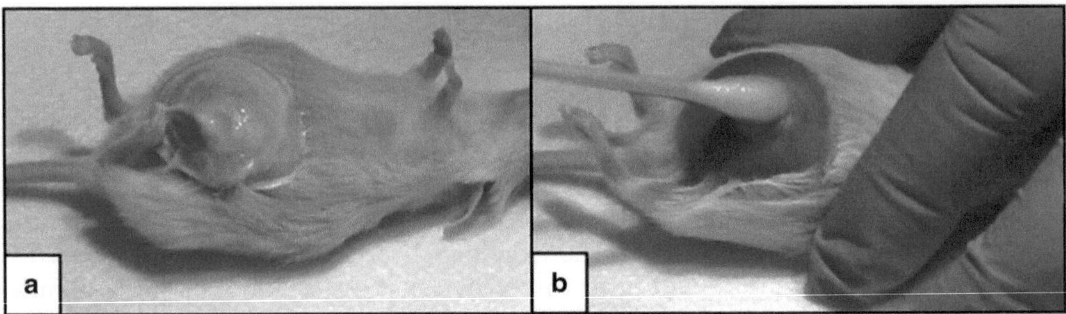

Fig. 1. (**a**) Chemical depilatory cream is applied for 60 s. (**b**) 0.5% chlorhexidine solution is applied to the entire hairless surface, starting from the center and working outward in a circular pattern.

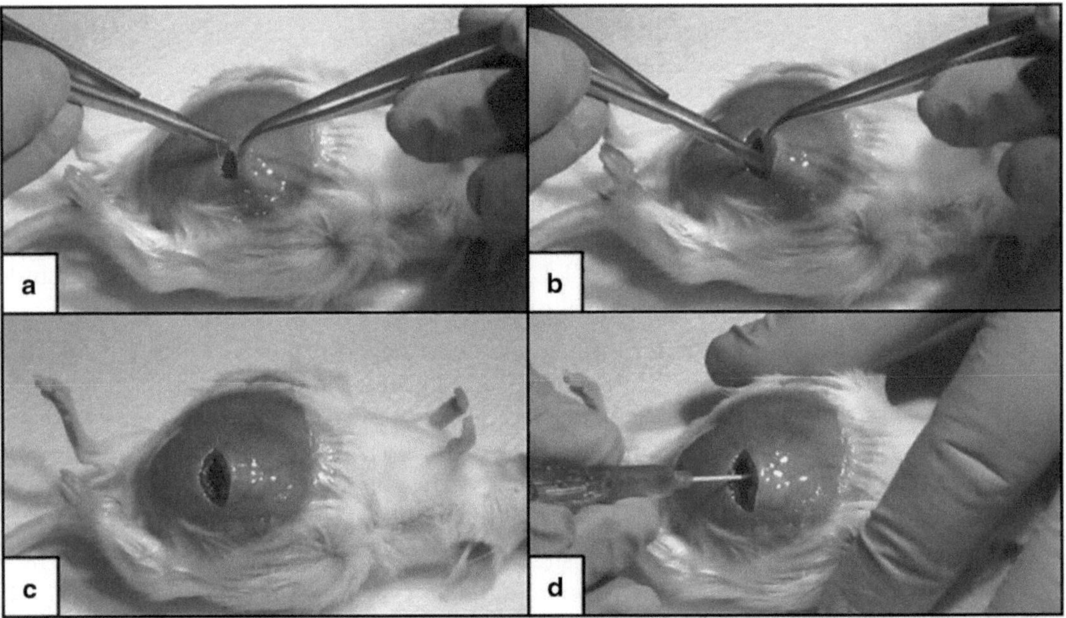

Fig. 2. (**a**) An 8-mm low transverse abdominal incision is made just lateral to the midline. (**b**) A 6-mm transverse cut is then made to divide the peritoneum. (**c**) The smaller elliptical opening of the peritoneum centered within the elliptical opening of the abdominal wall. (**d**) The bladder is punctured using a 24-gauge IV catheter.

catheter (Fig. 3b) and approximately 90% of the urine volume is aspirated (Fig. 3c). The urine is placed into 15-mL conical tubes. Sufficient urine is aspirated so that the animal no longer has bulging flanks; at this point, the abdomen should be flat, but not concave (see Note 4) (Fig. 3d).

5. At a distance 2-mm superior to the IV catheter entrance, an absorbable monofilament polydioxanone suture (6-0 PDS*II) is placed at the 12 o'clock position through the bladder wall, then through the peritoneum, and finally through the abdominal cutaneous layer. This is the first stitch of a four-quadrant fixation with interrupted sutures (Fig. 4).

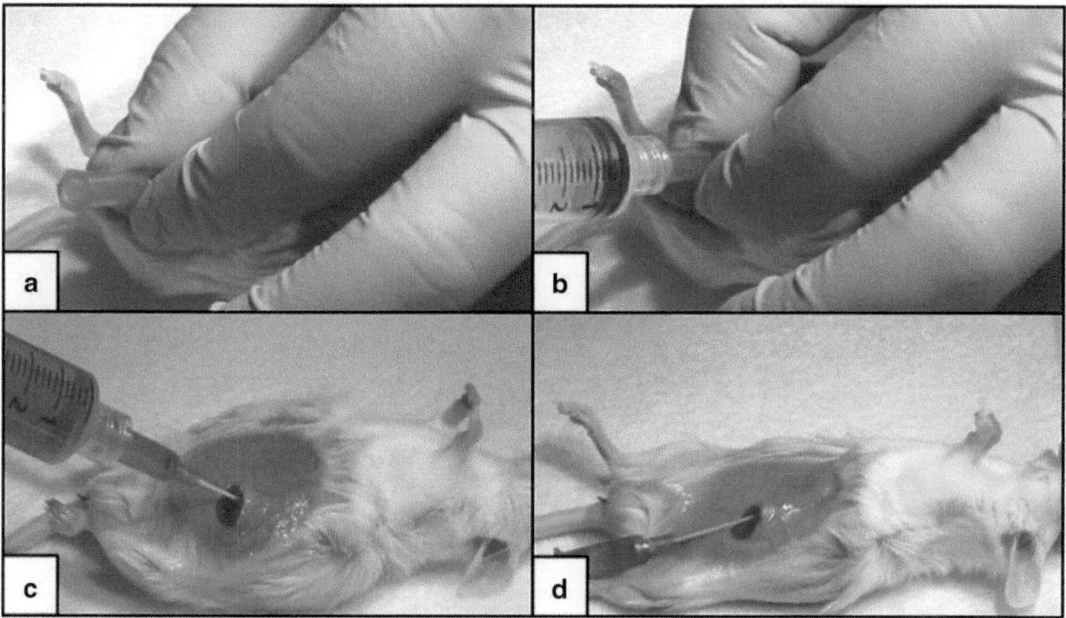

Fig. 3. (**a**) The stylet is removed from the plastic IV catheter. (**b**) A sterile 10-mL syringe is secured to the IV catheter. (**c**) Approximately 90% of the bladder urine volume is aspirated. (**d**) At this point, the abdomen is flat but not concave.

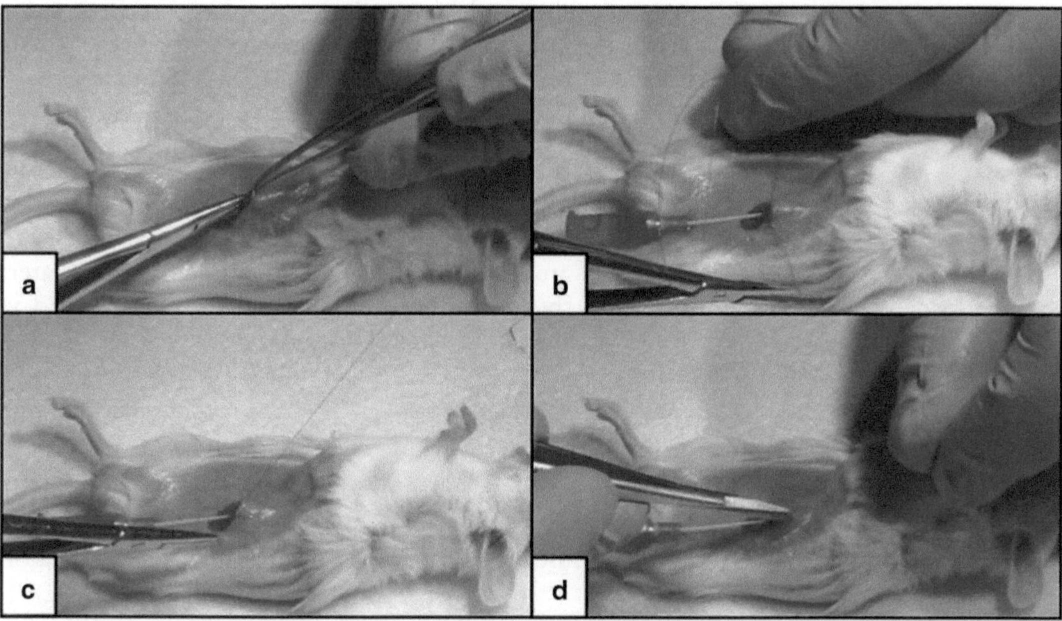

Fig. 4. (**a**) Suture needle piercing the bladder wall. The right hand is rotated into pronation to traverse the needle, directed anteriorly, through the bladder wall. (**b**) Formation of the loop of the first throw. (**c**) The superior end of the suture material and the needle holder are pulled in opposite directions to set the knot. (**d**) After additional throws, the suture is clipped to finish the first interrupted stitch.

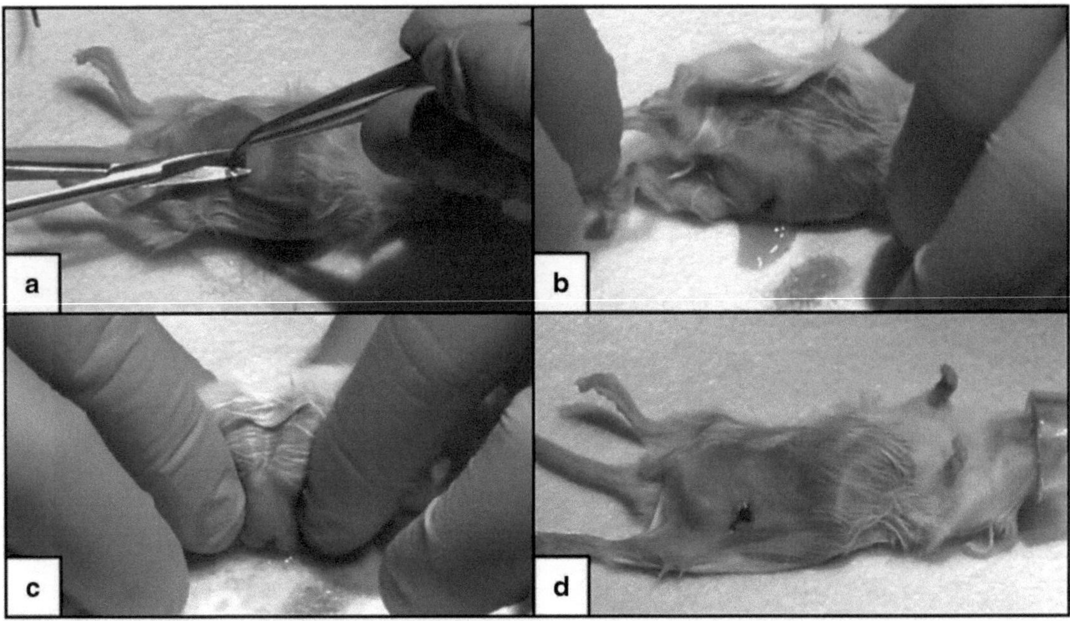

Fig. 5. (**a**) The stoma is enlarged by excising the bladder wall within the stoma. (**b**) The mouse is pulled from the nose cone, placed in the lateral position and the remaining 10% urine volume is drained via gravity. (**c**) Pressure is applied to the abdomen to evacuate remaining urine. (**d**) Decompressed bladder. At this point, the abdomen is concave.

6. The second, third, and fourth sutures are placed at the 3, 6, and 9 o'clock position in the same manner described, each being placed approximately 2-mm from the IV catheter entrance.
7. Once the four sutures are in place, the IV catheter is removed and the hole is enlarged using sharp dissection to form the stoma (see Note 5) (Fig. 5a).
8. Once complete, the elliptical stoma is ultimately 5 × 3 mm in size.
9. The mouse is pulled from the nose cone, placed in the lateral position and the remaining 10% urine volume is drained via gravity (Fig. 5b) and gentle abdominal pressure (see Note 6) (Fig. 5c).
   (a) At this point the abdomen is concave (Fig. 5d). The mouse is immediately reintroduced to the maintenance anesthesia nose cone, to inspect for organ prolapse and wound dehiscence.
10. Additional sutures can be placed as needed to complete fixation.

3.3. Immediate Postprocedural Care and Recovery

1. The hairless area near the surgical wound is blotted with a sterile gauze pad, rinsed with sterile saline and treated with a final swab of 0.5% chlorhexidine solution.
2. Triple antibiotic ointment is applied topically to the surgical site to prevent urine scald (see Note 7).

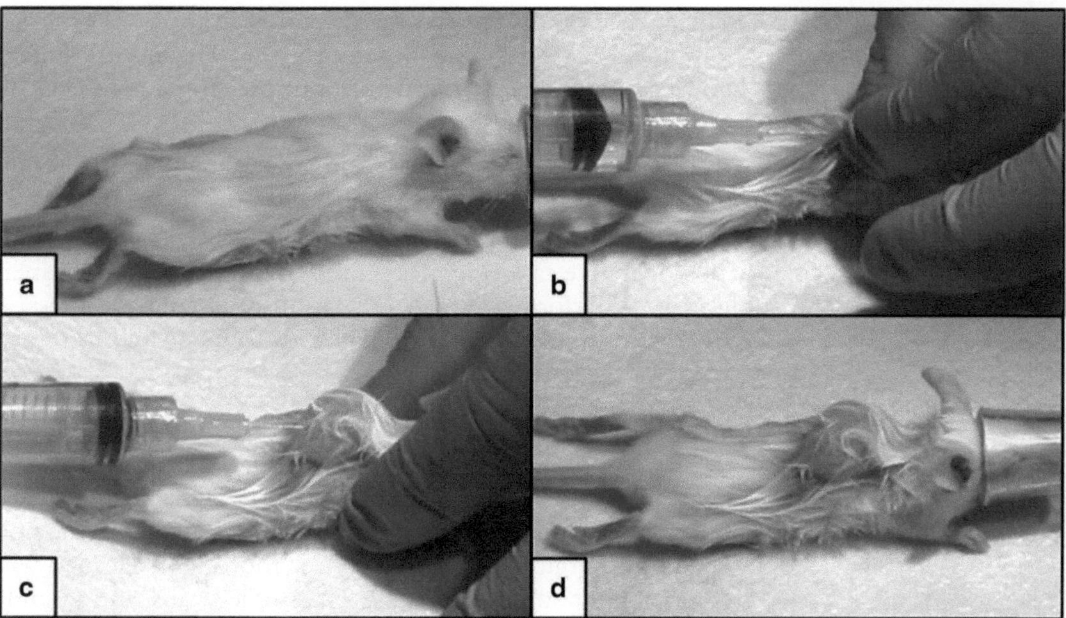

Fig. 6. (**a**) The animal is placed in the prone position. (**b**) The loose skin between the shoulder blades is lifted to form a tent. At the base of the tent, the needle is inserted directed anteriorly. (**c**) Sterile saline is injected into the subcutaneous space. (**d**) A 0.5-mL sterile saline bolus located between the shoulder blades in the subcutaneous space.

3. The animal is placed in the prone position, with the nose in the nose cone (Fig. 6a). A subcutaneous injection of sterile 0.9% NaCl is introduced to hydrate the mouse following the procedure. With the mouse remaining anesthetized, the loose skin between the shoulder blades is lifted to tent the skin. The entry site is prepped with a 70% Ethanol wipe, and a 26-gauge needle attached to a sterile syringe is inserted at the base of the skin tent (Fig. 6b). With the needle directed anteriorly, a 0.5-mL saline bolus is slowly injected into the subcutaneous space (Fig. 6c, d).
4. The mouse is then placed in a 37°C recovery chamber with constant oxygen flow, and monitored until fully conscious and ambulating normally (see Note 8).
5. The mouse is housed in a cage with paper bedding and allowed immediate access to a low-fat diet and water. The mouse is generally housed alone; however, in the case of a pup that is still nursing, the mouse is placed in a fresh, paper-bedded cage with its mother (dam).

3.4. Postoperative Care

1. The mouse is observed twice daily for the first 2 days following the CV procedure.
2. During each examination, topical ointment is applied using a sterile swab to protect the skin from urine scald.

3. The anchor points created by the suture fixation are observed for gaps that might allow organ prolapse. The animal remains housed alone or with the dam, until the stoma is healed and prolonged patency is confirmed.
4. If the stoma and surrounding skin are healing properly, topical ointment can be applied as needed until the hair grows.

3.5. Rare Postoperative Complications

Any postoperative care other than brief examination and ointment application is performed under inhalation isoflurane anesthesia as described. In some cases, the stoma needs to be dilated to remain patent.

1. Stoma dilation is performed by placing the mouse in the nose cone and using sterile forceps to gently stretch the opening (see Note 9).
2. If organ prolapse has occurred, the mouse is placed in the nose cone on a surgical pad. The organ is thoroughly cleaned with chlorhexidine solution using several sterile swabs, and carefully reinserted using blunt forceps. Sutures are placed, as described, where needed to seal the peritoneum to the abdominal wall.
3. In the case of bladder prolapse, the bladder wall is additionally anchored to the peritoneum and abdominal wall by increasing the number of fixation sites in the circumferential patterning as needed.

4. Notes

1. Chemical depilatory must be completely removed, as it is irritating to the skin. Following recovery, the animal will be weak and may not groom the surgical site. Multiple water-soaked gauze pads should be used as necessary. The body should be blotted with dry gauze pads to remove all water as a step towards retaining body temperature.
2. Chlorhexidine surgical scrub is applied in a circular pattern starting at the midpoint and working outward. It is important to work outward to the hair-covered surface, as it is the most contaminated surface.
3. The peritoneum of a severely dehydrated megabladder mouse is very thin, and precaution must be taken to keep from lifting and cutting through the bladder, as this would cause uroperitoneum and surgical demise.
   (a) The peritoneum is progressively difficult to grab with the forceps with increased bladder volume. In this case, it is necessary to take a bigger bite with the forceps, while still

making a 6-mm transverse incision at the midpoint of the abdominal opening.

(b) The transverse cut made to the peritoneum should be smaller than that made through the skin (Fig. 2c). Once the bladder volume is removed, the peritoneum and bladder wall will be difficult to discern. A large peritoneal opening will cause the peritoneum to be lost beneath the skin. A small incision will allow the surgeon to easily grab the peritoneum that will lie right on top of the bladder within the field of the skin opening.

4. The retained urine volume helps maintain the shape of the bladder for suture placement. The IV catheter is left in place as a point of reference for the stoma formation.
5. Sharp dissection: The bladder, peritoneum, and skin have been sutured in a circular fashion around the IV catheter entrance to the bladder. The IV catheter is removed and the bladder is lifted with forceps. Using sharp dissection, the bladder tissue within the suture fixation is removed. This forms a larger hole (stoma) to accommodate urine flow for the remainder of the animal's life. The stoma will heal and become smaller over time, but will allow urine evacuation if created correctly.
6. The surgeon's thumbs and forefingers are used to gently apply pressure from an anterior (left hand) and posterior (right hand) position towards the stoma. This pressure is to remove the remainder of the urine in the bladder, and will reveal weakness or incomplete fixation. Occasionally, underlying tissues will be visible following the application of gentle pressure. In this case, additional suture placement is required. If the stoma is not tested, the animal may prolapse due to normal gravity and movement overnight following recovery, in which case, the tissues would need thoroughly cleaned and reinserted prior to additional suturing.
7. Triple antibiotic ointment is not required; however, it is readily available in small volume disposable packets. Any petroleum-based ointment can be used as the urine will irritate unprotected abdominal skin. Once the animal has healed, and the hair has grown back, the hair will serve as the wick to protect the skin from scald.
8. Adequate oxygen flow, hydration, warmth, and stimulation will shorten the recovery time required for the animal to regain normal activity. The animal can be placed on a smooth recovery pad, and allowed access to moist food; however, the animal will regain normal function within minutes.
9. Occasionally, the stoma will close under scab formation. In this case, the mouse will need to be anesthetized, cleaned with dilute chlorhexidine solution and the stoma will need dilated using sterile forceps.

Acknowledgment

This work was supported by NIH grant DK070907 and DK085242.

References

1. Collins AJ, Foley RN, Herzog C et al (2010) Excerpts from the US Renal Data System 2009 annual data report. Am J Kidney Dis 55:S1–S420, A426–A427
2. (2010) North American Pediatric Renal Transplant Cooperative Study 2010 annual report. https://web.emmes.com/study/ped/annlrept/annlrept.html. Accessed 11 April 2010
3. Roth KS, Carter WH Jr, Chan JC (2001) Obstructive nephropathy in children: long-term progression after relief of posterior urethral valve. Pediatrics 107:1004–1010
4. Singh S, Robinson M, Nahi F et al (2007) Identification of a unique transgenic mouse line that develops megabladder, obstructive uropathy, and renal dysfunction. J Am Soc Nephrol 18:461–471
5. Ingraham SE, Saha M, Carpenter AR et al (2010) Pathogenesis of renal injury in the megabladder mouse: a genetic model of congenital obstructive nephropathy. Pediatr Res 68:500–507

Chapter 35

Ultrasound Imaging of the Murine Kidney

Ashley R. Carpenter, Brian Becknell, Susan E. Ingraham, and Kirk M. McHugh

Abstract

Ultrasound (US) is the most common and least invasive modality for clinical imaging of the kidney. One important application of US in nephrology is the detection and monitoring of structural changes in the kidney. Recent advances in US technology have facilitated the application of similar techniques to animal models of human disease. We have developed a simple US-based method of detection and quantitation of hydronephrosis in a mouse model of congenital obstructive nephropathy, the megabladder (*mgb*) mouse.

Key words: Ultrasound, Hydronephrosis, Congenital obstructive nephropathy, Mouse, Megabladder, Animal model of human disease

1. Introduction

Ultrasound (US) is the most common and least invasive modality for clinical imaging of the kidney. Neither ionizing radiation nor intravenous contrast agents are required for US, and serial studies can be obtained without concern for adverse or cumulative effects. Moreover, US serves a crucial role in the diagnosis and clinical management of patients with congenital anomalies of the kidney and urinary tract (CAKUT) as well as other renal conditions. These features of US have led researchers to adapt this modality to image murine kidneys.

Renal US studies in mice are distinct from those performed in human patients in several ways. First, the physiology of the mouse, including its size as well as rapid cardiac and respiratory rates, presents challenges to obtaining accurate, high-quality US imaging. As a result, most US devices designed for human assessments are inadequate for high-quality ultrasonography in the mouse. Small-animal imaging has been facilitated by the development of high-frequency, high-resolution US technology, which relies on

Odyssé Michos (ed.), *Kidney Development: Methods and Protocols*, Methods in Molecular Biology, vol. 886, DOI 10.1007/978-1-61779-851-1_35, © Springer Science+Business Media, LLC 2012

transducers that operate at frequencies in the 15–60 mHz range. Second, inhalation anesthesia is required to keep the animal immobilized and to slow the heart rate sufficiently in order to obtain a satisfactory image of the kidney. Third, complete removal of the overlying fur is necessary for clear images. Fourth, the cortex and medulla have similar echogenicity in the mouse kidney, making it difficult to distinguish between these compartments or to evaluate corticomedullary differentiation. Lastly, whereas the human kidney has six to ten calyces, the murine kidney has a single calyx. This difference facilitates quantification of renal pelvis dilatation in mice with hydronephrosis.

Recently, we have applied renal US to the megabladder (*mgb*) mouse model of congenital obstructive uropathy (1). When inherited as a recessive trait (*mgb–/–*), there is absent detrusor smooth muscle development *in utero*, leading to a nonfunctional, overdistended bladder and variable hydronephrosis. We have employed US to quantify the degree of hydronephrosis in postnatal *mgb–/–* kidneys *in vivo*, permitting us to stratify cohorts of mice on this key experimental variable (2). The US procedure can be completed in a small amount of time, and the animal can fully recover from inhalational anesthesia within minutes.

2. Materials

1. Vevo 2100 high-frequency US system (VisualSonics, Inc.), operating in B-mode.
2. MS-550D transducer (VisualSonics, Inc.), operated at 40 mHz frequency.
3. Visual Sonics Advanced Physiological Monitoring Unit (APMU) (VisualSonics, Inc.).
4. Anesthesia station (901808, VetEquip, Inc.).
5. Forane, isoflurane, USP (Baxter).
6. Ophthalmic lubricant (Dechra Veterinary Products).
7. Heat lamp (Thermo Fisher Scientific, Inc.).
8. Electrode gel (Parker Laboratories, Inc.).
9. Tape (Thermo Fisher Scientific, Inc.).
10. Animal clippers (78005010, Jarden Corporation).
11. Nair® depilatory cream.
12. Sterile cotton swab applicators (Thermo Fisher Scientific, Inc.).
13. 2″×2″ Sterile Gauze (Thermo Fisher Scientific, Inc.).
14. Sterile water.
15. US gel, warmed to 37°C (Parker Laboratories, Inc.).

3. Methods

Prior to US, mice are permitted unlimited access to low-fat diet and water.

3.1. Preparation

1. The mouse is anesthetized with inhaled isoflurane in an induction chamber at a rate of 3.5% isoflurane in 1 L/min (L/min) oxygen flow.
2. A heat lamp is used to keep the animal warm during anesthesia.
3. The animal is placed prone on the APMU with the nose placed in a mouse nose cone.
   (a) Anesthesia is maintained with 2.5% isoflurane in 1 L/min oxygen via nose cone, for the remainder of the imaging procedure.
4. Ophthalmic lubricant is applied with a cotton swab to prevent corneal dehydration (Fig. 1a).

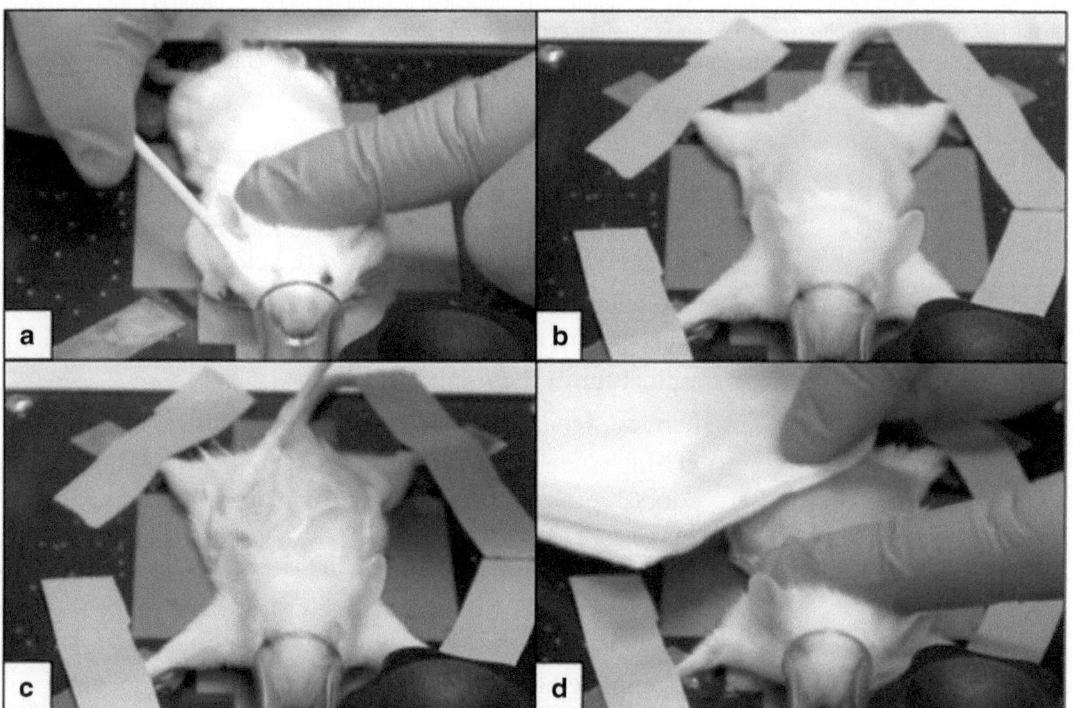

Fig. 1. (**a**) Following induction anesthesia, the mouse is placed prone on the APMU and ophthalmic lubricant is applied to prevent corneal dehydration. Ongoing anesthesia and oxygen are provided via nose cone. (**b**) The mouse is gently restrained by taping the paws of extended limbs to the electrodes of the mouse pad. (**c**) Nair® is applied to the paraspinal fur in the lumbar region after shaving. (**d**). After 90 s, Nair® is wiped away using sterile gauze.

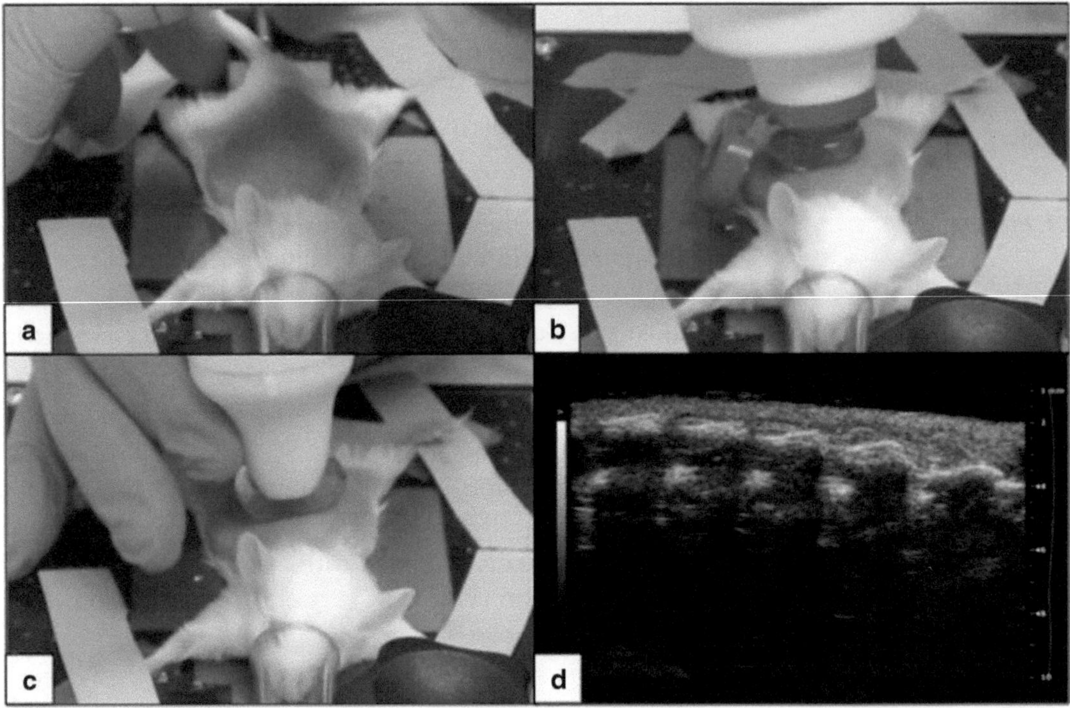

Fig. 2. (**a**) Complete depilation is required prior to imaging. The lubricated internal temperature probe is carefully inserted into the rectum. (**b**) Warm ultrasound (US) gel is carefully applied, taking care to avoid bubbles. Sufficient gel is required to permit manipulation of the transducer without directly contacting the skin. (**c**) The transducer is placed atop the spine. (**d**) An US view of the lumbar spine.

5. Electrode gel is blotted onto the plate electrodes of the APMU. Legs are gently extended and the anesthetized animal is gently restrained by taping the paws onto the electrodes (Fig. 1b).
   (a) This allows for heart rate monitoring during the procedure.
6. Animal clippers or electric razor is used to gently clip the paraspinal fur in the lumbar region.
7. A chemical depilatory is used to complete fur removal.
   (a) Using a sterile swab, depilatory cream is applied to the dorsal lumbar region for approximately 90 s (Fig. 1c).
   (b) The lumbar surface is wiped using sterile gauze to remove the fur and depilatory cream (see Note 1). This is followed by thorough wiping with sterile water-soaked gauze (Fig. 1d) and then blotting with dry sterile gauze.
   (c) Complete hair removal is necessary for clear imaging.
8. The rectal probe is lubricated and inserted into the rectum (see Note 2) (Fig. 2a).
   (a) This permits body temperature monitoring during the procedure.

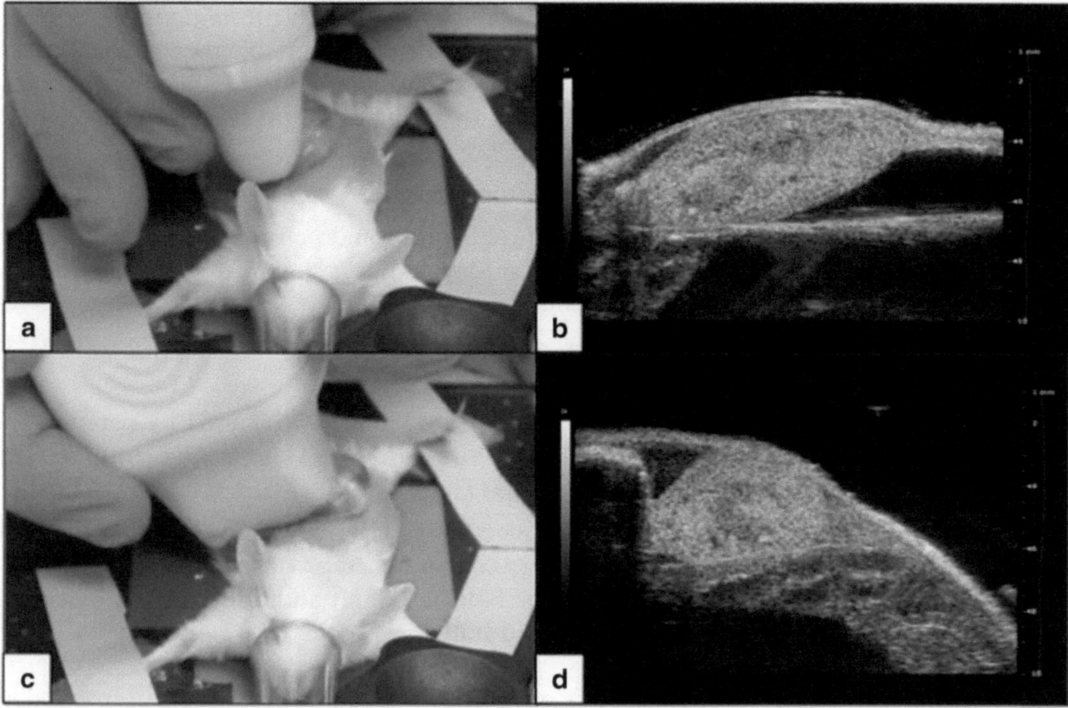

Fig. 3. (**a**) The transducer is moved laterally toward the right flank to obtain the longitudinal image. (**b**) A longitudinal image of the right kidney. (**c**) The transducer is rotated clockwise 90° to view the right kidney transversely. (**d**) A transverse image of the right kidney.

3.2. Imaging the Kidneys

The kidneys are located in the paravertebral retroperitoneal space, making the lumbar vertebral column a useful reference point.

1. US gel, prewarmed to 37°C, is generously applied directly to the depilated surface (Fig. 2b).
   (a) Care should be taken to minimize bubbles during gel application as air compromises image quality (see Note 3).
   (b) Sufficient gel must be applied to provide a layer on which the transducer can be manipulated without directly contacting the skin surface.
2. The transducer is placed atop the US gel along the spine (Fig. 2c). An US view of the spine is shown (Fig. 2d).
3. The transducer is moved laterally toward the right, to identify the right kidney (Fig. 3a), and then manipulated up and down to focus the kidney into the maximal longitudinal plane (Fig. 3b).
4. When the longitudinal axis is assessed, the renal papilla is identified in the center of the organ.
   (a) The papilla projects into the renal pelvis, which is a minimally echogenic space in the center of the kidney.

   (b) In normal animals, it may be difficult to identify the pelvis, as it is almost entirely occupied by the papilla. Papilla identification may be facilitated by manipulating the transducer, either gently lifting up or pressing down.
   (c) The hypoechogenic renal pelvis is easily identified in animals with hydronephrosis.
5. The image is captured and should be reviewed to confirm that it reflects the largest longitudinal plane, with papilla in the center of the organ.
   (a) Images are captured as B-mode images with a 40 MHz transducer.
6. A transverse image of the kidney is obtained by rotating the transducer clockwise 90° (Fig. 3c). This can be helpful to visualize the renal pelvis (Fig. 3d).
7. The transducer is next moved laterally to the left, past the midpoint of the spine, and a similar approach is utilized to visualize the left kidney (see Note 4). Apply additional US gel if needed, taking care to avoid bubbles.

3.3. Quantifying Hydronephrosis

Hydronephrosis is qualitatively recognized as distension and dilatation of the renal pelvis. As urological obstruction becomes more severe, there is cortical atrophy and loss of renal parenchyma. There is no standard scheme to quantify hydronephrosis of the murine kidney. Recently, we have devised a method to quantify hydronephrosis, based on the proportion of renal parenchyma in a longitudinal US image. Using this scheme, we have categorized kidneys with mild, moderate, or severe hydronephrosis.

1. The largest longitudinal plane of the kidney is identified, and an image is captured (see Note 5).
2. The longitudinal renal length (LRL) is measured by drawing a line from the most superior to the most inferior point in of the kidney.
   (a) This serves as a reference line for subsequent measurements.
3. Lines perpendicular to the LRL are placed for transverse renal width (TRW), renal pelvis diameter (RPD), and renal papilla width (RPW) (Fig. 4).
4. The percentage parenchyma in a two-dimensional plane is calculated as:

   % Parenchyma = ([TRW − RPD] + RPW)/TRW.
5. Hydronephrosis can be graded according to percent parenchyma:
   (a) If the renal papilla fully occupies the renal pelvis (i.e. RPD = RPW), then hydronephrosis is absent (Fig. 5a).
   (b) >67% Parenchyma = mild hydronephrosis (Fig. 5b).
   (c) 34–66% Parenchyma = moderate hydronephrosis (Fig. 5c).
   (d) <33% Parenchyma = severe hydronephrosis (Fig. 5d).

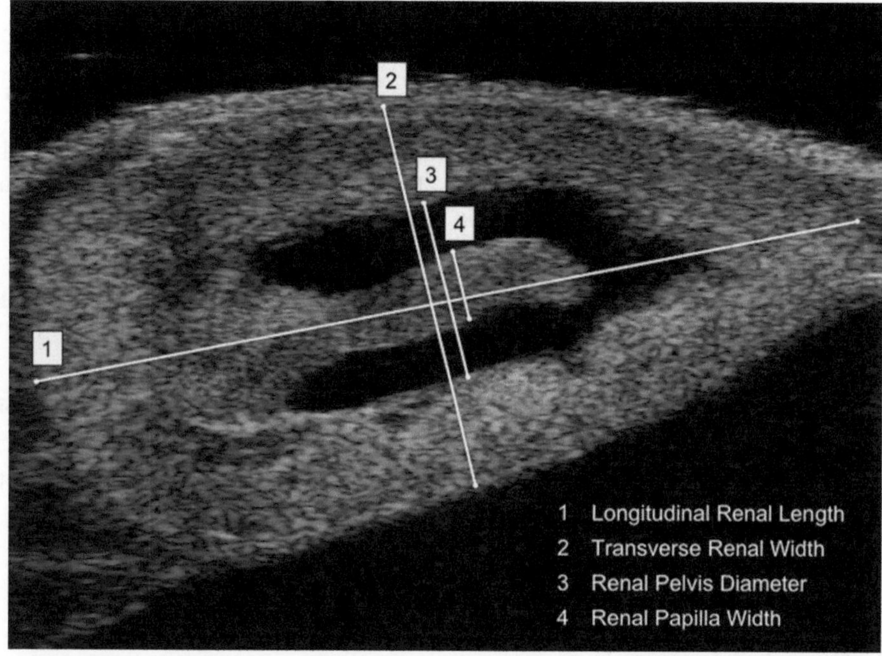

Fig. 4. Longitudinal image of a kidney with moderate hydronephrosis. Indicated measurements are shown. Note that transverse renal width (TRW), renal pelvis diameter (RPD), and renal papilla width (RPW) are all perpendicular to longitudinal renal length (LRL). The percentage of parenchyma is calculated as ([TRW – RPD] + RPW)/TRW.

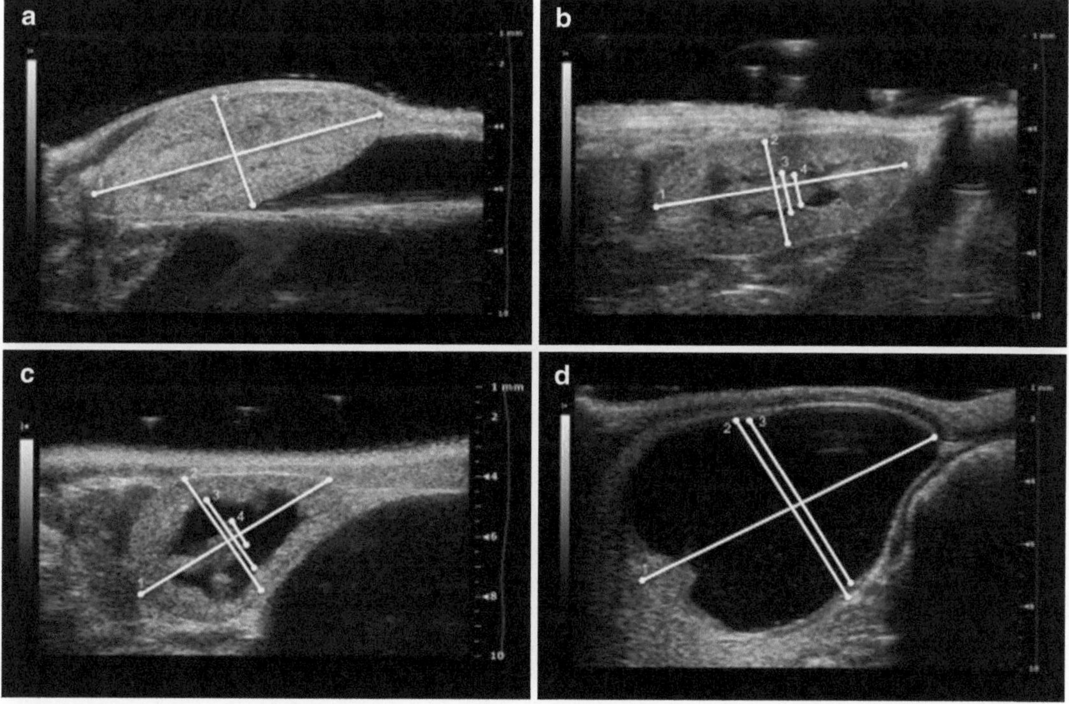

Fig. 5. Longitudinal images of healthy wild-type kidney (**a**), compared to mgb–/– kidneys with mild (**b**), moderate (**c**), and severe (**d**) hydronephrosis.

4. Notes

1. Chemical depilatory must be completely removed, as it is irritating to the skin. Multiple water soaked gauze pads should be used as necessary. The body should be blotted with dry gauze pads to remove all water as a step towards retaining body temperature.
2. The rectal probe must be secured to the AMPU using a small piece of tape. Care should be taken to avoid jostling the cord attached to the rectal probe.
3. If bubbles are present in the deposited US gel, it is best to wipe away the gel and reapply.
4. The left kidney is situated slightly more superiorly than the right.
5. It is best to capture images between heartbeats.

Acknowledgment

This work was supported by NIH grants DK070907 and DK085242.

References

1. Singh S, Robinson M, Nahi F et al (2007) Identification of a unique transgenic mouse line that develops megabladder, obstructive uropathy, and renal dysfunction. J Am Soc Nephrol 18:461–471
2. Ingraham SE, Saha M, Carpenter AR et al (2010) Pathogenesis of renal injury in the megabladder mouse: a genetic model of congenital obstructive nephropathy. Pediatr Res 68: 500–507

INDEX

Odyssé Michos (ed.), *Kidney Development: Methods and Protocols*, Methods in Molecular Biology, vol. 886, DOI 10.1007/978-1-61779-851-1, © Springer Science+Business Media, LLC 2012

P

Q

R

S

T

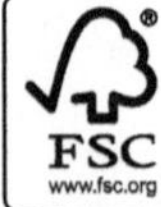

MIX
Papier aus verantwortungsvollen Quellen
Paper from responsible sources
FSC® C105338

If you have any concerns about our products,
you can contact us on
ProductSafety@springernature.com

In case Publisher is established outside the EU,
the EU authorized representative is:
Springer Nature Customer Service Center GmbH
Europaplatz 3, 69115 Heidelberg, Germany

Printed by Libri Plureos GmbH
in Hamburg, Germany